Application of Quantitative Methods in Veterinary Epidemiology

Application of Quantitative Methods in Veterinary Epidemiology

edited by:
J.P.T.M. Noordhuizen
K. Frankena
M.V. Thrusfield
E.A.M. Graat

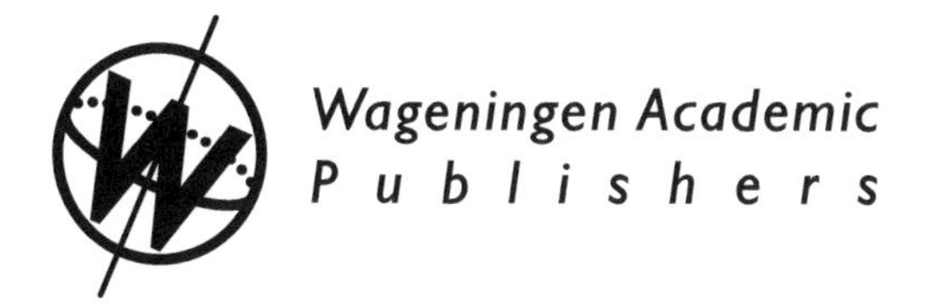

CIP-data Koninklijke Bibliotheek, Den Haag

ISBN: 9074134890

Subject headings: Veterinary epidemiology, Quantitative methods

Cover design: C.M. van der Hoofd

First published, 1997
Revised reprint, 2001
Second reprint, 2015
Third reprint, 2017

Preface

Within the health triad "animal-environment-man" the mutual relationships are very complex and variable in nature. The major areas of concern regard: public health (zoonoses; foodborne diseases), macro-economics (epidemics; endemics; international trade-related diseases), population dynamics of infection and transmission, and disease combat and prevention at farm level (including production diseases). Decision-making in all three areas has to be based on adequate information about animal health status, the respective farming conditions and risks involved, meaning that there is an increasing need for quantitative data, and for proper analysis and interpretation of such data. Animal production is the first link in the food production chain upto man. Society is also putting higher demand on professionals, who are active in the field of animal production, with regard to the quality of products of animal origin, animal health, production method, food safety, quality and animal welfare. Responsibilities of all professionals involved in the food production chain, therefore, are high.

This book describes tools which can help in better understanding of disease occurrence and disease patterns. Using such tools will result in more adequate disease control on the one hand, and in sound health care decision-making and preventive action through e.g., risk management on the other. Skills in handling quantitative epidemiological methods have been identified by the World Health Organization in the 90's as one of the domains in animal health care where more training of both professionals and undergraduates is needed.

The text you have in hand is a compilation of short theory lectures and many case study elaborations on quantitative epidemiological methods, used frequently in both international post-graduate courses for veterinarians and animal scientists and international undergraduate courses over the last few years. In addition to the core elements of quantitative methods, attention is also paid to other epidemiology-related issues such as food hygiene, economics, monitoring & surveillance, outbreak investigation and questionnaire design.

The main goal of this book is to further familiarize the reader with commonly applied methods in epidemiology and to provide hands-on for self-training in this field in order to increase knowledge and improve skills. Various chapters refer to statistical software, which can be obtained commercially or through Internet as public domain software. Ultimately, the knowledge and skills acquired should be applied in the field. This book can therefore not be regarded as a textbook in the classical sense. It is not meant that way either, because there are good textbooks about concepts and principles in veterinary epidemiology available.

We hope that the reader, or rather the active user, of this 2nd edition will obtain a new or better understanding of principles and applications (each with its opportunities and its limitations) for an optimal performance of professional tasks, now and in the future.

The Editors

J.P.T.M. Noordhuizen
K. Frankena
M.V. Thrusfield
E.A.M. Graat

Contents

Part II

The Design and Conduct of Clinical Trials ... 215

Chapter IX

Introduction To Theoretical Epidemiology ... 239

Chapter I

Introduction to Epidemiology

Michael Thrusfield
University of Edinburgh
Department of Veterinary Clinical Studies
United Kingdom

1. Definition of Epidemiology

Epidemiology is concerned with the prevention and control of disease in human and animal **populations**. Veterinary epidemiology additionally includes the investigation and assessment of other health-related events, notably productivity.

The word 'epidemiology' is derived from Greek roots, whose other constructs, such as 'epidemein' ('to visit a community'), give hints of the early association between epidemiology and infections that periodically entered a community (e.g., the great plagues such as foot-and-mouth disease, rinderpest and smallpox), in contrast to other diseases which were usually present in the population[1]. The related adjective is either 'epidemiological' or 'epidemiologic'[2].

2. Historical Perspective: Qualitative Epidemiology

Epidemiology is a practical discipline which has developed in the context of the diseases that afflict humans and animals at particular times. In early societies, the main health problems in man and his domesticated animals were **infectious**. The main goal of early epidemiological investigations was therefore an increase in an understanding of the mode of transmission and maintenance of infections, so that effective control measures could be instigated. Such investigations were *qualitative*.

Infectious diseases continued to be the main concern of human and veterinary medicine globally until the first part of this century. Rinderpest ravaged Europe during the 17th and 18th centuries, and provided impetus for the founding of many veterinary schools. However, the recognition of micro-organisms as causes of disease in the 19th century, and the subsequent development of antimicrobial drugs and vaccines, brought dramatic improvements in the control of infectious diseases, evidenced by changes in the league table of causes of human mortality over the last 150 years (Table 1.1). By the middle of this century, non-infectious (often termed 'chronic') diseases had assumed importance. In man, cancer, heart disease and stroke emerged as major causes of death, and chronic diseases also achieved greater significance than previously in companion animals. Moreover, the increase in livestock numbers and intensification of farm enterprises in developed countries, facilitated by control of the major epidemic infectious diseases, resulted in an increase in the importance of non-infectious production diseases in farm livestock (e.g., metabolic disorders in high-yielding dairy cows).

---

[1] Outbreaks of disease in human populations were called 'epidemics', and in animal populations were called 'epizootics', from which the term 'epizootiology' was derived (from the Greek ζωο- (*zoo-*) = animal). However, many infections (the zoonoses) affect both animals and man, and the semantic differentiation between studies involving human diseases and those concerned with animal diseases therefore is considered unwarranted. Thus, 'veterinary epidemiology' is now preferred to 'epizootiology', although the latter term still persists in some parts of the world.

[2] The English suffixes, '-ical' and '-ic', are virtually interchangeable, the former being more common in European English usage, and the latter more common in American usage.

Table 1.1. League table of causes of human mortality in the United Kingdom: 1860, 1900, 1970.

Year	*Rank*	*Disease*	*Percentage of total deaths*
1860	1	Tuberculosis	19.8
	2	Diarrhoea and enteritis	15.0
	3	Cholera	6.4
	4	Pneumonia/influenza/bronchitis	6.1
	5	Infantile convulsions	5.9
	6	Diphtheria and croup	2.7
		Dysentery	2.7
		Stroke	2.7
	9	Scarletfever	2.5
	10	Nephritis	2.4
1900	1	Pneumonia/influenza/bronchitis	14.4
	2	Tuberculosis	11.3
	3	Diarrhoea and enteritis	8.1
	4	Heart disease	8.0
	5	Nephritis	4.7
	6	Accidents	4.5
	7	Stroke	4.2
		Diseases of early infancy	4.2
	9	Cancer	3.7
	10	Diphtheria	2.3
1970	1	Heart disease	38.3
	2	Cancer	17.2
	3	Stroke	10.8
	4	Pneumonia/influenza/bronchitis	3.6
	5	Accidents (except motor vehicle), suicide	3.1
	6	Motor vehicle accidents	2.8
	7	Diseases of early infancy	2.3
	8	Diabetes	2.0
	9	Arteriosclerosis	1.7
	10	Cirrhosis	1.6

The emerging diseases frequently had unknown causes, and, when the causes were identified, they were often complex (Table 1.2). The **multifactorial** theory of cause, involving identification of factors associated with *host*, *agent* and *environment*, became a central dogma of epidemiology (Martin *et al.*, 1987; Thrusfield, 1997). Twentieth-century research by geneticists, in particular, has revealed the ubiquitous role of genes as causal factors, beginning with the identification of genetically determined diseases of the bones and joints in the 1920s, and currently involving genetic determinants of immunodeficiencies[3].

[3] This highlights the artificial nature of disciplinary boundaries: the geneticist and epidemiologist are both concerned with interactions between genetic and non-genetic factors - only the frequently indistinct time of the interaction may be used to classify an investigation as genetic or epidemiological.

Table 1.2. Some complex (multifactorial) diseases of animals.

Species	*Condition*	*Associated factors*	*Reference*
Cat	Diabetes mellitus	Breed, sex, age, body weight	Panciera *et al.* (1990)
Dog	Bladder cancer	Breed, sex, location (areas of industrial activity), passive smoking, environmental chemicals, insecticides, obesity	Hayes (1976), Hayes *et al.* (1981), Glickman *et al.* (1989)
Horse	Laryngeal hemiplegia	Breed, sex, age	Beard and Hayes (1993)
Ox	Cystic ovaries	Breed, parity, season, previous history of the condition, twinning, milk yield	Emanuelson and Bendixen (1991)
	Laminitis (in calves)	Breed, age, management, feeding, housing	Frankena *et al.* (1991)
Pig	Enzootic pneumonia	Sex, age, clinical disease, ventilation, herd size, replacement policy, diarrhoea	Aalund *et al.* (1976) Pointon *et al.* (1985) Willeberg *et al.* (1978)
Poultry	Hydropericardium syndrome	Location, management, broiler strain	Akhtar *et al.* (1992)
Sheep	Orf	Age, frequency of the disease, mammary lesions, infected pasture, animal density, nutritional deficiencies, lambing period	Ducrot and Cimarosti (1991)

Koch's postulates (Table 1.3), which had proved to be so successful in identifying causes of the 'simple' infectious diseases (e.g., tuberculosis), became inadequate criteria for identifying the causes of complex diseases because:

1. they were not applicable to non-infectious diseases; and:
2. they ignored the interactions that take place between infectious agents, hosts' genes, and the environment in diseases with a multifactorial cause.

Table 1.3. Koch's postulates.

An organism is causal if:

1. it is present in all cases of the disease;
2. it does not occur in another disease as a fortuitous and non-pathogenic parasite;
3. it is isolated in pure culture from an animal, is repeatedly passaged, and induces the same disease in other animals.

The postulates were therefore subsumed by a more comprehensive set formulated in the United States in the 1970s by Alfred Evans (Table 1.4). These can be applied to all types of disease, irrespective of complexity. An important characteristic of some of Evans' postulates is that they require the association between an hypothesized causal factor and the disease in question to be *statistically significant*. This involves comparing *groups* of animals, rather than investigating associations in the individual.

Table 1.4. Evans' postulates (rules) (from Evans, 1976).

1. the proportion of individuals with the disease should be significantly higher in those exposed to the supposed cause than in those who are not;
2. exposure to the supposed cause should be present more commonly in those with than those without the disease, when all other risk factors are held constant;
3. the number of new cases of disease should be significantly higher in those exposed to the supposed cause than in those not so exposed, as shown in prospective studies;
4. temporally, the disease should follow exposure to the supposed cause with a distribution of incubation periods on a bell-shaped curve;
5. a spectrum of host responses, from mild to severe, should follow exposure to the supposed cause along a logical biological gradient;
6. a measurable host response (e.g., antibody, cancer cells) should appear regularly following exposure to the supposed cause in those lacking this response before exposure, or should increase in magnitude if present before exposure; this pattern should not occur in individuals not so exposed;
7. experimental reproduction of the disease should occur with greater frequency in animals or man appropriately exposed to the supposed cause than in those not so exposed; this exposure may be deliberate in volunteers, experimentally induced in the laboratory, or demonstrated in a controlled regulation of natural exposure;
8. elimination (e.g., removal of a specific infectious agent) or modification (e.g., alteration of a deficient diet) of the supposed cause should decrease the frequency of occurrence of the disease;
9. prevention or modification of the host's response (e.g., by immunization or use of specific lymphocyte transfer factor in cancer) should decrease or eliminate the disease that normally occurs on exposure to the supposed cause;
10. all relationships and associations should be biologically and epidemiologically credible.

The various components of qualitative epidemiology are summarized in Table 1.5.

Table 1.5. Components of epidemiology.

Qualitative epidemiology	*Quantitative epidemiology*
The natural history of disease (e.g., transmission and maintenance of infection)	Measuring the amount of disease: *ad hoc* surveys, routine data-recording systems, monitoring and surveillance
Qualitative causal studies (e.g., public health investigations)	Observational studies: case-control, cross-sectional, and cohort
Characterization of microbes (e.g., sero-epidemiology and molecular epidemiology)	Modelling Clinical trials Economic assessment of disease and its control Risk assesment

3. Qualitative and Quantitative Epidemiology: A Transition?

Table 1.5 also shows that epidemiology has *quantitative* aspects. Sometimes, a temporal *transition* from qualitative to quantitative epidemiology has been identified. The former has been termed 'old', and the latter 'new', epidemiology (Gordon, 1950). However, this transition is illusory. There has been a shift in emphasis towards - rather than a change to - quantitative methods, which began (in both human and veterinary medicine) primarily as a *descriptive* exercise.

The structured recording of data on animal disease, which is the basis of modern **monitoring and surveillance systems**, was used in ancient Japan to identify farmers requiring financial assistance (Smithcors, 1957). John Graunt collected human mortality data in England in the 17th century (Graunt, 1662). In 18th century France, a rinderpest outbreak prompted the establishment of a commision on epidemics, headed by Felix Vicq d'Azyr, Marie Antoinette's personal physician. This evolved into the Royal Society of Medicine which pioneered the collection of statistical data on animal and human epidemics, and the weather. Accurate recording of animal disease status became necessary when disease certification and eradication programmes expanded during the early part of this century (e.g., tuberculosis eradication in the United Kingdom: MAFF, 1965). A strong case for the routine monitoring of animal disease was made in the last half of the last century (Hutton and Halvorsorn, 1974; Ingram *et al.*, 1975)[4], and some general **surveys** of animal disease had already been undertaken, a notable example being Gracey's (1960) survey of livestock diseases in Northern Ireland. Gradually, passive and active[5] systems of data **collection evolved**. For example, in the United Kingdom in the1960s, passively-collected data formed the basis of VIDA: a nationwide database of diagnoses conducted on submissions to government veterinary diagnostic laboratories (Hugh-Jones *et al.*, 1969). By the 1990s, active data-collection systems were being developed (e.g., NAHMS in the United States: Curtis and Farrar, 1990).

The scientific revolution which began during 16th century posited that the physical universe was orderly and could be explained mathematically (Dampier, 1948). This argument was extended to the biological world, where it was considered that 'laws of mortality' must exist. Graunt's mortality studies included attempts to formulate such laws by constructing life tables, and Daniel Bernoulli (1766) applied life-table methods to smallpox data, thereby demonstrating that inoculation was efficaceous in conferring lifelong immunity. A hundred years later, William Farr produced a simple **mathematical model** of the 1865 rinderpest epidemic in the United Kingdom (Brownlee, 1915).

---

[4] The development of animal disease monitoring is traced by Poppensiek and his colleagues (1966).

[5] Passive data collection uses existing sources of data, whereas actively-collected data are gathered to fulfil specific data requirements, and are often not available from pre-existing sets of data. Their respective merits and disadvantages are discussed by Davies (1990), in the context of the European Union. More recently, it has been suggested that these two terms should be replaced by ones reflecting the contemporary goals of modern animal-disease surveillance (Scudamore, 2000). Thus, *core surveillance* (using both passive and active methods) may be applied to the provision of baseline data on morbidity, whereas *strategic (targeted) surveillance* provides information on specific diseases that are the subject of control campaigns (e.g., bovine spongiform encephalopathy: Doherr *et al.*, 2000).

Quantification in the context of *analysis* of biological (including medical) events evolved in the 18th century, when the *Age of Enlightenment* saw a growth in literature dealing with the relationship between probability and the need for objectivity in science and society (the 'Probabilistic Revolution'). The mathematical foundation of probability was laid by Jakob Bernoulli (1713) and developed in a medical context by Pierre-Simon Laplace (1814). Bernoulli developed a theory of *inverse probability*, which stated that the frequency of an event would approach its probability of occurrence if the number of observations was large enough. Laplace argued that all rational judgement has a mathematical precision that can be captured by probability theory, which he related particularly to medical therapy, suggesting that a preferred method of treatment '*will manifest itself more and more in the measure that the number (of observations) is increased*'.

Emerging interest in probability theory resulted in controversy over whether medicine was an 'art' or a 'science'. The physician Cabanis, for instance, stated in 1788 that '*in medicine, all, or almost all, depends on ... a happy instinct, the certitude that is found most often in sensations similar to that of an artist*' (Lehec and Cazeneuve, 1956). This debate is sometimes still seen in discussions between clinicians, epidemiologists and statisticians. Controversies may arise because of a misunderstanding of the role of statistics - particularly of probability theory - in biological inquiry. The statistician uses a mathematical model to represent the basic stucture of nature (as we view it) and uses probability models to represent the 'uncertainty component' in order to accommodate discrepancies that occur between the model and the observations. If the discrepancies are too great, the model is modified, thereby moving closer to the truth. As such, statistical investigation is a fundamental part of scientific (and therefore clinical) inquiry, and aids clinical judgement, rather than conflicting with it. The recent field of 'evidence-based medicine' exemplifies this fact (Guyatt, 1991).

A pivotal move towards *comparative* statistical techniques occurred when Pierre-Charles-Alexander Louis developed his 'numerical method', requiring systematic record keeping and rigorous analysis of multiple cases. He documented typhoid in Paris, showing that the disease occurred predominantly in young adults, and that the average age of fatal cases was higher than that of survivors, suggesting that the younger patients had the best prognosis (Louis, 1836). He subsequently demonstrated that blood-letting was of no benefit to typhoid cases, and his calculation of average values was adopted by other early protagonists of **clinical trials** (e.g., Joseph Lister, who assessed the value of antiseptic surgery in the context of increased post-surgical survival: Lister 1870).

Application of probability theory to medicine was cautiously and tendentiously accepted by British and French medical statisticians, who were largely concerned with the descriptive statistics of the major public health issues (Table 1.1), rather than with statistical inference. Nevertheless, during the 19th century, strong links were forged between epidemiologists, mathematicians and statisticians through the common influence of Louis[6], and by the 20th century rigorous methods of statistical

[6] An interesting 'family tree', showing the links between 18th-20th century statisticians, public-health physicians and epidemiologists, is depicted by Lilienfeld and Lilienfeld (1980).

inference were developing (Stigler, 1986) and were being applied in medicine and agriculture. Some of these, such as significance tests, formed the basis of early **observational studies** of the cause of disease. (The first modern observational study was Lane-Claypon's' (1926) investigation of reproductive factors in relation to mammary cancer in women - see also Table 2.1).

Quantification in veterinary medicine therefore does not represent a major transition; it has *evolved,* increasing in complexity. An example of such evolution in a specific area is the development of clinical trials, whose modern history began with Lind's 18th century assessment of citrus fruit in the prevention of human scurvy (Lind, 1753), progressing through the first *placebo-controlled* trial at the end of the 18th century (Haygarth, 1800), Lister's use of *historical controls* in his work with antiseptics (Lister, 1870), Pasteur's enrolment of *concurrent controls* in his evaluation of an anthrax vaccine in sheep (Descour, 1922), and reaching maturity with the birth of the modern *randomized controlled clinical trial* in the 1940s (Doll, 1992).

The evolution of some other areas of epidemiology is summarized briefly in the next chapter, further demonstrating that modern quantitative epidemiology represents a *shift in emphasis,* reflecting the contemporary need for more rigorous evaluation of animal disease and factors associated with its occurrence.

References

Aalund, O.; Willeberg, P.; Mandrup, M.; Riemann, H. (1976) Lung lesions at slaughter: association to factors in the pig herd. Nordisk Veterinærmedicin, 28, 481-486.
Akhtar, S.; Zahid, S.; Khan, M.I. (1992) Risk factors associated with hydropericardium syndrome in broiler flocks. Veterinary Record, 131, 481-484.
Beard, W.L.; Hayes, H.M. (1993) Risk factors for laryngeal hemiplegia in the horse. Preventive Veterinary Medicine, 17, 57-63.
Bernoulli, D. (1766) Essai d'une nouvelle analyse de la mortalité causée par la petite vérole et des avantages de l'inoculation pour la prévenir. In: Histoire de L'Académie Royale des Sciences, 1760, Avec les Mémoires de Mathématique et de Physique. L'Imprimerie Royale, Paris. Translated in: Bradley, L. (1971) Smallpox Inoculation: An Eighteenth Century Mathematical Controversy. University of Nottingham Adult Education Department, Nottingham.
Bernoulli, J. (1713) Ars Conjectandi. Thurnisiorum, Basel.
Brownlee, J. (1915) Historical note on Farr's theory of the epidemic. British Medical Journal, II, 250-252
Curtis, C.R.; Farrar, J.A. (Eds) (1990) The National Animal Health Monitoring System in the United States. Preventive Veterinary Medicine, 8, 87-225.
Dampier, W.C.D. (1948) A History of Science and its Relations with Philosophy and Religion. 4th edn. Cambridge University Press, Cambridge.
Davies, G. (1993) Do we need a European surveillance system? In: Proceedings of the Society for Veterinary Epidemiology and Preventive Medicine, Exeter, 31st March-2nd April 1993. Ed. Thrusfield, M.V. Pp 153-163.
Descour, L. (1922) Pasteur and His Work. Wedd, A.F. and Wedd, B.H. (Translators). T. Fisher Unwin, Ltd., London.
Doherr, M.G.; Baumgarten, L.; Heim, D. (2000) The need for an active (targeted) surveillance system for BSE and scrapie in addition to the mandatory reporting of clinical cases. In: Proceedings of the Society for Veterinary Epidemiology and Preventive Medicine, Edinburgh, 29th-31st March 2000. Eds. Thrusfield, M.V. and Goodall. E.A, Pp 198-203.
Doll, R. (1992) Sir Austin Bradford Hill and the progess of medical science. British Medical Journal, 305, 1521-1528.

Ducrot, C.; Cimarotsi, I. (1991) Complementary aspects of the logistic model and of the correspondence analysis to investigate risk factors in animal pathology: application to the study of orf risk factors in sheep breeders. In: Proceedings of the Sixth International Symposium on Veterinary Epidemiology and Economics, Ottawa, 12th-16th August 1991. Ed. Martin, S.W. Pp 97-100.

Emanuelson, U.; Bendixen, P.H. (1991) Occurrence of cystic ovaries in dairy cows in Sweden. Preventive Veterinary Medicine, 10, 261-271.

Evans, A.S. (1976) Causation and disease. The Henle-Koch postulates revisited. Yale Journal of Biology and Medicine, 49, 175-195.

Frankena, K.; van Keulen, K.A.S.; Noordhuizen, J.P.; Noordhuizen-Stassen, E.N.; Gundelach, J.; de Jong, D.-J.; Saedt, I. (1991) Prevalence and risk indicators of digital laminitis in dairy breeding calves. Studievereniging voor Veterinaire Epidemiologie en Economie, Proceedings, Utrecht, 11 December 1991. Eds. Hogeveen, H. and Nielen, M. Pp. 41-52.

Glickman, L.T.; Schofer, F.S.; McKee, L.J.; Reif, J.S.; Goldschmidt, M.H. (1989) Epidemiologic study of insecticide exposures, obesity, and risk of bladder cancer in household dogs. Journal of Toxicology and Environmental Health, 28, 407-414.

Gordon, J.E. (1950) Epidemiology - old and new. Journal of the Michigan State Medical Society, 49, 194-199.

Gracey, J.F. (1960) Survey of Livestock Diseases in Northern Ireland. Her Majesty's Stationery Office, Belfast.

Graunt, J. (1662) Natural and Political Observations in a Following Index, and Made upon the Bills of Mortality. London. Reprinted 1939: Johns Hopkins Press, Baltimore.

Guyatt G.H. (1991) Evidence-based medicine. (Editorial) American College of Physicians Journal Club, A-16 (Annals of Internal Medicine 114,. Suppl. 2).

Hayes, H.M. (1976) Canine bladder cancer: epidemiologic features. American Journal of Epidemiology, 104, 673-677.

Hayes, H.M.; Hoover, R.; Tarone, R.E. (1981) Bladder cancer in pet dogs: a sentinel for environmental cancer? American Journal of Epidemiology, 114, 229-233.

Haygarth, J. (1800) Of the Imagination, as a Cause and as a Cure of Disorders of the Body; exemplified by Fictious Tractors, and Epidemical Convulsions. R.Cruttwell, Bath.

Hugh-Jones, M.E.; Ivory, D.W.; Loosmore, R.M.; Gibbins, J. (1969) Veterinary Investigation Diagnosis Analysis. Veterinary Record, 84, 304-307.

Hutton, N.E.; Halvorson, L.C. (1974) A Nationwide System for Animal Health Surveillance. National Academy of Sciences, Washington.

Ingram, D.G.; Mitchell, W.R.; Martin, S.W. (Eds) (1975) Animal Disease Monitoring. Thomas, Springfield .

Lane-Claypon, J.E. (1926) A further report on cancer of the breast. Reports on Public Health and Medical Subjects, 32. His Majesty's Stationery Office, London.

Laplace, P.-S. (1814) Essai Philosophique sur les Probabilitiés. Translated as: A Philosophical Essay on Probabilities. Truscott, F.W. and Emory, F.L. (translators) (1951). Dover Publications, New York.

Lehec, C.; Cazeneuve, J. (Eds) (1956) Oeuvres Philosophiques de Cabanis. Vol. 1. Presses Universitaires de France, Paris.

Lilienfeld, A.M.; Lilienfeld, D.E. (1980) Foundations of Epidemiology. 2nd edn. Oxford University Press, New York.

Lind, J. (1753) A treatise of The Scurvy in Three Parts: Containing an Inquiry into the Nature, Causes and Cure of That Disease, together with a Critical Chronological View of what has been published on the subject. Murray and Cochran, Edinburgh.

Lister, J. (1870) On the effects of the antiseptic system of treatment upon the salubrity of a surgical hospital. Lancet, 1, 4-6, 40-42.

Louis, P.-C.-A. (1836) Anatomical, Pathological and Therapeutic Researches upon the Disease Known under the Name of Gastro-Enterite Putrid, Adynamic, Ataxic, or Typhoid Fever, etc., compared with the Most Common Acute Diseases. Bowditch, H.I. (translator). Vol. 1 Hilliard Gray, Boston; Vol. 2 Isaac R. Butts, Boston.

MAFF (1965) Animal Health: A Centenary 1865-1965. Her Majesty's Stationery Office, London.

Martin, S.W.; Meek, A.H.; Willeberg P. (1987) Veterinary Epidemiology: Principles and Methods. Iowa State University Press, Ames, Iowa.

Panciera, D.L.; Thomas, C.B.; Eicker, S.W.; Atkins, C.E. (1990) Epizootiologic patterns of diabetes mellitus in cats: 333 cases (1980-1986). Journal of the American Veterinary Medical Association, 197, 1504-1508.

Pointon, A.M.; Heap, P.; McCloud, P. (1985) Enzootic pneumonia of pigs in South Australia - factors relating to incidence of disease. Australian Veterinary Journal, 62, 98-101.
Poppensiek, G.C.; Budd, D.E.; Scholtens, R.G.(1966) A Historical Survey of Animal-Disease Morbidity and Mortality Reporting. National Academy of Sciences, Washington DC Publication No. 1346.
Scudamore, J.M. (2000) Surveillance – past, present and future. In: Proceedings of the Society for Veterinary Epidemiology and Preventive Medicine, Edinburgh, 29th-31st March 2000. Eds. Thrusfield, M.V. and Goodall. E.A. S.W. Pp xi-xx.
Smithcors, J.F. (1957) Evolution of the Veterinary Art. Veterinary Medicine Publishing Company, Kansas.
Stigler, S.M. (1986) The History of Statistics: The Measurement of Uncertainty Before 1900. The Belknap Press of Harvard University Press, Cambridge, Mass. and London.
Thrusfield, M. (1997) Veterinary Epidemiology. Revised 2nd edn. Blackwell Science, Oxford.
Willeberg, P.; Gerbola, M-A.; Madsen, A.; Mandrup, M.; Nielsen, E.K.; Riemann, H.P.; Aalund, O. (1978) A retrospective study of respiratory disease in a cohort of bacon pigs: I Clinico-epidemiological analyses. Nordisk Veterinærmedicin, 30, 513-525.

Chapter II

Current Areas of Application of Epidemiology and Perspectives

Michael Thrusfield
University of Edinburgh
Department of Veterinary Clinical Studies
United Kingdom

J.P.T.M. Noordhuizen
Department of Farm Animal Health
Faculty of Veterinary Medicine
University of Utrecht
The Netherlands

1. Introduction

Chapter I demonstrated that veterinary epidemiology has been regarded historically as a microbiological discipline, dealing with the transmission and maintenance of infections, and therefore relying heavily on a knowledge of the pathogenesis of infectious diseases. This emphasis was logical because of the widespread occurrence of major infectious diseases such as foot-and-mouth disease, contagious bovine pleuropneumonia, tuberculosis and rinderpest. However, now that these frequently highly contagious diseases have been brought under control in many countries, and multifactorial - often endemic - diseases, with or without an infectious component (e.g., mastitis and hypocalcaemia, respectively) are becoming more important, the need for quantitative information on disease occurrence, and on the factors associated with it, is increasing.

In addition to a fuller understanding of the development of complex, multifactorial diseases in the animal production sector, the impact of modern production systems on human health - in terms of the zoonotic infections and food safety - is receiving attention. Thus, quality control at all points in the food-production chain (the animal producers, animal transporters, slaughterhouses, product plants, and product distributors) is receiving more attention than hitherto. This attention is being demanded by consumers' awareness of product quality, animal production systems and animal welfare. This puts considerable responsibility on primary animal producers and those who are directly involved in animal health, notably veterinarians and animal-production scientists.

These groups therefore need to be better equipped than previously: first with information on health and disease, and secondly with skills to apply methods for providing sufficient reassurance about animal health and welfare, and the safety and quality of animal products. These methods require analysis and interpretation of data on disease and other health-related events in animal production systems so that problems can be reduced, eliminated or prevented cost-effectively. Thus, in recent years, there has been a rapid expansion of **quantitative** techniques and studies. These are introduced below, and some will be considered in detail in this book.

2. Improving Animal Health

2.1. Disease diagnosis

Accurate diagnosis is central to modern control and eradication campaigns. For instance, it is extremely important that the clinical diagnosis of suspect cases of highly contagious diseases is confirmed (or ruled out) by laboratory tests (e.g., serological examination) as soon as possible so that control or eradication procedures can be implemented rapidly. The proportion of false-positive and false-negative test results influence the applicability of such tests: for example, it might be very costly to slaughter false-positive cases unnecessarily; whereas it would be imprudent to rule out false-negative cases unjustifiably because infection could remain in a herd or region. Using clinical epidemiological techniques, the extent of false results can be quantified. This facilitates identification of the most appropriate tests and test strategies for the task in hand (e.g., initial identification of suspect cases *vs.* surveillance during an established control campaign). These issues are addressed in detail in Chapter IV.

2.2. Sampling populations

Diagnostic tests (and other techniques such as clinical examination) are also enlisted to estimate the amount of disease in a population or to declare freedom from clinical disease or infection. Sometimes whole populations must be screened (e.g., tuberculosis or bovine leucosis eradication). In other situations, a **sample** of the population is tested. This approach is less labour-intensive, quicker and less costly than testing all animals, and, if properly conducted, can provide results of adequate precision. Examples are: "How many animals need to be sampled to estimate disease prevalence?" and "If all samples are test-negative, what is the chance that at least one diseased/infected animal remains in the herd?". Methods and examples are given in Chapter III.

2.3. Observational studies

Observational studies investigate associations between disease and putative risk factors, using formal statistical techniques[7] to estimate the degree of risk associated with exposure to the factors (a well-known example is the study of the association between smoking and lung cancer in man). Rigorous quantitative investigations date from the second quarter of this century. Since then, there has been a gradual progression in their complexity, culminating in modern multivariate techniques which can identify multiple risk factors and their interactions (Table 2.1). Modern veterinary studies identify risk factors associated with host, agent and environment in both livestock and companion animals, and can also provide valuable insights into the pathogenesis of human diseases (Thrusfield, 1988).

Table 2.1. Some landmarks in observational studies.

First modern case-control study (reproductive factors in relation to breast cancer)	Lane-Claypon, 1926
Demonstration of relative risk estimation in case-control studies	Cornfield, 1951
Control of extraneous variables by direct standardization	Wynder *et al.*, 1954
Relative risk estimation from stratified data	Mantel and Haenszel, 1959
Application of multivariate methods to study many variables	Cornfield *et al.*, 1961
Causal postulates including quantitative hypothesis testing	Evans, 1976

[7] Recall that Evans' postulates (Chapter I) notably include demonstration of statistical associations as indicators of underlying *biological* associations.

One of the major objectives of observational studies is to identify the determinants of disease and health, and to *quantify* the contribution that these determinants make to disease occurrence. These quantified risk factors help to identify high risk" groups and specific causes of disease. For instance, if factors such as a long walking distance, the use of chalk in the boxes, the height of the shoulder rail above the floor, and the distance between shoulder rail and wall, increase the risk of lameness in dairy cattle by 5.4, 1.3, 1.8 and 2.0 times, respectively (relative to none of these factors being present), then the aggregate risk on a particular farm where all of these factors are present is 25 times greater than on farms where these factors are absent. Further details and methods relating to observational studies are described in Chapter V.

2.4. Clinical trials

In the past, the efficacy of prophylactic and therapeutic procedures has not been evaluated objectively - judgements often being based on the subjective impressions of individual veterinarians and physicians. The frequently subtle differences between new and established therapies demand rigorous, objective assessment, and attention is now being paid to properly designed **clinical trials** (e.g., Noordhuizen *et al.*, 1993), and marks an increasing awareness of a subject which has evolved over the past 200 years (Table 2.2). Such trials are statistically similar to observational studies.

Table 2.2. Some landmarks in clinical trials.

Assessment of effect of citrus fruit on scurvy	Lind, 1753
First placebo-controlled trial (Perkins' tractors)	Haygarth, 1800
Trials using historical controls (antiseptic surgery)	Lister, 1870
Trials using concurrent controls (ovine anthrax vaccine)	Pasteur, 1890
Randomized controlled trials (whooping cough vaccine)	Bradford-Hill, 1945

Clinical trials can be applied to intervention programmes, such as a mastitis control programme. The design, group selection, execution, analysis and interpretation of such trials must be undertaken carefully. On the other hand, scientific rigour may have to be compromised under field conditions. Many reports in the literature about field trials are deficient in their basic design (Noordhuizen *et al.*, 1993). Now that resources are limited and registration of products is important from a technical, public health and environmental point of view, it is important that clinical trials conducted in the field follow strict protocols. Special attention will be given to this in Chapter VIII.

2.5. Databases, and monitoring and surveillance systems

Detection of new diseases, risk factors, and changing trends in disease occurrence require collection of relevant information. Questionnaire-based surveys often have been used, but can be laborious and time-consuming. However, computerised data recording is expanding rapidly, and provides an efficient means of storing and analyzing data. Structured collections of data - **databases** - exist for clinical, laboratory, and field data. For example, the North American *Veterinary Medical Data Base* (*VMDB*: Warble, 1994) - formerly the *Veterinary Medical Data Program* (*VMDP*: Priester, 1975) - records data from several North American veterinary schools, and has provided valuable data for observational studies. Computer software for supporting herd health programmes has been produced too (e.g., Noordhuizen and Buurman, 1984). Recently, in the United States, *NAHMS* (the *National Animal Health Monitoring System*: Curtis and Farrar, 1990) has been developed at the national level to include information on livestock disease and productivity, including data for economic assessment. This system is indicative of the trend towards accurate, regular recording of animal disease and productivity at sector-level.

With the increasing need for information about health and disease in animals by both the animal production sector and public health authorities, disease **monitoring** systems are becoming more important than previously. These may be incorporated into formal disease **surveillance** systems as part of specific control and eradication campaigns. Figure 2.1. summarizes the potential application of monitoring systems for pig health.

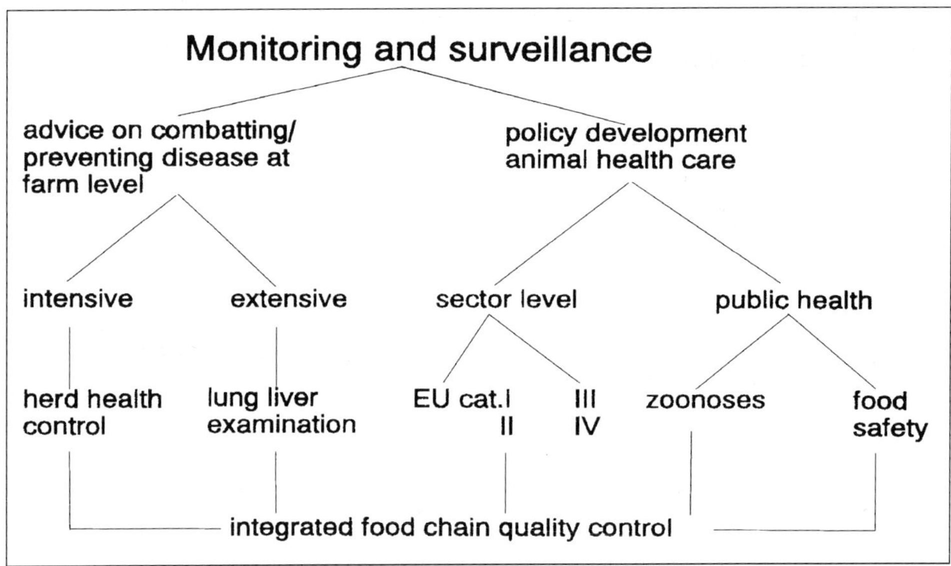

Figure 2.1. Overview of areas for application of monitoring pig health (from Noordhuizen, 1993).

EU category I diseases are those that threaten large areas of the EU such as 'foot-and-mouth' disease, classical swine fever, Newcastle disease.
EU category II diseases are less epidemic but are a threat to regions; examples are tuberculosis, brucellosis.
EU category III diseases are those that can be eradicated on a voluntary basis, if the EU approves the programme. Examples are IBR, Aujeszky's disease; these diseases are important from an economic point of view: export.
EU category IV refers to diseases that can be controlled through breeding farms at the top of the production pyramid. Examples are atrophic rhinitis and *Salmonella enteritidis*.
EU category V diseases are related to fish and aquaculture.

Monitoring systems gather information on animal health and disease (occurrence and spread) which is otherwise unavailable. Systems may use parts of existing databases (passive data collection) or may require *ad hoc* data collection (active data collection) and now may be used together as constituent parts of either core surveillance or strategic surveillance (*see* Chapter I). However, it is important that the data requirements are clearly identified *before* data collation or gathering begins, so that time and effort are not wasted. The information that is gathered can be used to follow spatial and temporal trends in disease, to predict disease occurrence and to formulate epidemiologically and economically sound alternatives for disease control.

Monitoring systems commonly use 'sentinel' stations, that is, veterinary practices, farms or herds/flocks which are chosen according to a pre-set protocol and are located in a region according to sound sampling procedures (e.g., by proportional allocation) and are representative too. A monitoring system may incorporate diagnostic tests for disease detection and determination of disease freedom. In addition to collecting disease/health data, it may also gather data on animals' environment to determine risk factor profiles so that high risk groups can be defined, and action programmes to combat and prevent disease can be constructed. Table 2.3 lists the main questions to be answered before setting up a monitoring system. Only after such preparatory work can a monitoring system be considered to be practically, economically, technically and politically feasible.

Table 2.3. Main questions to be answered before constructing a formal monitoring system.

1.	What is the major objective of monitoring and why?
2.	Which and what type of sentinel stations are needed?
3.	How are these stations selected?
4.	How are the regions incorporated in the system selected?
5.	To what extent is representativeness needed and why?
6.	How is the number of samples determined, and what types of samples are required?
7.	How reliable are the diagnostic tests that will be applied?
8.	How reliable is the expected information to be gathered?
9.	What type of analytical methods should be used?
10.	What are the expected costs of monitoring, and what are the benefits?

From Table 2.3 several conclusions can be drawn. First, the objectives should be clear and well defined. Secondly, sampling procedures and diagnostic test evaluation play key roles. Thirdly, the analytical procedures need to be defined in advance of implementation of a system.

Vermunt (1990) has estimated the costs for monitoring farms for the prevalence of salmonellosis in The Netherlands to be 3 to 9 million US dollars per year, respectively, for (1) swine breeder and multiplier herds only, and (2) all swine and poultry farms. It is obvious that, if disease monitoring is economically relevant to the animal production sector, then the sector itself should build the system (investment costs are likely to be recouped). However, it becomes more costly when monitoring is imposed on the sector by public health authorities, as in the case of zoonoses (e.g., salmonellosis). In this situation, a monitoring system could burden the sector with costs that it could not recoup. The consumer, too, could have a large influence through public attitudes to 'wholesome' food.

For European Union disease categories I and II (see note to Figure 2.1), it appears impractical to develop new systems. Instead, existing systems are likely to be adapted to contemporary demands by being linked to modern identification and registration systems for tracing back cases. For other categories, monitoring is of value (1) to the sector itself, for improving the health status of farms, and the public image of their products, and (2) to quality assurance as the consumers demand "safer" products. Monitoring and surveillance is addressed in more detail in Chapter XII.

2.6. Modelling

Modelling is the representation of physical processes, designed to increase appreciation and understanding of them. In veterinary medicine, **mathematical models** are constructed to attempt to predict patterns of disease occurrence and what might happen if various alternative control strategies are adopted (Hurd and Kaneene, 1993). They frequently rely on the power of modern computers, simulating disease as computer models. Examples include models of alternative control strategies for trypanosomiasis (Habtemariam *et al.*, 1983), genetic resistance to the African brown ear tick (Gettinby *et al.*, 1988) and *Eimeria acervulina* infection in broilers (Henken *et al.*, 1994).

The risk parameters derived from observational studies can be used to model the risk of disease developing by describing the probabilities of transition from one health state (e.g., susceptible) to another (e.g., immune or infected) according to exposure to a variety of risk factors.

A particular type of computer model is the **expert system**, which includes the opinion of experts in its parameters. An example is the expert system, ECFXPERT, for predicting the transmission and maintenance of East Coast fever for various host and parasite parameters (Gettinby and Byrom, 1989).

A modelling procedure, particularly suited to infectious diseases, utilizes the parameter, the **basic reproduction ratio, R_0**, (Anderson and May, 1985; Jong, de and Diekmann, 1992). The parameter, R_0, represents the average number of susceptible animals that will be infected by one infectious animal. If $R_0 < 1$ then the infection will die out, and if $R_0 > 1$ then a major outbreak could be expected. Examples of applying R_0 are Aujeszky's disease in pigs (Bouma *et al.*, 1995) and mastitis in dairy cows (Lam *et al.*, 1996).

Although modelling has expanded recently, its evolution has (like clinical trials) spanned over 200 years (Table 2.4), and is marked by increasing complexity. Currently, several models may be linked together to produce large-scale **systems models**. These include **decision support systems**, which assist veterinarians in planning disease control policies. An example is EpiMAN (Morris *et al.*, 1993): a decision support system for managing outbreaks of foot-and-mouth disease which includes a model of airborne transmission of the virus and an expert system for tracing animals and scheduling farm patrols.

Table 2.4. Evolution of mathematical modelling.

Smallpox vaccination (simple life table)	Bernouilli, 1766
Smallpox mortality (curve fitting)	Farr, 1840
Rinderpest (curve fitting)	Farr, 1866
Simple epidemic models	McKendrick, 1926
	Reed and Frost, 1928
	Greenwood, 1931
Comprehensive mathematical theory of infectious epidemics	Bailey, 1957
Practical models of disease control strategies	1970s - 1980s
Decision support systems (expert systems)	1980s - 1990s
System and population dynamics models	1990s -

3. Statistical Packages

The increased availability of relatively inexpensive microcomputers has provided the epidemiologist with powerful means of storing and analyzing data. General statistical packages have been available for many years. Recently, however, packages have become available specifically for epidemiological use. These include *EPISCOPE* (Frankena *et al.*, 1990), recently converted to run under WINDOWS and named *WINEPISCOPE 2.0*[8] (Thrusfield *et al.*, 2000), and *EPI INFO* (Dean *et al.*, 1990) which contain programs aiding design of field surveys and observational studies, and for evaluating diagnostic tests; and *POWERSIM*[9] which is a general modelling package. Other useful general statistical packages are *STATA*[10] and *MINITAB*[11].

4. Economic Assessment of Animal Disease

Veterinary interest in economics has increased because of the need for government veterinary services in western countries to justify budgets in the face of declining agricultural output, and because of the economic consequences of animal disease limiting or preventing international trade in livestock and livestock products. Initially, economic assessment of animal disease related simply to the financial loss caused by wastage (e.g., by the death of the animal or condemnation of its organs). This narrow interpretation of economic assessment is being expanded (McInerney, 1988a). A major

[8] To be downloaded from any of the following Websites:
(1) http://www.zod.wau.nl/qve
(2) http://infecepi.unizar.es/pages/ratio/soft_uk.htm
(3) http://www.clive.ed.ac.uk/winepiscope/

[9] Powersim AS, PB 642, Bergen, Norway.

[10] STATA Corporation, Stata Statistical software, release 6.0, College Station Texas, USA.

[11] Minitab. Inc. 3081 Enterprise Drive, State College, PA 16801 - 2756, USA.

area of veterinary involvement has been in **social cost-benefit analysis** (SCBA), where the costs of disease control are weighed against the benefits that accrue from its control. A more comprehensive approach involves considering disease in terms of its impact on the physical transformation of animals (and other associated resources, such as feed and grassland) into products such as milk, meat and wool. In such an economic model, an economic investigation is concerned with identifying the optimum disease control strategy in the context of society's needs (McInerney, 1988b).

5. Risk Analysis

Current political pressures in the world favour movement towards free trade, and the *unquantified* risk of introduction of a disease can now no longer be presented as a trade barrier. There is therefore a need to assess *objectively* the risks associated with particular diseases (rather than relying on the somewhat subjective judgements of individual scientists or individual parties).

This has resulted recently in the application of formal quantitative **risk analysis** to animal health problems (Morley, 1993). This comprises different stages of action: (1) risk analysis (involving hazard and risk factor identification, risk quantification, risk modelling which comprises economic evaluation and presentation of alternative strategies); (2) risk management (decision-making about the best possible and acceptable choices - both technically, socially and politically - and the implementation of the appropriate strategy); and (3) risk communication (where all parties involved meet at an early stage to discuss perceived risk and its acceptability). This procedure relies considerably on epidemiological techniques. For example, an assessment of the risk associated with the unrestricted importation of animals or animal products would consider the prevalence of pathogens in the source population, the probability of the pathogens surviving during importation, and the probability of the pathogens coming into contact with local livestock after importation (MacDiarmid, undated) . Examples include the risk of disease transmission by bovine embryo transfer (Sutmoller and Wrathall, 1995) and the risk of introduction of *Aeromonas salmonicida* into salmon fisheries via frozen ocean-caught salmon fillets).

Risk modelling is often complex. The basic idea can be presented by the risk chain concept given by Merkhofer (1987), and is outlined in Figure 2.2. This shows how elementary disease information such as prevalence and knowledge about risk factors is used for modelling change in health state and evaluation of outcomes. The effects of interventions such as treatment, vaccination or management adaptation can be investigated, too.

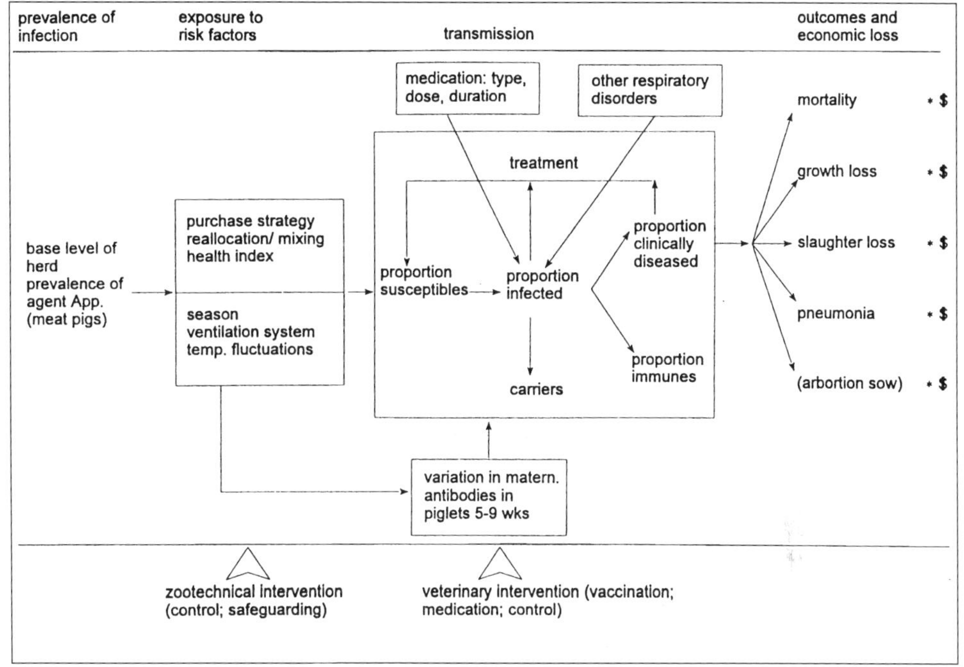

Figure 2.2. The risk chain concept after Merkhofer (1987) simplified and adapted for *Actinobacillus pleuropneumoniae* infections in meat pigs.

From Figure 2.2 it can be deduced that risk factor profiles can be incorporated into this type of investigation. Hence, various epidemiological methods (e.g., diagnostic test evaluation and observational studies) can be integrated into a larger programme. However, much of the information that is required for risk modelling is not available in many countries because an infrastructure is required to produce relevant data, both nationally and internationally. A potential further application of the risk chain concept is in implementing the HACCP (Hazard Analysis Critical Control Point) procedure at farm level, to identify weak links in the production process. This is discussed further in Chapter X. The wider range of modelling techniques (e.g., simulation modelling) are not explored, but an introduction to these can be found in Chapter IX and in Thrusfield (1997).

6. Public Health

Currently, the quality and safety of food of animal origin are major concerns of public health. The animal production sector is addressing these issues, for example, through the introduction of integrated food chain control programmes. Outbreaks of food-borne diseases, however, still occur in man. Examples are salmonellosis after consumption of contaminated eggs or egg products, listeriosis after soft cheese consumption, and *Escherichia coli* $O_{157}H_7$ infections acquired from beef products.

The coupling of sanitary, veterinary and public health databases (i.e., 'networking' data), would be a major step forward in the early detection and joint control of food-borne diseases. Additionally, there is a growing interest in adapting meat inspection to the modern need for safeguarding products of animal origin against residues and contamination, and Veterinary epidemiology (specifically, risk analysis) has now become of considerable importance to the development of meat hygiene and public health (Sutmoller, 1997; Ahl and Sutmoller, 1997). Certification programmes for animal products meeting the requirements for quality assurance will need further development (Noordhuizen and Welpelo, 1996). Moreover, intervention strategies to cope with hazards and risks must be designed. Thus, the integration of animal health and production with the demands of public health is becoming an important way of meeting the requirements of society.

7. The Role of Qualitative Epidemiology

Qualitative epidemiology is still an important part of modern epidemiology. Although there was a decline in the occurrence of many infectious diseases during the late nineteenth and early twentieth centuries (see Chapter I and James; 1988), some remain and are recrudescing (e.g., human tuberculosis in the wake human immunodeficiency syndrome: Cook, 1997). Infectious diseases continue to be major problems in many developed countries, where complex ecological relationships (particularly involving arthropod vectors and feral hosts) need to be elucidated. Although there have been notable successes in the control of many infectious diseases of animals (e.g., tuberculosis and brucellosis in many developed countries), some are refractory and are actually spreading (Table 2.5). Additionally, new infectious diseases, such as bovine spongiform encephalopathy and porcine reproductive and respiratory syndrome, continue to appear (Table 2.6) and need to be studied using both established microbiological, pathological and parasitological techniques and the newer molecular epidemiological methods.

New qualitative tools for identifying diseases have been provided by the recent rapid emergence of molecular biology. Control campaigns aimed at infectious diseases have traditionally used microbiological and serological investigations to identify diseased and immune animals. The recent 'explosion' of molecular biology has provided tools for improved identification of infectious agents and genetic defects (Goldspink, 1993). Microbes can be identified by unique sequences of nucleic acids within their genome. These techniques provide more refined diagnostic methods than conventional serology. Their application to animal disease control is now being realized. An example is the use of nucleotide sequence determination to identify strains of foot-and-mouth disease (Beck and Strohmaier, 1987); this has demonstrated that most European outbreaks in the last twenty years were probably caused by escape of virus from a vaccine production plant, or from the use of inadequately inactivated vaccine, rather than by natural outbreaks. New tests have been developed for diseases for which no suitable, rapid tests were previously available (e.g., a DNA probe for *Mycobacterium paratuberculosis* infection of cattle: Murray *et al.*, 1989). The application of these molecular techniques to epidemiological studies has been termed **molecular epidemiology** (Oxford, 1985).

Table 2.5. Current trends in the distribution of some infectious diseases of animals (Based on Mulhern et al. (1962), Knight (1972), Blaha (1989), West (1988) and Radostits et al. (1994).

Disease	Host	Trends
Anthrax	All animals, particularly devastating in cattle	World-wide range; now contracting to mainly tropics and sub-tropics
Tuberculosis	Many species, especially serious in cattle	Eradication has proved problematic but some success has been achieved. No country is totally free from tuberculosis.
Swine vesicular disease	Pigs	Decreased significance since 1982
Contagious bovine pleuropneumonia	Cattle	Eradicated from much of Europe
Rift Valley fever	Cattle	Spread to much of East Africa
Bluetongue	Sheep	Spreading for past 100 years
Sheep pox	Sheep	Eradicated from Europe in 1951. Present in Africa, Middle East and India
Aujeszky's disease	Pigs	Spreading; recently entered Japan
Johne's disease	Cattle, sheep, goats	World-wide distribution with increasing prevalence in some countries, and spreading in Europe
Bovine brucellosis	Cattle	Eradicated from many developed countries, and spreading in Europe
Glanders	Horses	Eradicated from many developed countries
Rabies	All mammals, some birds	Eradication is problematic. Geographically isolated areas are generally free, although most countries experience rabies to some extent.

Table 2.6. Some emergent and novel infectious diseases of animals in the 20th century, (mainly abridged from Thrusfield, 1997).

Year	Country	Infection
1907	Kenya	African swine fever
1912	Kenya	Rift Valley fever
1918	USA	Swine influenza
1926	Java	Newcastle disease
1929	South Africa	Lumpy skin disease
1939	Colombia	Venezuelan equine encephalomyelitis
1946	Canada	Mink enteritis
1953	USA	Bovine mucosal disease
1972	USA	Lyme disease
1977	Worldwide	Canine parvovirus
1978	Iraq	Pigeon paramyxovirus-1
1986	UK	Bovine spongiform encephalopathy
1987	USA	Porcine reproductive and respiratory syndrome
1990	The Netherlands	Bovine birnavirus
1994	Australia	Equine morbillivirus

8. Perspectives

In several countries, for example, in the European Union, animal health care at the national level is considered by government to need improvement with regard to both epidemic and endemic diseases. Given the wide variation between countries and also between regions and farms within countries, authorities may strive for a system of certification of farms. Such a system will most probably comprise a whole spectrum of diseases, ranging from epidemic to endemic diseases.

First of all, farms should be free from the highly contagious diseases, named in the EU categories I and II. This state of freedom has to be checked regularly. If outbreaks occur, the infected area will be closed and measures such as slaughter and follow-up screening to detect residually infected herds will be taken; a temporary trade block will be part of this procedure, too.

Secondly, there is a category of "intermediate" diseases such as Aujeszky's disease and bovine herpesvirus I (IBR) which may influence trade between countries. Several countries importing animals from other countries require health certificates to accompany animals. There is a growing tendency to expand these certificates from clinical disease to subclinical infection. Thus, serological examination - including the ability to distinguish between field and vaccinal strains of microbes - is an important component of such an approach. Moreover, properly evaluated tests and correct sampling protocols are pivotal to success.

Health certificates will ultimately lead to access to the widest possible markets: from only a local market for low-health category animals to international markets for those with high-health certification.

It should be borne in mind that, where certification is based on clinical or subclinical freedom from disease or infection, there is still the risk of disease following build up of infections within a herd. It might therefore be worthwhile to consider a system of certification of farms based on risk factor profiles" for a range of diseases. These profiles originate from epidemiological studies of risk factors, as mentioned above. "Health-risk classes" may then be defined through the aggregate risks identified by the different disease studies. The HACCP technique could also be implemented at farm level (Noordhuizen and Welpelo, 1996). This approach would be much more valuable than certification based on "proven" freedom from clinical or subclinical diseases at certain times.

9. Conclusions

From the preceding paragraphs it can be concluded that veterinary epidemiology is directly relevant to both the animal production and public health sectors. Moreover, various developments are forecast in several fields where epidemiology could play a substantial role.

However, undergraduate and post-graduate education at universities should be adapted to these new requirements. Furthermore, in-service training should be encouraged so that professionals in the field are prepared for their changing tasks. Additionally, veterinary epidemiological research needs to be targeted at current problem areas; and administrators and regulators may need to change their perspectives to cope with the new requirements of animal health and consumer's concern for food safety. The succeeding chapters in this book are designed to familiarize readers with veterinary epidemiological techniques which can then be applied in veterinary medicine, animal production and related fields to improve the health of animal and human populations.

References

Ahl, A.S.; Sutmoller, P. (Coordinators) (1997). Contamination of animal products: prevention and risks for public health. Revue Scientifique et Technique, Office International des Épizooties, 16 (2) 307-715

Anderson, R.M.; May, R.M. (1985). Vaccination and herd immunity to infectious diseases. Nature, 318, 323-329.

Beck, E.; Strohmaier, K. (1987). Subtyping of European foot and mouth disease virus strains by nucleotide sequence determination. Journal of Virology, 61, 1621-1629.

Bernoulli, M.D. (1766). Essai d'une nouvelle analyse de la mortalité causée par la petite vérole et des avantages de l'inoculation pour la prénir. In: Histoire de l'Académie Royal des Sciences, 1700, Avec les Mémoires de Mathématique et de Physique. L'Imprimerie Royale, Paris. Translated in: Bradley, L. (1971). Smallpox Inoculation: An Eighteenth Century Mathematical Controversy. University of Nottingham Adult Education Department, Nottingham.

Blaha, T. (Ed.) (1989). Applied Veterinary Epidemiology. Elsevier, Amsterdam.

Bouma, A.; Jong, M.C.M. de; Kimman, T.J. (1995). Transmission of pseudorabies virus within pig populations is independent of the size of the population. Preventive Veterinary Medicine, 23, 163-172.

Cook, A.J.C. (1997). Human and bovine tuberculosis in the HIV era. In: Society for Veterinary Epidemiology and Preventive Medicine, Proceedings, Chester, 9-11th April 1997. Goodall, E.A.; Thrusfield, M.V. (Eds.). pp. 36-46.

Cornfield, J. (1951). A method of estimating comparative rates from clinical data: applications to cancer of the lung, breast and cervix. Journal of the National Cancer Institute, 11, 1269-1275.

Curtis, C.R.; Farrar, J.A. (Eds.) (1990). The National Animal Health Monitoring System in the United States. Preventive Veterinary Medicine 8, 87-225.

Dean, A.D.; Dean, J.A.; Burton, A.H.; Dicker, R.C. (1990). Epi Info Version 5: A word processing, database, and statistics program for epidemiology on micro-computers. USD Incorporated, Stone Mountain, Georgia.

Evans, A.S. (1976). Causation and disease. The Henle-Koch postulates revisited. Yale Journal of Biology and Medicine, 49, 175 -195.

Farr, W. (1840). Appendix to Second Annual Report of the Registrar-General of Births, Deaths and Marriages in England. pp. 3-22. William Clowes and Sons, London. In: House of Commons Parliamentary Papers, Vol. XVII. Reports from Commissioners, 2. Births; Deaths; Marriages; Poor Laws, Session 16 January - 11 August 1840, pp. 39-58.

Frankena, K.; Noordhuizen, J.P.; Willeberg, P.; Voorthuysen, P.F. van; Goelema, J.O. (1990). EPISCOPE: Computer programs in veterinary epidemiology. Veterinary Record, 126, 573-576.

Gettinby, G.; Byrom, W. (1989). ECFXPERT: A computer model for the study of East Coast Fever. In: Proceedings of the Simulation Society of Australia Inc., affiliated with the International Association for Mathematics and Computers in Simulation - 8th Biennial Conference and Bushfire Dynamics Workshop, Canberra, 25-27th September 1989. Australian National University, Canberra, pp. 123-127.

Gettinby, G.; Newson, R.M.; Calpin, M.M.J.; Paton, G. (1988). A simulation model for genetic resistance to acaricides in the African brown ear tick, *Rhipicephalus appendiculatus*. Preventive Veterinary Medicine, 6, 183-197.

Goldspink, G.E. (1993). The impact of recombinant DNA techniques on veterinary diagnosis and genetic screening. In: The Advancement of Veterinary Science. The Bicentenary Symposium Series. Volume 1: Veterinary Medicine Beyond 2000. Michell, A.R. (Ed.). CAB International, Wallingford, pp. 59-71.

Habtemariam, T.; Ruppanner, R.; Riemann, H.P.; Theis, J.H. (1983). Evaluation of trypanosomiasis alternatives using an epidemiological simulation model. Preventive Veterinary Medicine, 1, 147-156.

Haygarth, J. (1800). Of the Imagination, as a Cause and as a Cure of Disorders of the Body; exemplified by Fictious Tractors, and Epidemical Convulsions. R. Cruttwell, Bath.

Henken, A.M.; Graat, E.A.M.; Ploeger, H.W.; Carpenter, T.E. (1994) Description of a model to simulate effects of *Eimeria acervulina* infection on broiler production. Parasitology, 108, 513-518.

Hurd, H.S.; Kaneene, J.B. (1993). The application of simulation models and systems analysis in epidemiology: a review. Preventive Veterinary Medicine, 15, 81-99.

James, W. (1988). Immunization: the Reality Behind the Myth. Bergin and Garvey, Massachusetts.

Jong, M.C.M. de; Diekmann, O. (1992). A method to calculate for computer simulated infections - the threshold value R_0 that predicts whether or not the infection will spread. Preventive Veterinary Medicine, 12, 269-285.

Knight, H.D. (1972). Bacterial and spirochetal diseases: other bacterial infections. In: Equine Medicine and Surgery - A Textbook and Reference Work. 2nd edn. Catcott, E.J.; Smithcors, J.F. (Eds.). pp. 108-110. American Veterinary Publications, Wheaton, Ill., pp. 85-113.

Lam, T.J.G.M.; Jong, M.C.M. de; Schukken, Y.H.; Brand, A. (1996). Mathematical modelling to estimate efficacy of postmilking teat disinfection in split-udder trials of dairy cows. Journal of Dairy Science, 79, 62-70.

Lane-Claypon, J.E. (1926). A Further Report on Cancer of the Breast. Reports on Public Health and Medical Subjects, 32. His Majesty's Stationery Office, London.

Lind, J. (1753). A Treatise of the Scurvy in Three Parts: Containing and Inquiry into the Nature, Causes and Cure of that Disease, together with a Critical Chronological View of what has been published on the Subject. Murray and Cochran, Edinburgh.

Lister, J. (1870). On the effects of the antiseptic system of treatment upon the salubrity of a surgical hospital. Lancet, 1 (4-6), 40-42.

MacDiarmid, S.C. (1993). The risk of Introducing *Aeromonas salmonicida* into New Zealand salmon fisheries through the vehicle of frozen fillets of ocean-caught Canadian salmon. Ref. I-CAN-135. Ministry of Agriculture and Fisheries, Wellington

MacDiarmid, S.C. (undated). Quantitative Methods for Assessing Risks Posed by Importations of Animals and Their Products. Ministry of Agriculture and Fisheries, Wellington

Mantel, N.; Haenszel, W. (1959). Statistical aspects of the analysis of data from retrospective studies of disease. Journal of the National Cancer Institute, 22, 719-748.

Mclnerney, J.P. (1988a). The economic analysis of livestock disease: the developing framework. Acta Veterinaria Scandinavia Supplement, 84, 66-74.

Mclnerney, J.P. (1988b). Economics in the veterinary curriculum: further dimensions. In: Proceedings of the Society for Veterinary Epidemiology and Preventive Medicine, Edinburgh, 13-15th April 1988. Thrusfield, M.V. (Ed.). pp. 20-29.

Merkhofer, M.W. (1987). Decision Science and Social Risk Management. D. Riedel Publushing Company, The Netherlands.

Morley, R.S. (Coordinator) (1993). Risk analysis, animal health and trade. Revue Scientifique et Technique, Office International des Epizooties, 12, 1001-1362.

Morris, R.S.; Sanson, R.L.; McKenzie, J.S.; Marsh, W.E. (1993). Decision support systems in animal health. In: Proceedings of the Society for Veterinary Epidemiology and Preventive Medicine, Exeter, 31 March-2 April 1993. Thrusfield, M.V. (Ed.). pp. 188-199.

Mulhern, F.J.; Mott, L.O.; Shahan, M.S.; Anderson, R.G. (1962). Eradication of animal diseases. In: After a Hundred Years, The Yearbook of Agriculture 1962. The US Department of Agriculture. The US Government Printing Office, Washington DC, pp. 313-320.

Murray, A.; Moriarty, K.M.; Scott, D.B. (1989). A cloned DNA probe for the detection of Mycobacterium paratuberculosis. New Zealand Veterinary Journal, 37, 47-50.

Noordhuizen, J.P.T.M.; Buurman, J. (1984). Veterinary automated management and production control programme for dairy farms (VAMPP): the application of MUMPS for data processing. Veterinary Quarterly, 6, 62-77.

Noordhuizen, J.P.T.M. (1993). Monitoring and surveillance systems in pig husbandry: sense and nonsense. Tijdschrift voor Diergeneeskunde, 118, 405 - 408 (in Dutch).

Noordhuizen, J.P.T.M.; Frankena, K.; Ploeger, H.; Nell, T. (Eds.) (1993). Field Trial and Error. Proceedings of the International Seminar with Workshops on the Design, Conduct and Interpretation of Field Trials, Berg en Dal, The Netherlands, 27-28th April 1993. Epidecon, Wageningen.

Noordhuizen, J.P.T.M; Welpelo, H.J. (1996). Sustainable improvement of animal health care by systematic quality risk management according to the HACCP concept. Veterinary Quarterly, 18, 121-126.

Oxford, J.S. (1985). Biochemical techniques for the genetic and phenotypic analysis of viruses: 'Molecular Epidemiology'. Journal of Hygiene, 94, 1-7.

Priester, W.A. (1975). Collecting and using veterinary clinical data. In: Animal Disease Monitoring. Ingram, D.G.; Mitchell, W.F.; Martin, S.W. (Eds.). Charles C. Thomas, Springfield, pp. 119-128.

Radostits, O.M.; Leslie, K.E.; Fetrow, J. (1994). Herd Health: Food Animal Production Medicine. 2nd edn. W.B. Saunders Company, Philadelphia.

Sutmoller, P. (Coordinator) (1997). Contamination of animal products: prevention and risks for public health. Revue Scientifique et Technique, Office International des Épizooties, 16 (1) 9-270

Sutmoller, P. and Wrathall, A.E. (1995). Quantitative Assessment of the Risk of Disease Transmission by Bovine Embryo Transfer. Scientific and Technical Monograph Series No. 17. Pan-American Foot-and-Mouth Disease Center (PAHO/WHO), Rio de Janeiro

Thrusfield, M.V. *et al.* (2000). Accepted by The Veterinary Record.

Thrusfield, M.V. (1988). Companion animal epidemiology: its contribution to human medicine. Acta Veterinaria Scandinavia Supplement, 84, 57-65.

Thrusfield, M. (1997). Veterinary Epidemiology. Revised 2nd edn. Blackwell Science, Oxford.

Vermunt, E.M.C. (1990). A monitoring system for *Salmonella* in poultry and pigs. Report of COVP Het Spelderholt, Beekbergen, The Netherlands (in Dutch).

Warble, A. (1994). Veterinary Medical Data Base (VMDB) update. American Veterinary Computer Society Newsletter, September-October 1994, pp. 8-10.

West, G.P. (Ed.) (1988). Black's Veterinary Dictionary. 18th edn. A and C Black, London.

Chapter III

Principles and Methods of Sampling in Animal Disease Surveys

E.A.M. Graat
Wageningen University
Department of Animal Sciences
Quantitative Veterinary Epidemiology Group
The Netherlands

K. Frankena
Wageningen University
Department of Animal Sciences
Quantitative Veterinary Epidemiology Group
The Netherlands

H. Bos
Dronten Agricultural College
Department of Animal Husbandry
The Netherlands

1. Introduction and Definitions

Sampling implies that not all individuals of a population are investigated, but that the data are collected on a part (subset) of the population. The investigation of a subset instead of the complete population is attractive because it reduces needed laboratory capacity, labour and financial input. There are two major reasons why a planned sample is often used in epidemiology: first, to describe population characteristics (e.g., disease prevalence) and secondly to determine relationships between exposure to certain factors and a specified disease.

In an ideal situation, the investigator has a ***sampling frame*** (a complete list of all ***sampling units***) of the ***target population*** (population from which information is required). Then, the ***study population*** (population from which the sample is drawn) is identical to the target population. However, this is often not the case. For example, individual identification of animals is not always possible and hence a complete sampling frame cannot be constructed when the animal is the unit of concern. Additionally, some herds may not be located. Thus, these herds/animals will never appear in a sampling frame and the study population is not representative for the target population. This reduces the validity of the outcome of the study for extrapolation to the target population. Finally, the ***sampling fraction*** is the ratio of sample size to the size of the study population.

By investigating a subset of the population, part of the information present in the total population is lost and the true value of the parameter of interest in the population is not obtained as such, but it is ***estimated***. Now the precision and accuracy of the estimate depend on the way the subset is obtained (sampling design) and on the number of units in the subset (sample size). Sources of error in measurement may be classified as either random or systematic. A high precision indicates lack of random error, while a high accuracy indicates lack of systematic error. A small sample size leads to low precision. Non-representativeness of the study population with regard to the target population results in a lowered accuracy. For example, it is unlikely that disease prevalence can be estimated accurately from data obtained by laboratories of animal health services or equivalent institutes, because diseased animals have a higher probability of being submitted to these organizations. Even if all animals are within the sampling frame, errors might occur due to:

- lack of cooperation of the animal-holder
- information is obsolescent
- sampling units are untraceable (e.g., lost ear tags)

These errors cannot be compensated by increasing the sample size.

In the following, sampling designs and formulae for calculating sample sizes will be described.

2. Sampling Designs

Six major types of sampling methods can be discriminated:

1. non-probability sampling,
2. simple random sampling,
3. systematic random sampling,
4. stratified random sampling,
5. cluster sampling,
6. multistage sampling.

2.1. Non-probability sampling

Non-probability methods do not rely on random techniques to decide whether or not units are included in the sample. One example is 'convenience sampling': results are obtained from units that are easily accessed by the investigator, for example because he knows that those farmers will cooperate. This often leads to biased results because farmers that are willing to cooperate might have the problem being studied and they hope/expect that this research will show results that will reduce their problem. Also, the opposite might be true: farmers having the problem will not cooperate because the outcome will be harmful to their position. The same holds for farms that are thought to be free of the disease; farmers cooperate because they learn from the study (how do I keep free in future?) or they refuse to cooperate because there is a possibility that the disease will be detected during the study.

Example: a veterinarian wants to know how many dairy cows are infected with bovine herpesvirus 1 (BHV-1) in his practice. Because it is too expensive and too laborious to sample all animals, he decides to investigate all animals on 10 well-managed herds that are always cooperating in his research studies. Knowing the history of these farms, he expects that 5 of these herds will be free of disease and 5 others are positive, assuring a balance between possibly infected and uninfected herds. Give your opinion about this method of sampling. If you were one of the farmers, would you cooperate? (Though the method of sampling will not give the correct answer to the question, farmers might cooperate because they get information about their own herd).

2.2. Simple random sampling

Using this method, the units included in the sample are selected by means of a random process. For example, if you want to select 50% of all units, you can flip a coin per unit and if the result is 'head' then the unit is included in the sample and if it is 'tail', it is not selected. Another possibility is drawing numbers from a hat. More sophisticated methods are available like random number tables, randomizers on pocket calculators, and random number generators within software packages. When the study population is representative of the target population, random procedures assure that the sample is representative for the target population. However, in practice random sampling is often difficult. The first reason for this is that not all elements of the population are in the sampling frame (e.g., not all farms/animals are registered). Secondly, in most cases the investigator depends on the willingness of the owner to cooperate in the study.

Example: you want to know the percentage of cows that is infected with BHV-1 virus. The first step is to list all the cows (N). Secondly, you draw randomly n (sample size) numbers from the list. The n selected cows are representative for the total population (N). The required value of n can be calculated beforehand (see paragraph 4).

2.3. Systematic random sampling

This type of sampling implies that units are selected at regular intervals from the sampling frame. For example, given the outcomes of sample size calculations, you need to select 1% of the animals. Firstly, you draw a ***random*** number between 1 and 100, suppose it is 73. Then, animal 73, 173, 273, ... etc. are selected, ending up with a 1% sample size. In this way it is assured that the animals are evenly distributed over the total population. Bias might occur, if the sampling frame is organized in a systematic way. Suppose that each farm has 100 animals and that the animals appear per farm and in order of age in the sampling frame. In case of systematic sampling you will select a specific age group! Systematic sampling is often conducted when there is no sampling frame. An example of this might be when, because of some reason, only at Tuesdays carcasses at the slaughterhouse are sampled and not at other days. Some farmers may send their animals to slaughter always at Wednesday and therefore they will never will be present in the sample.

2.4. Stratified random sampling

Stratification means that the sampling frame is divided into strata (groups) before selection. Next, systematic or simple random sampling is performed within ***each*** group. Stratification is applied if the population is heterogeneous concerning the variable of interest, e.g., seropositivity increases with age. Then, by creating more homogeneous groups (age groups) a more robust estimate for the characteristic of interest is obtained. A major advantage of this method is that it is possible to draw unequal percentages per stratum. This is very attractive in case it is known that the variance of the outcome differs between strata. By sampling larger percentages of animals from strata with higher variances, the precision of the estimate will improve. A disadvantage is that ***a priori*** information must be available to determine to which stratum each element belongs.

Example: you want to determine the percentage of N cows that is infected with BHV-1 virus and it is estimated by drawing a sample of 10%. It is also known that 80% of the cows are in the North and 20% are in the South. Due to the higher density of cows in the North the prevalence of the BHV-1 is higher (estimate by experts: 80%, compared to 50% in the South). Now a stratified analysis might consist of sampling in both regions 10% of all animals to be sure that both regions are sampled proportionally. Would it be reasonable to select unequal proportions per region?
Answer: yes, relatively more samples from the South, because the variance of a prevalence of 50% is higher than the variance of a prevalence of 80% (see paragraph 4.3).

2.5. Cluster sampling

In cluster sampling, clusters of animals (e.g., litters or herds) are randomly selected while the unit of concern is the animal. All animals in a cluster are then examined. These clusters might be selected by any of the former mentioned random methods. Cluster sampling might be used when not all animals can be listed in the sampling frame (due to non-registration), but all clusters are registered.

Example: you want to know the percentage of N cows that is infected with BHV-1 virus. It is not possible to list all cows due to lack of individual registration. The first step is to list all the M herds. Secondly, you draw randomly m (sample size) herds from the list. The m selected farms are representative for the total population (M) and m can be calculated beforehand. The third step is to determine per selected farm whether BHV-1 virus is present or not. In this third step you take blood from all animals in the herd. Thus, the ultimate sample size n depends on the sizes of the selected herds.

2.6. Multistage sampling

This method is a more complex type of cluster sampling, with sampling also occurring at the second (and following) level(s). It means that not all elements (animals) within a cluster are selected. This type of sampling has practical advantages. The number of clusters (n_1 primary units) and the number of elements per cluster (n_2 secondary units) can be varied in order to obtain a higher precision of the estimate (=minimize variance, if variability between clusters does exist) or to reduce costs (if costs vary between sampling primary versus secondary units).

An example of multistage sampling is that you first select n_1 farms, secondly you select n_2 litters within each farm and lastly you select n_3 piglets within each selected litter on which you measure the parameter of interest. Thus the total number of observations is then $n_1 * n_2 * n_3$.

3. Biostatistic Intermezzo

Prior to sample size calculations, some basic knowledge about types of data and statistics needs to be addressed.

3.1. Data

Data can be either qualitative or quantitative in origin. Qualitative data describes to which category an animal belongs, e.g., is it male or female. Hence these data are also called categorical data. Categorical data are scored on a nominal or ordinal scale. Nominally scaled data makes use of symbols to put animals into a category. Thus, sex might be coded as 0 (or M) or 1 (or F), 0 being the males and 1 being the females. The coded value (0 or 1) has no quantitative meaning. Every animal in a category has the same characteristic (same breed, same sex). A measurement on the ordinal scale has a very weak quantitative meaning in that it represents groups of animals that can be compared to each other in terms of 'better than' or 'worse than'. Thus, animals with a demeanour score of 3 (moribund) are more sick than animals that score a value of 2 (apathy) or 1 (normal activity). Note that the coding might be reversed (1 being moribund and 3 being normally active).

Quantitative data imply some kind of measurement, e.g., temperature or body weight which both might show a large range of values (hence these data are also termed continuous data). Quantitative data might be discrete as well, indicating that it can not take any value on a continuous scale. Discrete data in fact are counts (like litter size or herd size).

3.2. Data description

Tables, graphs and calculations might be used to describe and summarize the data. Frequency tables or histograms are useful for summarizing categorical data (or continuous data that are processed to categories by making intervals with specified width). Data derived from Campbell (1974) on spermatozoa concentrations in semen of 45 bulls serve as an example.

Observed concentrations (in sorted order) in units of 10^7 sperms/ml:

75	86	90	93	95	96	97	97	102	104	104	105
110	110	110	113	117	118	120	120	121	122	122	123
123	124	125	126	127	128	129	132	133	138	138	139
139	142	142	142	143	143	148	150	159			

A histogram can be made by making classes of specified width and count the number of observations per class. If a width of 15 units is specified then 7 classes can be created:

Class	Frequency
65 - 79	1
80 - 94	3
95 - 109	8
110 - 124	14
125 - 139	11
140 - 154	7
155 - 179	1

In a histogram these data look like as in Figure 3.1.

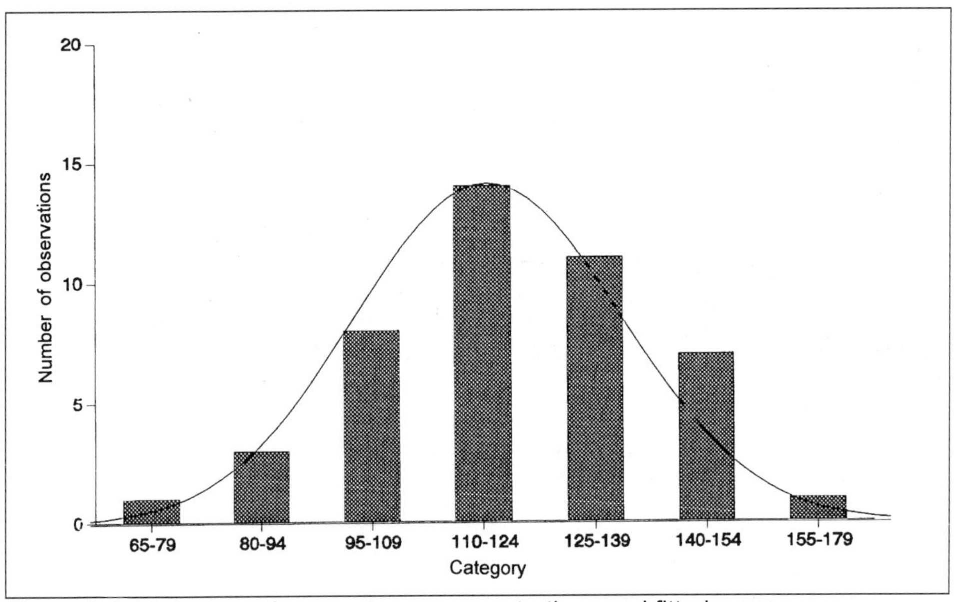

Figure 3.1. Histogram of spermatozoa concentrations and fitted curve.

The most frequently occurring category is called the 'mode' (Mo). The mode is at the peak value of the frequency distribution. The difference between the highest and lowest observed value is called the 'range' (R). Thus the mode is the category 110 to 129 and the range is 159 - 75 = 84. If many observations are made and the width of the interval is more and more decreased, the frequency distribution will look like a smooth curve that would represent much better the distribution of the continuous measurement.

Two types of figures can be calculated to describe the data: measures of position and measures of dispersion. The mean and the median are measures of position. The mean is simply the sum of all observations divided by the number of sample observations. The symbol used for the sample mean isx and for the population mean μ (mu). The median is that value that divides the observations in 2 parts of equal size. Thus 50% of all observations lie below this value and 50% of the observations show higher values. In case of an even number of observations the median is computed as the average of the 2 most central observations. If the observations are split in 4 categories, the term quartile is used. The lower quartile (Q_1) represents the value below which 25% of the observations lie. Then the median is Q_2 and Q_3 is the value above which 25% of the observations lie. In the semen concentration example the mean is calculated as (75 + 86 + ... + 159)/45 = 120.4 and the median (Q_2) is 122, Q_1 = 104.5 and Q_3 = 138.

Measures of dispersion (or spread) are the range, the semi-interquartile range (SIR), the variance and the standard deviation. The range has been defined before as the difference between the highest and lowest value. The SIR indicates how close the data are to the median and is calculated as $(Q_1+Q_3)/2$. In the semen example the SIR amounts to (104.5+138)/2 = 121.25. The variance and standard deviation (SD) indicate how close the data are to the mean. The variance and the SD are closely related because the SD is the square root of the variance. The variance in the semen example is 367.7 and the SD is 19.2. How the variance and the SD are calculated depends on the shape of the frequency distribution. Two distributions will be discussed: the Normal distribution and the Binomial distribution.

Normal distribution

Returning to the sperm concentration example, it is obvious that there is variation in sperm concentration between samples. Figure 3.1 shows the distribution of sperm concentration. If we had a very large number of samples, the width of the bars can be decreased further and further and the bell shaped curve would describe the distribution. If the distribution has this shape, it is a called a Normal distribution. The curve is unimodal (has one peak) and symmetric around the mean. Typical for a Normal distribution is that the mean and median are about equal. A Normal distribution can be described by the quite complicated looking function:

$$Y = f(x) = \left[\frac{1}{\sigma\sqrt{(2\pi)}}\right] e^{\frac{-(x-\mu)^2}{2\sigma^2}} \qquad \textbf{(3.1)}$$

e is the base of natural logarithm (a constant: 2.7183) and π equals 3.1416. Then, function f(x) is completely determined by **μ** (mu) and **σ** (sigma) with **μ** being the **mean** and **σ** the **standard deviation**.

The mean **μ** can be calculated from equation 1 by taking the first derivative, f'(x), of f(x) and solve it for f'(x)=0 (in mathematical terms, the solution will give the maximum of f(x)). Solving this equation is very complicated. However, the mean can also be obtained in a much easier way:

sum all the sperm concentrations and divide it by the number of samples measured = $\Sigma x_i/n$.

The parameter σ can be calculated by taking the second derivative, f"(x), of f(x) and solve it for f"(x) = 0 (in mathematical terms, the solution will give the point of reflection of f(x)). Fortunately, σ^2 can be approximated from the data using the formula:

$$\sigma^2 = \sum_{i=1}^{n} \frac{(x_i - \bar{x})^2}{(n-1)}$$

and of course σ is then the square root.

In the special case that **μ**=0 and σ=1, the curve is called a ***standard Normal distribution***, denoted as N(0,1), and this is the yard stick in statistical analyses on Normally distributed data with mean μ and standard deviation σ: N(**μ**,σ).

It is obvious that in the example the **μ** of sperm concentration is not equal to 0. The value of σ is not easily read from the curve. To compare the curve with the N(0,1), one needs to rescale the sperm concentration by $Z = (x - \mu)/\sigma$. After this transformation, the N(0,1) table (Appendix) can be used and the probabilities of certain outcomes can be determined.

For example, if one sperm sample is selected randomly then the probability that its rescaled concentration is between 0 and 1.0 equals 0.3413. As the curve is symmetric, the same probability holds for rescaled concentrations between -1 and 0. Thus, for rescaled concentrations between -1 and +1, the probability is 2 ∗ 0.3413 = 0.68 (see Figure 3.2).

Also and complementary, the probability of a Z smaller than -1 or larger than 1 equals 1-0.68 = 0.32. In the following table (according to Snedecor and Cochran (1980)) it is shown how probabilities can be calculated from the Appendix (A is the value directly read from Appendix).

Probability of a rescaled value:	To be calculated as:
1. Lying between 0 and Z	A
2. Lying between -Z an Z	2A
3. Lying outside the interval (-Z,Z)	1 - 2A
4. Less than Z and Z is positive	0.5 + A
5. Less than Z and Z is negative	0.5 - A
6. Greater than Z and Z is positive	0.5 - A
7. Greater than Z and Z is negative	0.5 + A

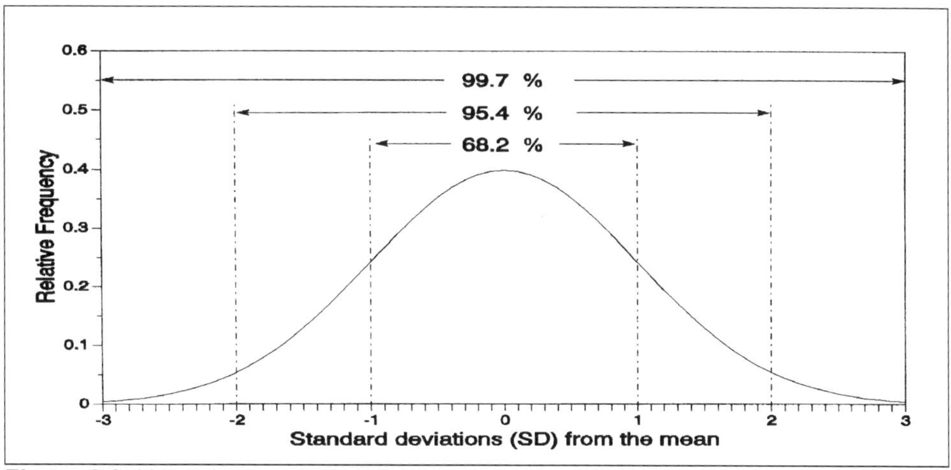

Figure 3.2. Normal curve and probabilities.

Case 3 in the table above corresponds to a 2-sided (or 2-tailed) test. Cases 4-7 are 1-sided tests. A confidence level of 95% ($P < 0.05$) is often used in statistics and especially in cases 3, 5 and 7. Which Z-value corresponds to this probability?

In case 3: $1 - 2A = 0.05$; A is 0.475 and $Z = 1.96$.
In case 5: $0.5 - A = 0.05$; $A = 0.45$ and $Z = -1.64$ (Z is negative!).
In case 7: Z yields +1.64

Typical values for Z at commonly used confidence levels are in Table 3.1.

Table 3.1. Values of Z at commonly used confidence levels as derived from the standard Normal distribution.

	80%	90%	95%	99%
2-sided test:	1.28	1.64	1.96	2.58
1-sided test:	0.84	1.28	1.64	2.33

Binomial distribution

The Binomial distribution is suited for categorical data. The parameters that characterize this distribution are the number of observations (denoted by n) and the probability of being a member of a category, for example the animal is diseased or healthy. Then the probability of being diseased is p, the probability of being healthy is q and p + q = 1.

Suppose a litter consists of 10 piglets and the expected ratio between boars and sows is 1:1. Thus p=0.5 and q=0.5. It is most likely that the litter consists of 10∗p = 5 boars and 10∗q = 5 sows. However, the litter might consist of 4 boars and 6 sows as well and with a very small probability all piglets might be males or females. The probability of each outcome is:

No. of sows	No. of boars	Probability
10	0	0.0010
9	1	0.0098
8	2	0.0439
7	3	0.1172
6	4	0.2051
5	5	0.2461
4	6	0.2051
3	7	0.1172
2	8	0.0439
1	9	0.0098
0	10	0.0010

These probabilities were derived using the formula:

$$Pr(s) = \frac{n!}{s!*(n-s)!} * p^s * q^{n-s}$$

where s equals the number of sows and n-s the number of boars (n=10). n! equals 10*9*8*.....*1 and n!/(s!*(n-s)!) gives the number of combinations that will lead to a certain outcome. By definition 0!=1. Thus for n=10 and s=9, the number of combinations is 10!/(9!*1!) = 10 as the single boar might have been the first in the litter, the second, the third,.... or the tenth.

If p = 0.5, the distribution is symmetric. Other values for p will result in skewed distributions (Figure 3.3). The shape of the distribution is solely determined by n and p. When n increases, the skewness decreases and under certain conditions (n*p greater than 5 and n*q greater than 5) the distribution approximates a Normal distribution. The advantage of this is that the Z-values of the Normal distribution can be used for further statistical calculations, e.g., calculation of confidence intervals. If the approximation is not allowed, exact confidence intervals should be calculated.

In Binomial distributions, the measure of position is given by E = n*p and a measure of dispersion is given by SD = $\sqrt{(p*q)}/\sqrt{(n)}$.

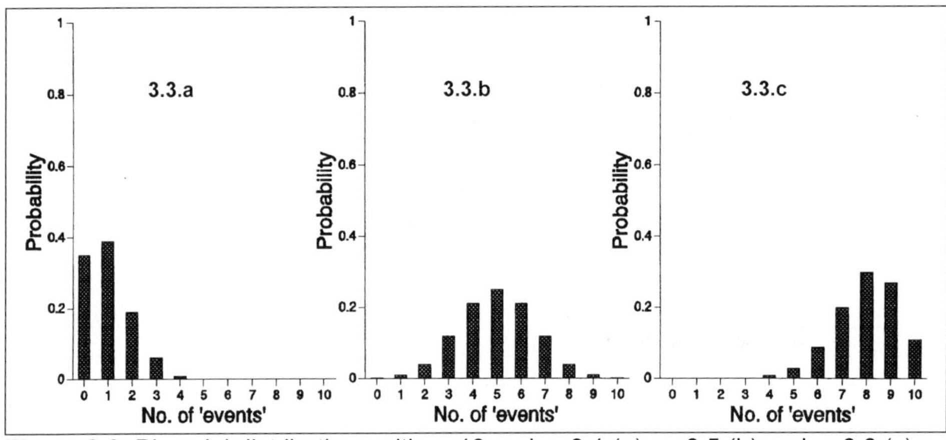

Figure 3.3. Binomial distributions with n=10 and p=0.1 (a), p=0.5 (b) and p=0.8 (c).

Confidence intervals and power

In sampling, parameters of interest are calculated from a subset of the population. The sample mean is then used as an estimate of the population mean. Each sample can be regarded as a drawing from a $N(\mu,\sigma)$ distribution and the standard deviation of the ***sample mean*** - not for the single drawing! - (often referred to as the standard error) is $\sigma/\sqrt{n}$, in which n is the number of drawings. Strictly spoken, the formula $\sigma/\sqrt{n}$ is valid only for random sampling ***with*** replacement. When n/N (sampling fraction) is large (larger than 0.1, rule of thumb) then $\sigma/\sqrt{n}$ should be multiplied by: $\sqrt{(1 - n/N)}$. A confidence interval (CI) for the sample meanx can be written as:

$$\bar{x} \pm \frac{Z * \sigma}{\sqrt{n}} \qquad \textbf{(3.2)}$$

In case we choose a 95% CI, Z equals 1.96. This confidence interval is interpreted as: if one should repeat this process of taking a random sample from the population a hundred times then the sampling mean would be in 95 out of 100 samplings within the assessed interval.

Sometimes one is not interested in the mean of the population but in a difference of that mean with a pre-defined value or in differences between parts of the population, e.g., production differences between healthy and diseased animals.

The parameter of interest is rather the magnitude of the difference between the means than the means on their own. The null hypothesis is stated as: the difference (D) is equal to 0. If in the total population the true difference is equal to or larger than D, the null hypothesis should be rejected. The probability of rejecting the null hypothesis when it is false, is called the ***power*** of the test (Table 3.2).

Table 3.2. Power and confidence.

		True Difference	
		Present	Absent
Conclusion of Statistical Test	Different (reject null hypothesis)	(a) Correct ($1 - \beta$, power)	(b) Incorrect (Type I or alpha error)
	Not Different (accept null hypothesis)	(c) Incorrect (Type II or beta error)	(d) Correct ($1 - \alpha$, confidence)

The power is a rather complicated quantity, because it depends on D, n, σ and the type (1-sided or 2-sided) and significance level of the test. It can be shown that the power of a test is the probability that:

$$Z_{\beta} > \left(\frac{-\sqrt{n}}{\sigma}\right) * D + Z_{2\alpha}$$

This probability can again be read from the table in the Appendix.

In the next part of this session, formulae will be shown to solve n when we know σ, fix Z_{α} to a specific value and eventually specify Z_{β} and D as well.

4. Sample Size Estimation

The formulae for sample size estimation depend on the type of data and the design of the study. One cannot use the same formula for estimation of milk yield and for estimating disease prevalence or to detect whether a herd is diseased or not. In this paragraph, the following sample size calculations will be explained:

1. to estimate a mean;
2. to estimate differences between means;
3. to estimate a proportion (e.g., prevalence);
4. to estimate differences between proportions;
5. to detect a disease in a population;
6. to estimate the relationship between exposure and disease.

Sample size calculations are necessary before carrying out a survey or experiment. Outcomes of these calculations are ***guidelines*** to about how many units should be included in the study. Calculations can be done by using a hand-calculator, or software such as EPISCOPE (Frankena *et al.*, 1990) or WINEPISCOPE[12], the public domain version under WINDOWS.

4.1. Sample size formula to estimate a mean

To calculate sample sizes for a mean obtained from a Normal distribution, it is needed to estimate both the mean and its standard deviation (SD). Secondly, the interval L should be defined, indicating that with a probability of x% the true population mean will be within the interval of the sample mean ± L. This interval is therefore an indication of the precision of the estimate. Thirdly, we have to decide on x. There is no general rule for this decision, but 95 is commonly used. From x we can determine the corresponding number (Z) of units of SD. For example, if x=95 then the significance level is 5% and $Z_{0.05}$=1.96, which means that 95% of all the observations will fall within the interval: mean ± 1.96∗SD/√n

Now the confidence interval (CI) for a mean, obtained by drawing elements from a Normal distribution, can be written as:

$$CI = \bar{x} \pm \frac{Z_{\alpha} * SD}{\sqrt{n}}$$

[12] To be downloaded from the Website: http://www.zod.wau.nl/qve

If the part after the ± sign is denoted as L, n is calculated as:

$$n = \frac{Z_{\alpha}^{2} * SD^{2}}{L^{2}} \quad \textbf{(3.3)}$$

Example: suppose you want to estimate growth/day in veal calves. Growth should be around 1000 grammes/day and an estimate of the SD is 250 grammes. How many calves should be weighed to check whether or not the mean growth of a large unit is between 950 and 1050 grammes/day? A confidence level of 95% is required. (If you want more practice: determine also numbers needed in case (1) SD increases with 50%, (2) the confidence level decreases to 90 %, or (3) L is changed from 50 to 100). Answers: 97; 217; 68; 25.
Note: as we cannot sample animals partially, the calculated sample size should be rounded upwards.

If a relatively large part of a population with size N is sampled, i.e., the sampling fraction (n/N) is large, the standard deviation is generally overestimated. Suppose you have all elements of the population sampled (n=N), then the 'sample' mean is exactly equal to the population mean and the standard deviation should be 0. Therefore, a correction of the SD is necessary if more than 10% (rule of thumb) of the population is sampled. This correction consists of multiplying the SD with $\sqrt{(1-f)}$, where f = n/N is the sampling fraction (1 - f is also called the finite population correction). If n equals N then the SD indeed becomes 0. The finite population correction can also be applied directly in formula (3.3) through dividing the calculated n by 1 + f.

$$n_a = \frac{n}{\left(1 + \frac{n}{N}\right)}$$

Example: suppose the number of sampled veal calves in the previous exercise originated from a population of 750 animals. Calculate the adjusted sample size. Suppose the sampled veal calves originated from a population of 10,000 animals. Calculate the adjusted sample size. Answers: 85; 95.

4.2. Sample size to estimate differences between means

Sometimes an investigator is interested in differences between groups of animals, e.g., differences in milk production between mastitic cows and healthy cows. Suppose milk production is a Normally distributed parameter. Now we can perform a ***one-tailed*** test, because we know that mastitic cows will show a ***reduced*** milk production. This has an impact on the value of Z_{α}: the one-sided value of $Z_{0.05}$ is equal to the two-sided $Z_{0.10}$ (see Table 3.1.).

In order to make the sample size calculation we need:

- an estimation of the difference between both groups δ
- the standard deviation of the trait
- the significance level α
- the power of the test, i.e., the probability (1-β) of obtaining a significant result if the true difference equals δ

The sample size formula is written as (Snedecor and Cochran, 1980):

$$n = \frac{2 * (Z_\alpha + Z_\beta)^2 * SD^2}{\delta^2} \qquad \textbf{(3.4)}$$

Z_α, Z_β	=	values of the standard Normal distribution at specified levels of confidence and power
SD	=	standard deviation
δ	=	estimated difference

The constant, 2, in formula (3.4) arises from the assumption that the SD is equal in both groups. The calculated sample size is the number of animals per group.

Example: suppose daily milk production in healthy cows is 25 litres and in mastitic cows it is assumed to be reduced with 10%. Thus δ = 2.5 litres. The standard deviation of daily milk production is known to be 6 litres. Given a one-sided α of 0.05, $Z_{0.05}$ = 1.64 and a power of 80%, $Z_{0.20}$ = 0.84 (Table 3.1), determine the sample size ***per group***. For more practice vary the value of SD, δ and α to your liking. Answer: 71 per group.

4.3. Sample size to estimate a proportion (e.g., prevalence)

In the previous sample size calculations, it was assumed that the traits were recorded as continuous measurements that were Normally distributed. However, when one wants to investigate presence of disease, one deals with a yes/no (binomial) situation because each selected element is either healthy or diseased. One property of the Binomial distribution is that the variance of the mean (e.g., the prevalence) equals p∗(1 - p) when p is expressed as a proportion (or it is p∗(100 -p), when p is expressed as a percentage). Of course, the standard deviation is the square root of p∗(1 - p). Then, formula (3.3) can be used again for determining the sample size. A striking property of the SD of a proportion is that it is symmetric around its maximum at p = 0.5 (or 50%). Hence, the sample size is maximal when p is estimated to be 50% and this value should be used when there is no idea of the actual proportion (see Table below). The finite population correction is also applicable in the binomial situation.

Sample sizes given L=0.05, Z_α=1.96 and infinite N at varying estimated prevalences:											
Prev.	0	0.10	0.20	0.30	0.40	0.50	0.60	0.70	0.80	0.90	1.0
SD	0	0.30	0.40	0.46	0.49	0.50	0.49	0.46	0.40	0.30	0
n	0	139	246	323	369	385	369	323	246	139	0

It should be noticed that L is the ***absolute*** precision. It is often more convenient to take a lower absolute precision at low or high prevalences. For example, one is not interested whether or not the prevalence equals 4% ± 10%, but 4% ± 2%.

Example: a farmer raising veal calves asks you to determine the prevalence of salmonellosis due to *Salmonella dublin* in veal calves. It is a large unit with 1000 calves. The prevalence on this farm is known to range from 0 to 80%. It is prudent to put the estimated prevalence at 50%, because nothing is known about the actual prevalence except that it is between 0 and 80%. By choosing 50%, you will end up with the largest possible sample size for a desired value of L and Z. Secondly, you need to put values on L and Z, and you choose 5% and 1.96. The ultimate result obtained is that the actual prevalence is with a probability of 95% between 45 and 55%. Now, calculate n. Determine whether the finite population correction is needed. If so, determine the adjusted n. Answers: 385; 278.

After you have done the sampling, it shows that the prevalence is 10%, which is much lower than your initial estimate of 50%.

In fact, more than enough animals have been sampled to fulfil the initial conditions (L = 0.05 and Z = 1.96) and the values of these can be recalculated (the adjusted n equals 278). For example:

$$L = \frac{Z_\alpha * SD}{\sqrt{n}} = \frac{1.96 * \sqrt{0.1 * 0.9}}{\sqrt{278}} = 0.035 \text{ (or } 3.5\,\%)$$

Taking the finite population correction into account, the SD equals $\sqrt{(0.1 * 0.9)} * \sqrt{(1 - 278/1000)} = 0.255$ and, subsequently, $L = 1.96 * 0.255/\sqrt{278} = 0.03$. The actual prevalence is, with a probability of 95%, within the interval 10 ± 3.0%.

4.4. Sample size to estimate differences between proportions

Suppose you want to compare two antibiotics. Two groups of animals are infected with an appropriate pathogen and the percentages of recovery in both groups are compared. Question: how many animals should be included in each group? The following formula can be used (Snedecor and Cochran, 1980):

$$n = \left(\frac{Z_\alpha + Z_\beta}{p_1 - p_2}\right)^2 * \left(p_1 q_1 + p_2 q_2\right) \qquad \textbf{(3.5)}$$

Z_α, Z_β =	values of the standard Normal distribution at specified levels of confidence and power
p_1, p_2 =	estimated proportions of recovery in group 1 and 2
q_1, q_2 =	1 - p_1, 1 - p_2, respectively

Example: a pharmaceutical company has developed a brand new antibiotic against pathogen X. No other antibiotics are available, so no comparison can be made with existing antibiotic treatments. However, it is known from field data that 70% recovers from the disease (although effects on production are tremendous). It is expected (hoped) that after use of the antibiotic 95% of the animals will cure and that the duration of the disease will be shorter as well. Thus, p_1 = 0.70 and p_2 = 0.95. Choosing a one-sided (!) confidence of 95% and a power of 80%, it shows that the values for Z_α and Z_β are 1.64 and 0.84, respectively. Using formula 3.5, calculate n per group. Is it justified to choose a one-sided hypothesis here or should a two-sided hypothesis be chosen? Can the second aspect, the duration of disease, be taken into account? Answers: 26; one-sided will do as it is expected that the antibiotic is better than doing nothing; no.

4.5. Sample size to estimate equality of proportions (or means)

Suppose an antibiotic cures 95% of the animals. This figure is hard to beat for a new antibiotic and the researcher might be content to prove that the new antibiotic is about as effective as the existing one. How many animals should be treated in a comparative experiment? Formula (3.5) (or (3.4)) can be used again, but now $p_1 - p_2$ (or δ) is defined as the ***permitted difference***. In case of equivalence testing α and β are the mirror images of those used for difference testing. Thus, a typical value for the confidence level 1 - α is now 0.8 and a typical value for the power 1 - β is 0.95. In general, testing for equivalence needs a larger sample size than testing for a difference. This is due to the fact that the power is always one-sided while the confidence level might be defined either as one-sided or two-sided. Table 3.3 shows the sample sizes per treatment group to show equivalence.

Table 3.3. Observations per treatment group for various proportions cure in the treatment groups and a number of values for the permitted difference d using a one-sided test (assuming 1 - β = 0.95, 1 - α = 0.8).

	Expected proportion cure in both groups						
d	0.30	0.40	0.50	0.60	0.70	0.80	0.90
0.05	1038	1187	1236	1187	1038	790	445
0.10	260	297	310	297	260	198	111
0.15	116	133	138	133	116	88	49
0.20	66	75	78	75	66	49	28

4.6. Sample size to detect a disease in a population

Suppose one is interested in the percentage of ***farms*** that is infected by pathogen X (prevalence based on whether or not the pathogen is present at a farm). A farm is considered to be infected when at least one of its animals is infected. First the appropriate number of farms as units of concern is randomly chosen (see paragraph 4.3 for sample size calculation) and secondly the status of the farm (infected or not) is determined. The proportion of infected animals per farm is not of major interest. Ideally, one would screen ***all*** the animals on a farm, but often this is not necessary and one can stand with a selected number of animals. Suppose that it is known that if the disease is present, about 50% of the animals are likely to be positive. By sampling one animal you have 50% probability to test a truly positive farm as positive. In general, one aims at a higher probability to classify a positive farm correctly (e.g., 95%). By selecting 2 animals, the probability is increased up to 75% (25% of drawings show two negatives), 3 animals yield 87.5%, 4 animals 93.75% and 5 animals 96.875%. Thus, between 4 and 5 animals should be sampled to detect positive farms with a probability of 95%, if 50% of the animals is truly diseased.

These calculations can be put into a general formula (Cannon and Roe, 1982):

$$n = \left(1 - (1-P)^{\frac{1}{d}}\right) * \left(N - \frac{(d-1)}{2}\right) \qquad \textbf{(3.6)}$$

n = sample size
P = probability of finding at least one case (= confidence level, e.g., 0.95)
d = number of (detectable) cases in the population
N = population size

If the test that is used to evaluate the status of the animals has not a 100% sensitivity (see Chapter IV, paragraph 3), d is equal to the number of diseased or infected animals multiplied by the sensitivity of the test. It is assumed that no false-positives are present or that they are ruled out by confirmatory tests.

Example: suppose you want to detect whether or not a flock of N = 1000 animals is positive with regard to pathogen X. If X is present, you suspect that about 50% of the animals will be infected, thus d = 500. Setting *P* to 0.95, n equals: $(1 - 0.05^{1/500}) * (1000 - 499/2) = 4.48$ (rounded as 5). Is this number much affected by N? (No, because the prevalence is rather high).

About the same formula can be used to determine the maximum number of positives (d) in a population given that **all** samples (n) were tested negative:

$$d = \left(1 - (1-P)^{\frac{1}{n}}\right) * \left(N - \frac{n-1}{2}\right) \qquad \textbf{(3.7)}$$

Example: suppose that 1,000 slaughter cows were tested negative on *E. coli* $O_{157}:H_7$ and the total number of cows slaughtered amounted to 1 million. What is the maximal prevalence in the 'population' of slaughter cows? What is the maximum prevalence if the sensitivity of the test is only 85%? Answers: if p is set to 0.95 then d equals 2990 which is about 0.3%; 0.3/0.85 = 0.35.

4.7. Sample size to estimate the relationship between exposure and disease

As pointed out in the introduction, there are two major reasons why a planned sample is often used in epidemiology. Firstly, to describe population characteristics (e.g., disease prevalence or presence, see previous paragraphs) and secondly to determine relationships between exposure to certain factors and a specified disease. The relation between exposure to a factor (or a set of factors) and the development of disease is expressed by measures of associations like the relative risk (RR), or its estimator the odds ratio (OR). How these parameters are calculated and how they should be interpreted will be shown in Chapter V. For the time being, it is sufficient to know that diseased animals are compared to non-diseased animals regarding to the status of the exposure (yes or no). Also, for estimation of the RR (OR) a sample size formula does exist. The following values have to be assumed/stated:

- the relative frequency p_0 of exposure among non-diseased animals
- the minimal magnitude (R) of the risk measure that is of interest
- the ratio c between non-diseased/diseased animals (number of controls per case)
- Z_α, corresponding to the level of confidence, $1 - \alpha$
- Z_β, corresponding to the level of the power, $1 - \beta$

To calculate the appropriate sample size for risk estimators, the following formula can be used (Schlesselman, 1982):

$$n = \frac{\left[z_\alpha \sqrt{\left(1+\frac{1}{c}\right)\overline{p'}\,\overline{q'}} + z_\beta \sqrt{p_1 q_1 + \frac{p_0 q_0}{c}} \right]^2}{(p_1 - p_0)^2} \qquad \textbf{(3.8)}$$

in which

$$\overline{p'} = \frac{(p_1 + c\,p_0)}{(1+c)} \text{ and}$$

$$\overline{q'} = 1 - \overline{p'}$$

p_1 is the relative frequency of exposure among cases and is calculated as:

$$p_1 = \frac{p_0 R}{1 + p_0 * (R-1)}$$

$\overline{p'}$ = average exposure weighted for numbers of cases and controls.

Example: you want to investigate the relation between type of ventilation and the occurrence of salmonellosis in poultry. Two types of ventilation are evaluated: mechanical and natural. p_0 is estimated to be 30%; R is interesting if it is at least about 2.5; c, Z_α, Z_β are set to 1, 1.96 and 0.84 respectively.

Using the formulae, it shows that the sample size ***per group*** equals:

$$p_1 = \frac{0.30 * 2.5}{1 + 0.30 * 1.5} = \frac{0.75}{1.45} = 0.52$$

$$\overline{p'} = \frac{0.52 + 1 * 0.3}{2} = 0.41$$

$$n = \frac{\left[1.96 * \sqrt{2 * 0.41 * 0.59} + 0.84 \sqrt{0.52 * 0.48 + \frac{0.30 * 0.70}{1}} \right]^2}{(0.52 - 0.30)^2} = 77$$

Thus, given the assumptions, about 77 cases and 77 controls should be investigated.

5. Concluding Remarks

In this chapter several sampling designs were described. Formulae do exist to estimate sample sizes on beforehand and these should always be applied in prospective studies. These sample size calculations are only guidelines to how many units should be investigated. It is not a strict number as the assumptions underlying the calculations will almost never exactly mirror the true values. To detect small differences you will need large samples. So, if your resources are not sufficient to use the calculated sample size, the decision might be not going to start with the experiment or survey. To be sure, you should calculate the power of the study on beforehand when having a limited sample size.

Besides the described ones, many other formulae for calculation of sample sizes do exist (e.g., for a different hypothesis, a somewhat different design or different types of data). However, the general principle is always the same and, therefore, only the most basic and most frequently used sample size formulae were presented here.

References

Campbell, R.C. (1974). Statistics for biologists. 2nd edn. Cambridge University Press, Cambridge.

Cannon, R.M.; Roe, R.T. (1982). Livestock Disease Surveys: a Field Manual for Veterinarians. Australian Government Publishing Service.

Frankena, K.; Noordhuizen, J.P.; Willeberg, P.; Voorthuysen, P.F. van; Goelema, J.O. (1990). EPISCOPE: Computer programs in veterinary epidemiology. Veterinary Record, 126, 573-576.

Schlesselman, J.J. (1982). Monographs in Epidemiology and Biostatistics - volume 3: Case Control Studies: Design, Conduct, Analysis. Oxford University Press, New York/Oxford.

Snedecor, G.W.; Cochran, W.G. (1980). Statistical Methods. 7th edn. Iowa State University University Press, Ames, Iowa.

Further Reading

Martin, S.W.; Meek, A.H.; Willeberg, P. (1987). Veterinary Epidemiology: Principles and Methods, Iowa State University Press, Ames, Iowa.
Thrusfield, M. (1995). Veterinary Epidemiology. 2nd edn. Blackwell Science, Oxford.

6. Exercises

6.1. Sample size for detection of disease in a population

Detection of positive animals

Suppose a farmer has 100 cows, 30 calves and 20 ewes. He is interested whether or not animals on his farm are infected with *Leptospira hardjo*. In general, 10% of the animals is infected if the disease is present on a farm. As the farmer knows a little bit about statistics, he wishes a confidence level of 95%.

1a. Calculate the number of samples that is needed to investigate whether or not the disease is present on the farm (solve n from N, d and *P*).
1b. Calculate the number of samples that is needed to investigate whether or not the disease is present in a each category of animals.
1c. How many samples should be taken in case the total population size is 1,000 resp. 10,000 animals?
1d. Repeat questions 1a, 1b and 1c in case the minimum prevalence is 20% and explain the difference.

Maximum number of positives when all samples are negative

Coccidiosis infection is a serious problem in broiler flocks. Treatment of the flock is based on a sample of 3 animals out of 10,000: if one of these animals is positive the flock is treated, if all are negative, the flock is left untreated.

2a. If *P* is set to 0.95, solve d.
2b. Give your comment about this method using the answer of the previous question.
2c. Undoubtedly, you have given a negative comment! Now, suppose that production losses only occur when 65% of the broilers is positive. How many samples should be taken to conclude whether or not more than 65% of the broilers is positive? Reconsider your comment.

Screening

A screening programme for the infectious disease Y in pigs is developed. Disease Y is known to be present at rather low prevalences in a herd (in general less than 20%). One of the goals is to estimate the number of farms that is positive. In total 10,000 farms of 100 animals each must be screened. One million dollar is available. Collection of one sample costs 5 dollars, the subsequent analysis 15 dollars.

3a. To keep things easy, the same number of samples is taken on all farms. From a financial point of view, how many samples can be collected on each farm?
3b. Is that number sufficient to detect a disease at the 20% level?
3c. If you had to decide about a 'stop or go' of the screening programme, what would be your conclusion?
3d. Suppose that the disease is present at a level of 50%. Repeat questions 3b and 3c.

Trouble shooting

A farmer of a 95 cow herd runs into trouble: some cows abort, others have a lower production than expected and so on. He calls for the practitioner who sends 5 randomly taken blood samples to the Animal Health Service for detection of antibodies against virus X. All samples show negative results. The practitioner tells the farmer that the probability of presence of X in his herd is minimal and that there should be another reason for the troubles.

4a. Give your comment about this conclusion, e.g., by calculating the maximum number of positive animals (solve d from n, N and p).
4b. Was it reasonable to take the samples ***at random***?

6.2. Sample size to estimate a proportion

Effect of population size

1a. A fictive population consists of 100 animals. How many samples are needed to confirm a prevalence of 50% ± 5% at a 95% confidence level, using the unadjusted sample size? What is the sampling fraction and what is the adjusted sample size?
1b. Repeat question 1a for population sizes of 1,000, 10,000, 100,000 and 1 million animals.
1c. A rule of thumb is that the adjusted sample size should be used when the sampling fraction exceeds 5 or 10% of the population size. Do you agree with this rule considering the answers of question 1b?

Effect of (estimated) prevalence

The prevalence of disease X is unknown and it is decided to perform a survey to estimate that prevalence. Three experts are asked to give their opinion about their expectation of the prevalence. Expert 1 estimates the prevalence as high as 75%, expert 2 as 50% and expert 3 as 25%.

2a. Calculate the needed sample sizes according to the expert opinions. (assume: pop. size = 1 million, precision = 5% and the conf. level = 95%)
2b. The sample sizes using the opinion of expert 1 and 3 are exactly equal. Explain why.
2c. When a prevalence is unknown and there is absolutely no idea about it, which prevalence would you use for the sample size calculation and why?

Effect of precision

3a. In the previous exercise (2a) the precision was set to 5%. Recalculate the sample size when the precision is set to 10%.
3b. Recalculate the sample sizes of question 3a., setting the ***relative*** precision to 10%.

Effect of confidence level

4a. What do you expect with regard to the sample size when the confidence level decreases?
4b. Confirm your expectation by computing the sample size using a population of 1000 animals, estimated prevalence = 50% and the precision = 10%. The confidence level is set to 97.5%, 95% and 90%, respectively.

Fattener claim

A fattener unit consists of 1500 pigs. The farmer notices that several pigs show clinical signs of atrophic rhinitis. This disease may cause severe economic losses, and thus he claims the losses from the multiplier. As it is too cumbersome to check all animals individually, it is decided to take a random sample and use the percentage of positives in this sample to calculate the total number of diseased animals.

The fattener takes 20 samples and sends them to the Animal Health Service for analysis. It appears that 50% of the samples is positive, and thus the fattener claims losses for 750 pigs.

5a. How many samples are needed to measure a prevalence of 50% in a 1500 pig herd?
5b. What is the achieved precision of the estimation of the prevalence?
5c. If you were the multiplier and you knew all about statistics and sample sizes, what would be your answer to the claim?

National prevalence of infected herds

The government of country X is interested in the prevalence of leptospirosis on both the herd level and the animal level. In country X agriculture is very structured: there are 100,000 farms with 100 animals each. You are asked to develop a project to estimate both prevalences. This exercise concerns a very important part of every project: the number of observations that is planned. Preliminary studies show that about 20% of the cows on positive farms is positive.

6aI. Describe how you will determine the number of farms that is needed to estimate the percentage of ***herds*** that is infected. How do you select these herds?
6aII. Give values to the parameters of interest and calculate the number of herds to estimate the percentage of herds that is infected.
6aIII. Give values to the parameters of interest and calculate the number of animals that is needed to ***detect*** the disease on a farm. How do you select these animals?

6bI. Describe how you will determine the number of animals that is needed to estimate the percentage of ***animals*** that is infected, assuming that all animals form a homogeneous population.

6bII. Give values to the parameters of interest and calculate the needed sample size.

6c. Suppose country X consists of 2 counties, the North (80% of all farms) and the South (20% of all farms). It is assumed that within each county, the animals form a homogeneous population. In the South co-grazing with sheep is very common, while it is not in the North. Co-grazing with sheep is known to be a risk factor for leptospirosis in cattle. Does this knowledge have any consequences for the way you select the herds in question 6aI?

6.3. Sample size to estimate a difference between proportions

Effect of magnitude of difference

1aI. It is expected that 20% of all cows suffering from coli mastitis will recover without any treatment. When using antibiotic X, it is expected that 70% will recover. Calculate the number of animals in each 'treatment'-group (one group is treated with a placebo) for a statistical evaluation that the antibiotic has a positive effect on the percentage of animals recovering. Set the confidence level to 95% and the power to 90%.

1aII. Do you prefer the 'one-tailed' or 'two-tailed' sample size? Explain!

1bI. Recalculate 1a when comparing antibiotic X to antibiotic Y, the latter is expected to cure about 50%.

1bII. Explain why the sample size in 1bI is much larger than in 1aI.

Effect of proportion level

2aI. You need to compare 2 anthelmintics. Anthelmintic 1 is supposed to suppress the faecal egg output with 95%, anthelmintic 2 suppresses it with 85%. Calculate the number of animals in each treatment group for a statistical evaluation that anthelmintic 1 is more effective than anthelmintic 2. Set the confidence level to 95% and the power to 90%.

2aII. Give your opinion about the following statement: "The numbers calculated in 1a are sufficient to conclude that anthelmintic 1 gives 10% more egg output suppression when compared to anthelmintic 2".

2bI. Recalculate question 1 when anthelmintic 1 suppresses the egg output with 75% and anthelmintic 2 with 65%.

2bII. Explain the difference between 2aI and 2bI.

Effect of type I error

3. Take the figures of exercise 1aI. Change the confidence level to 90% and 99% and compare the answers. Explain the difference.

Effect of type II error

4. Take the figures of exercise 1al. Change the power level to 80% and 95% and compare the answers. Explain the difference.

7. Answers

7.1. Sample size for detection of disease in a population

Detection of positive animals

1a. The total number of animals is 150. It is assumed that all animals are equally susceptible for the disease and that the animals are kept together.
The percentage diseased is 10%, so if the disease is present, 15 animals will be infected. The sample size to detect the disease is 26 (formula (3.6)).

1b. Cows: 25
Calves: 19
Ewes: 16
When the population is very small and the disease is present at rather low levels, almost the total population should be sampled.

1c. 29 samples in both cases. Under the specified conditions the formula its limit in infinity is 29.

1d. 13; 13, 11, 10; 14. If the prevalence is higher, the sample size needed to detect at least one positive animal decreases.

Maximum number of positives when all samples are negative

2a. From formula (3.7): d = 6316. In words, when the 3 samples are negative there might be at maximum about 63% (6316) of all animals infected!

2b. Of course you have answered that it is of no sense to base the decision about treatment of the flock on this very unreliable method.

2c. It appears that you need ... 4 animals (3.11 to be exactly, and as we cannot sample a 0.11 part of the animal, it is rounded to 4)! To detect whether or not the production loss limit will be reached needs only very few animals. This is caused by the fact that this limit is set to a very high level (65%).

Screening

3a. One sample costs 20 dollars, so 50,000 samples can be collected. This is 5 samples per farm.

3b. No, you need 13 samples (formula (3.6)) to detect the disease at the herd level (if the prevalence level equals 20%).

3c. Stop.

3d. Now, you need 5 samples. The programme can start.

Trouble shooting

4a. 42 cows might be positive, which is about 44% (formula (3.7)). Thus the conclusion of the practitioner is only correct under the condition that if virus X is present, more than 45% of all cows will be seropositive.

4b. No! To enlarge the possibility of sampling a positive animal, he should have taken samples from ***suspected*** cows. However, then it is not possible to use formula (3.6) any more as it assumes random sampling. Secondly, we do not know how good the practitioner is in selecting suspected animals.

7.2. Sample size to estimate a proportion

Effect of population size

1a. The sample size is 385 animals (formula (3.3)), using SD of a proportion of 50%), which means that 385% of the population is sampled. This of course is not possible. The corrected sample size is 80 (due to the finite population correction).

1b. The unadjusted sample size is always 385.

population size	adj. sample size	sampling fraction
1,000	278	27.8
10,000	370	3.7
100,000	383	0.38
1,000,000	384	0.0038

1c. Take the figures of question 1b. as an example. In case of a population of 10,000 animals 370 samples are needed. According to the rule of thumb, the finite population correction is not needed and thus 385 samples should be taken. This means an oversampling of 15 animals. It depends on the costs per sample whether or not this oversampling is cumbersome.

The rule of thumb has been developed for ease of calculation. By hand, the unadjusted sample size is calculated first, then the sampling fraction and, if this exceeds 10%, the adjusted sample size. Computer programmes mostly compute the adjusted sample size simultaneously and of course the adjusted value will be used in all cases.

Effect of (estimated) prevalence

2a. Expert 1: 289 (formula (3.3)), using SD of a proportion of 25%),
Expert 2: 385 (formula (3.3)), using SD of a proportion of 50%),
Expert 3: 289 (formula (3.3)), using SD of a proportion of 75%),

2b. The sample size depends on the standard deviation of the (estimated) prevalence. This standard deviation is equal to the square root of PREV∗(100 - PREV). For expert 1 the SD equals SQRT(75 ∗ 25), while it is SQRT(25 ∗ 75) for expert 3. The SD's are equal and thus the obtained sample sizes are equal.

It can also be explained in the following way. Estimation of a 'disease prevalence' of 25% is exactly equal to estimation of a 'health prevalence' of 75%! For sample size considerations it does not matter whether the proportion of healthy or the proportion of diseased is determined.

2c. 50%. At this level the sample size is maximal. If the expected prevalence was not correct and the prevalence is closer to 50% than expected, the sample size would be too small to get the desired precision.

Effect of precision

3a. 25% and 75%: 73
50%: 97
The less precise one wants to be, the less samples one needs.

3b.

Estim. prevalence	Rel. precision	Abs. precision	Sample size
25	10	2.5	1153
50	10	5	385
75	10	7.5	129

Be aware of the difference between ***absolute*** and ***relative*** precision. The formula always uses the absolute precision.

Effect of confidence level

4a. When the confidence level is set to a lower level the sample size will decrease.

4b. 112 - 88 - 64: these are the adjusted sample sizes. The unadjusted sample sizes are respectively 126 - 97 - 68 with sampling fractions of 11%-9%-6%.

Fattener claim

5a. To estimate a prevalence in a 1500 pig herd needs 91 animals (at a precision of 10% and a confidence level of 95% after finite population correction-formula (3.3)). With a 5% precision and 95% confidence these figures are respectively 306 (adjusted) and 385 (unadjusted).

5b. This question can be solved directly from the formula $L = (Z*SD)/\sqrt{n} = 1.96*50/\sqrt{20} = 21.9\%$. It is not necessary to take the finite population correction into account in the SD because the sampling fraction is only 1.3% (20/1500). For completeness: if that correction had been applied the precision equals $Z*SD*\sqrt{(1 - n/N)}/\sqrt{n} = 21.8\%$.

5c. The precision is too low, the prevalence might be 50 - 21.9 = 28% as well as 50 + 21.9 = 72%. Tell the fattener that you are willing to pay for 0.28∗1500 = 420 pigs or that he should sample more pigs to estimate the prevalence more precisely.

National prevalence of infected herds

6aI. In the worst case, at least for sample size considerations, 50% of all farms is infected. Thus the estimated prevalence is set to 50%. The precision and the confidence level are set to 'reasonable' values (e.g., 10% and 95%). The sample size can be calculated from these figures.
When nothing is known about the disease, simple random sampling is best.

6aII. 97 (or 385 when the precision is set to 5%).

6aIII. Using the formula for the detection of a disease in a 100 cow herd, it appears that 13 animals per herd are needed. For detection of disease it is common to sample those animals that are suspected of having the disease. If you do not know anything about the disease: use random sampling. In total 97∗13 = 1261 animals are sampled.

6b. The percentage of positive farms is unknown. In the worst situation, it is 100%. In that case, 20% of all animals turns out to be positive. To estimate a prevalence as high as 20% in an infinite homogeneous population one needs 62 animals (at a precision of 5%: 246).
These animals should be randomly spread over all farms. In fact, we have oversampled the population (n = 1261) for this purpose.

6c. Due to random error it is possible to select more herds from the South than from the North and vice versa. To estimate the prevalence in a proper way it is needed to select the farms in a stratified way: from all farms selected 80% should be in the North and 20% should be in the South. In that case, the greater risk of leptospirosis in the South does not have an adverse effect on the prevalence estimations. But this is only true if expected prevalence within strata is equal.

7.3. Sample size to estimate a difference between proportions

Effect of magnitude of difference

1a. Using formula (3.5): n = 13 per group. The one-tailed number per group is sufficient because you want to know whether or not the treatment is **better** than doing nothing.

1bI. One-tailed: 99, two-tailed: 121 per group. As it is expected that X is better than Y, a one-tailed test will be sufficient.

1bII. The difference between the proportions is 50 and 20 in question 1a and 2a, resp. The smaller the difference, the more samples you will need to show that this difference is statistically significant.

Effect of proportion level

2aI. 150 animals each (use formula (3.5)).

2aII. Most likely you have answered that it is a correct statement. Just solve question 2bI and reconsider your opinion, if necessary.

2bI. 356 animals each (use formula (3.5)). The difference between egg output suppression is still 10%!

2bII. The number of samples needed depends on the difference between both proportions and on the proportion level itself. When this level is closer to 50%, the sample size increases. Thus the statement in 2aII is **not** correct; it should also mention the proportion level.

Effect of type I error

3. If the power is set to 90%:

Conf. level	Sample size
90	10
95	13
99	20

If the confidence level increases, the number of samples increases. The more you want to exclude the possibility that a difference is due to random error, the more samples you will need.

Effect of type II error

4. If the confidence level is set to 95%:

Power	Sample size
80	10
90	13
95	16

If the power increases, the number of samples increases. The more you want to exclude the possibility that an existing difference is not detected, the more samples you will need.

APPENDIX (from Snedecor and Cochran, 1980)

Table Cumulative Normal Frequency Distribution

(area under standard normal curve from 0 to Z)

N (0,1)

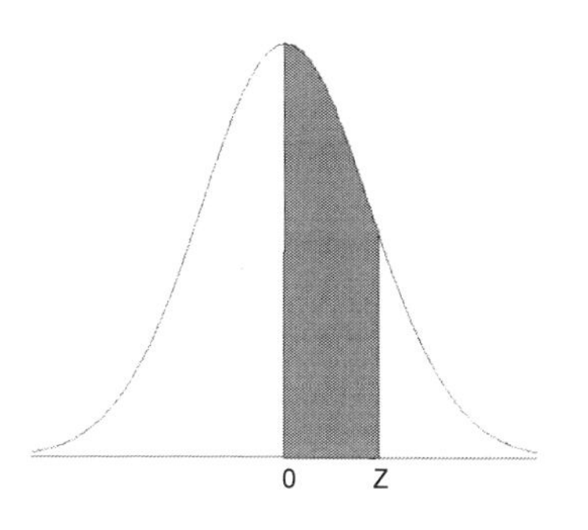

Z	0.00	0.01	0.02	0.03	0.04	0.05	0.06	0.07	0.08	0.09
0.0	.0000	.0040	.0080	.0120	.0160	.0199	.0239	.0279	.0319	.0359
0.1	.0398	.0438	.0478	.0517	.0557	.0596	.0636	.0675	.0714	.0753
0.2	.0793	.0832	.0871	.0910	.0948	.0987	.1026	.1064	.1103	.1141
0.3	.1179	.1217	.1255	.1293	.1331	.1368	.1406	.1443	.1480	.1517
0.4	.1554	.1591	.1628	.1664	.1700	.1736	.1772	.1808	.1844	.1879
0.5	.1915	.1950	.1985	.2019	.2054	.2088	.2133	.2157	.2190	.2224
0.6	.2357	.2291	.2324	.2357	.2389	.2422	.2454	.2486	.2517	.2549
0.7	.2580	.2611	.2642	.2673	.2704	.2734	.2764	.2794	.2823	.2852
0.8	.2881	.2910	.2939	.2967	.2995	.3023	.3051	.3078	.3106	.3133
0.9	.3159	.3186	.3212	.3238	.3264	.3289	.3315	.3340	.3365	.3389
1.0	.3413	.3438	.3461	.3485	.3508	.3531	.3554	.3577	.3599	.3621
1.1	.3643	.3665	.3686	.3780	.3724	.3749	.3770	.3790	.3810	.3830
1.2	.3849	.3869	.3888	.3907	.3925	.3944	.3962	.3980	.3997	.4015
1.3	.4032	.4049	.4066	.4082	.4099	.4115	.4131	.4147	.4162	.4177
1.4	.4192	.4207	.4222	.4236	.4251	.4265	.4279	.4292	.4306	.4319
1.5	.4332	.4345	.4357	.4370	.4382	.4394	.4406	.4418	.4429	.4441
1.6	.4452	.4463	.4474	.4484	.4495	.4505	.4515	.4525	.4535	.4545
1.7	.4554	.4564	.4573	.4582	.4591	.4599	.4608	.4616	.4625	.4633
1.8	.4641	.4649	.4656	.4664	.4671	.4678	.4686	.4693	.4699	.4706
1.9	.4713	.4719	.4726	.4732	.4738	.4744	.4750	.4756	.4761	.4767
2.0	.4772	.4778	.4783	.4788	.4793	.4798	.4803	.4808	.4812	.4817
2.1	.4821	.4826	.4830	.4834	.4838	.4842	.4846	.4850	.4854	.4857
2.2	.4861	.4864	.4868	.4871	.4875	.4878	.4881	.4884	.4887	.4890
2.3	.4893	.4896	.4898	.4901	.4904	.4906	.4909	.4911	.4913	.4916
2.4	.4918	.4920	.4922	.4925	.4927	.4929	.4931	.4932	.4934	.4936
2.5	.4938	.4940	.4941	.4943	.4945	.4946	.4948	.4949	.4951	.4952
2.6	.4953	.4955	.4956	.4957	.4959	.4960	.4961	.4962	.4963	.4964
2.7	.4965	.4966	.4967	.4968	.4969	.4970	.4971	.4972	.4973	.4974
2.8	.4974	.4975	.4976	.4977	.4977	.4978	.4979	.4979	.4980	.4981
2.9	.4981	.4982	.4982	.4983	.4984	.4984	.4985	.4985	.4986	.4986
3.0	.4987	.4987	.4987	.4988	.4988	.4989	.4989	.4989	.4990	.4990
3.1	.4990	.4991	.4991	.4991	.4992	.4992	.4992	.4992	.4993	.4993
3.2	.4993	.4993	.4994	.4994	.4994	.4994	.4994	.4995	.4995	.4995
3.3	.4995	.4995	.4995	.4996	.4996	.4996	.4996	.4996	.4996	.4997
3.4	.4997	.4997	.4997	.4997	.4997	.4997	.4997	.4997	.4997	.4998
3.6	.4998	.4998	.4999	.4999	.4999	.4999	.4999	.4999	.4999	.4999
3.9	.5000									

Chapter IV

Measurement of Disease Frequency

A.M. Henken
National Institute for Public Health and The Environment, Bilthoven
The Netherlands

E.A.M. Graat
Wageningen University
Department of Animal Sciences
Quantitative Veterinary Epidemiology Group
The Netherlands

J. Casal
Universidad Anatomía de Barcelona
Facultad de Veterinaria
Departamento Patología i Producción de Animales
Spain

1. Introduction

Measurement of disease frequencies at the population level can be performed for several reasons. A first reason might be that one is interested in the presence or absence of a disease in the population. E.g., in The Netherlands all dairy herds are routinely screened on *Brucella abortus* infections in order to maintain the free-status. Secondly, knowledge about the level of a disease might be important in deciding how the optimal design of an eradication programme would look like. If the level is low, it might be decided to use a stamping-out policy, while at higher levels it might be decided to use a vaccination programme first in order to reduce that level. Thirdly, disease levels might vary between regions or herds giving indications that environmental or managerial factors play a role in the transmission. Also for calculations of national economic losses due to a specific disease, it is necessary to have an estimate of the level of that disease. Whatever the reason may be to investigate the frequency of a disease, the main principle is that the number of diseased animals is assessed or estimated. Because epidemiologists normally would like to make comparisons between different populations, it is better to express the specific numbers in terms relative to each population. Hence, the counts are expressed as a fraction[13] of the number of animals biologically capable of experiencing the event. This latter group is called the *population at risk*.

To determine the frequency of a disease, the disease status of individual animals needs to be assessed. Most frequently, a diagnostic test is used for this. Such a test might consist of detection of antibody or pathogen in the animal, detection of an abnormal level of e.g., enzymes or hormones, or a diagnosis from a clinician (e.g., in case of lameness). Almost all diagnostic tests are imperfect and this has consequences for how these tests should be used and interpreted (Thrusfield, 1995).

Though frequency measures are most interesting for an epidemiologist, this chapter mainly deals with characteristics of diagnostic tests, because this basic tool needs to be fully understood for a good interpretation of the outcomes.

2. Frequency Measures

Occurrence of disease, can be measured in a 'static' way (did the cow ***have*** mastitis or not at the moment of measurement) or in a 'dynamic' way (did the cow ***get*** mastitis during the study perod). Both measurements have an external time component, which is the day, year, or season in which the study is performed. Measurements of static situations theoretically do not have an internal time component, because the

[13] A fraction is a specific type of ratio in which the numerator is a subset of the denominator, for example: a/(a+b) is a fraction or proportion, while a/c would be a ratio. A fraction has a lower limit of zero and an upper limit of 1.0 (or 100 when expressed as a percentage). A ratio has a lower limit of zero and an upper limit of infinity (like feed conversion ratio). A rate is a specific type of ratio, i.e., the denominator is mostly 'per time-unit' (like growth rate) indicating the change occurring in the numerator when the denominator changes with one unit.

length of the study period theoretically is infinitely small (a snapshot). If occurrence of disease is measured as a dynamic event, then there is also an internal time component, which at maximum equals the length of the study period. An essential element is that the event of interest, like occurrence of disease, can only occur once per internal time period. So, if one wants to study the occurrence of mastitis and one wants to be able to count the event more than once per cow, one should choose as internal component not the whole lactation period but, for instance, periods of 4 weeks each. The combination of population at risk and internal time component provides the basis for calculation of denominators such as animal-years-at-risk.

With respect to disease, prevalence is the static situation analogue, and incidence is the dynamic analogue.

2.1. Prevalence

Prevalence represents the fraction (proportion) of existing cases in a population and is defined as:

> *the ratio (a/(a + b)) between the number of diseased animals (a) at a certain moment and the total number of animals at risk including the diseased ones (a + b) at that moment.*

In other words, prevalence (P) can be described as the probability that a randomly selected animal suffers from that disease at a certain moment. If the prevalence of a certain disease is 0.01% (0.0001), then 1 out of each 10,000 animals is affected and the probability of a randomly selected animal being affected at that moment equals 0.0001. The prevalence of a disease will depend on how many new cases arise per time-unit and the duration of disease, as is described later.

2.2. Incidence

Incidence describes the number of ***new*** cases that arise in a population over a specified period of time. There are two parameters describing incidence:

- cumulative incidence (CI);
- incidence rate (IR).

The *cumulative incidence* is:

> *the ratio between the number of animals that contracted the disease in a certain period and the number of healthy animals at risk in the population at the start of that period*

Thus, the cumulative incidence is a proportion and can be regarded as the average risk of animals developing the specific disease in a certain period. Cumulative incidence takes values between zero and one and has no dimension.

Example: Suppose that 20 out of 100, initially uninfected, pigs develop pseudorabies in a one-week period. The cumulative incidence in that week then amounts to: 20/100 = 0.2. When in the subsequent week another 15 pigs get pseudorabies, the cumulative incidence over the 2-week period amounts to 0.35 (see Table).

Week	Number of new cases	CI
1	20	0.20
2	15	0.35
3	10	0.45
4	5	0.50
5	1	0.51

The cumulative incidence over the entire 5-week period is 0.51. The chance of a randomly chosen pig contracting the disease in that 5-week period is 51%.

The length of the period has a large influence on the cumulative incidence: the longer the period, the higher the cumulative incidence. The animals, all initially healthy, should enter the study at the same time. If animals are lost to follow up (due to mortality or culling) one may use the average number of animals as denominator (number of animals at risk at start plus animals at risk at end divided by 2, which is identical to the number at risk at start minus half the number of withdrawals).

The *incidence rate* is defined as:

> *the ratio between the number of new cases of disease in a population during a certain period and the sum of the time-units at risk for all animals in the population at risk*

The time-units can be represented as animal-years, animal-weeks, or any other suitable time-unit. In the above example there were 51 new cases. The number of weeks at risk can be calculated as follows. The 20 animals that became infected in the first week contribute 20 times 0.5 = 10 animal-weeks, assuming that on average they contracted the disease halfway that week. The 15 animals that contracted the disease in the second week contribute 15∗1.5 = 22.5 animal-weeks, those from week 3: 10∗2.5 = 25, those from week 4: 5∗3.5 = 17.5, and those from week 5: 1∗4.5 = 4.5 animal-weeks. The 49 animals that remained healthy throughout contribute 49∗5 = 245 animal-weeks. In total, there were 324.5 animal-weeks at risk. It should be realized that only healthy animals contribute to the denominator because only healthy animals are at risk of getting the disease. The incidence rate equals 51/324.5 = 0.157 animals per animal-week at risk. This rate is also called the 'force of morbidity', it is the 'velocity' with which new cases arise in the population and its dimension is 'per time-unit'. In contrast to the other parameters, the incidence rate cannot be interpreted in terms of probability of having or contracting a disease, because it has no upper limit. For instance, expressing 0.157 animals per animal-week at risk on a yearly basis will give a value above unity: 0.157 ∗ 52 = 8.164.

The *relation between CI and IR* is:

$$CI_{(t)} = 1 - e^{(-IR * t)} ,$$

where e is the base of the natural logarithm, and t indicates the time-unit of concern. When the expected CI is smaller than 0.10 then the formula is approximately equal to:

$$CI_{(t)} = IR * t$$

Example: Suppose you have a population of 1000 healthy animals at start. Each week, 10% of the (remaining) healthy animals contract a disease and the study period is 5 weeks.

What is the CI?
What is the number of animal-weeks at risk?
What is the IR?
What are the real and via IR estimated CI per week?
How do you explain the fact that real and estimated CI are the same?

The number of cases in 5 weeks will be 410 (100 + 90 + 81 + 73 + 66). The CI will be 410/1000 = 0.41, which represents the chance of a randomly selected animal to contract the disease in the period of 5 weeks. The number of animal-weeks at risk amounts to 3890 (= 590∗5 + 100∗0.5 + 90∗1.5 + 81∗2.5 + 73∗3.5 + 66∗4.5). The IR then equals 410/3890 = 0.1054 animal per animal-week at risk. The comparison between real and estimated CI is:

week	# new cases	real CI	estimated CI[1]
1	0.1 ∗ 1000	0.100	0.100
2	0.1 ∗ 900	0.190	0.190
3	0.1 ∗ 810	0.271	0.271
4	0.1 ∗ 729	0.344	0.344
5	0.1 ∗ 656	0.410	0.410

[1] $1 - e^{-0.1054}$; $1 - e^{-0.2108}$; $1 - e^{-0.3162}$; etc.

Because the frequency of disease occurrence (10%) is constant per week, there is no difference between real and estimated CI.

The relation between IR and prevalence P is:

$$\frac{P}{(1-P)} = IR * D$$

The term P/(1 - P) represents the proportion of cases expressed against the healthy population (1 - P: only healthy animals can get the disease!). When an animal contracts a disease it can be designated as diseased for D time-units, where D is the duration of the disease. So, new cases contribute to P during only D time periods. When P is small (<0.05), the above formula reduces to:

$$P = IR * D$$

When prevalence, cumulative incidence or incidence rate are calculated for an entire population at risk, then the prefix 'crude' is used. When the parameter is calculated for a specific subgroup the prefix 'specific' is used (like sex-specific mortality).

3. Detection of Disease

3.1. Sensitivity and specificity

Diagnostic tests are imperfect, that is, the outcomes are not always correct. It should therefore be realized that also the classification into healthy and diseased is imperfect, leading to false-positives and false-negatives. The degree of misclassification can be quantified by comparing diagnostic methods available with a golden standard or to what is considered to be the best method at hand. Such a 'best' method might not be the best suited method in practice because it might be expensive, complex, or time-consuming. However, it might be suitable as a reference for the less perfect method.

For example, the best method to prove the presence of the nematode *Trichinella spiralis* in pigs is digestion of a diaphragmatic sample which is time-consuming and needs slaughter of the animal. The alternative method is to use an ELISA (Enzyme-Linked-ImmunoSorbent Assay) to demonstrate the presence of antibodies against *Trichinella* antigen. With this latter method, a large number of samples from live animals can be tested. The validity of the alternative method is expressed as its ***sensitivity*** and ***specificity***. The term 'validity' refers to the degree to which the test measures what it is supposed to measure in the long run. The terms 'sensitivity' and 'specificity' are tools to judge this validity and are characteristics of the test. The sensitivity of a test, SE, is the probability that a truly diseased animal indeed will be classified as diseased using the test. In formula:

$$SE = \frac{\text{(Number of diseased animals classified by the test as diseased)}}{\text{(Total number of diseased animals)}}$$

The specificity of a test, SP, is the probability that a truly non-diseased animal will be classified as non-diseased with the test. In formula:

$$SP = \frac{\text{(Number of healthy animals classified by the test as non - diseased)}}{\text{(Total number of healthy animals)}}$$

The value of SE and SP can be easily calculated when presented in a 2x2 table (Table 4.1):

Table 4.1. Contingency table for evaluation of sensitivity and specificity.

		Golden standard test		
		Diseased	Non-diseased	
Test	Diseased	a	b	a+b
	Non-diseased	c	d	c+d
		a+c	b+d	N

Sensitivity (SE) = a/(a + c)
Specificity (SP) = d/(b + d)

If a golden standard test is not available and the comparison is made using another imperfect test, sometimes the terms **relative sensitivity** and **relative specificity** are used. However, in this case it might be more appropriate to calculate the level of agreement as expressed by *kappa* (see paragraph 3.6). Crucial in the interpretation of the SE and SP is the panel (e.g., a collection of sera) that is used to evaluate the validity of the test. This panel should be representative for the population the test is going to be used in. Imagine a panel to validate a test on detection of antibodies to pathogen X. Unknown was that antibodies to pathogen Y do cross-react with those to pathogen X. If animals infected with Y were not in the panel and the test is used in a population where Y is present, then quite many animals might be false-positive and the test will be useless despite its, for this population invalid, high specificity.

Reasons for lack of sensitivity (false-negative results):

- Natural or induced tolerance: animals which do not produce antibodies in contact with a specific antigen (e.g., exposure to *bovine virus diarrhoea virus* (BVDV) during the first months of gestation gives rise to calves that do not recognize BVDV as antigen).
- Improper timing
  - the time between infection and sampling is too short to produce a measurable antibody response.
  - period close to parturition. The high amount of immunoglobulin (Ig) in colostrum causes a lower level of Ig in serum, that cannot be detected with low-sensitivity tests (e.g., Agar-Gel-ImmunoDiffusion (AGID) test for bovine leucosis). Note that "sensitivity" in immunologic or pharmacologic usage has a different meaning. It refers to the ability of a test to detect a small amount of antibody or drug. A test could be sensitive in an immunologic sense, but its sensitivity in an epidemiologic sense could be very poor and *vice versa*.
- Non-specific inhibitors:
  - e.g., anticomplement activity of serum (contaminated or haemolized)
- Blocking antibodies
  - e.g., an excessive amount of IgG_1 antibodies might block or mask the reaction of IgG_2 antibodies
- Immunosuppression
- Laboratory errors

Reasons for lack of specificity (false-positive results):

- Cross reactions with other infectious agents sharing similar antigens.
  - e.g., *Mycobacterium paratuberculosis* cross-reacts with *Mycobacterium tuberculosis*
- Non-specific reactions: e.g., haemagglutination inhibitors.
- True exposures unrelated to the present disease status:
  - Vaccination
  - Passive immunization (colostral antibodies)
  - Previous exposure
- Laboratory errors

In general, the SE and SP are inversely correlated: the higher SE, the lower SP. Strictly, this is only true for continuous and ordinal data (e.g., single serial dilution antibody titres or absorbency values). The reason for this negative association is the overlap that exists between results of negative and positive animals. This is demonstrated in Figure 4.1, which represents data from an ELISA-test against *Dictyocaulus viviparus* (lungworm) of cattle (Boon *et al.*, 1982). The reference method (golden standard') was the presence or absence of lungworm larvae in sputum and/or faeces. The average titre (as a result of the ELISA) was 3.86 for the sputum/faeces positive herds and 2.76 for the negative ones.

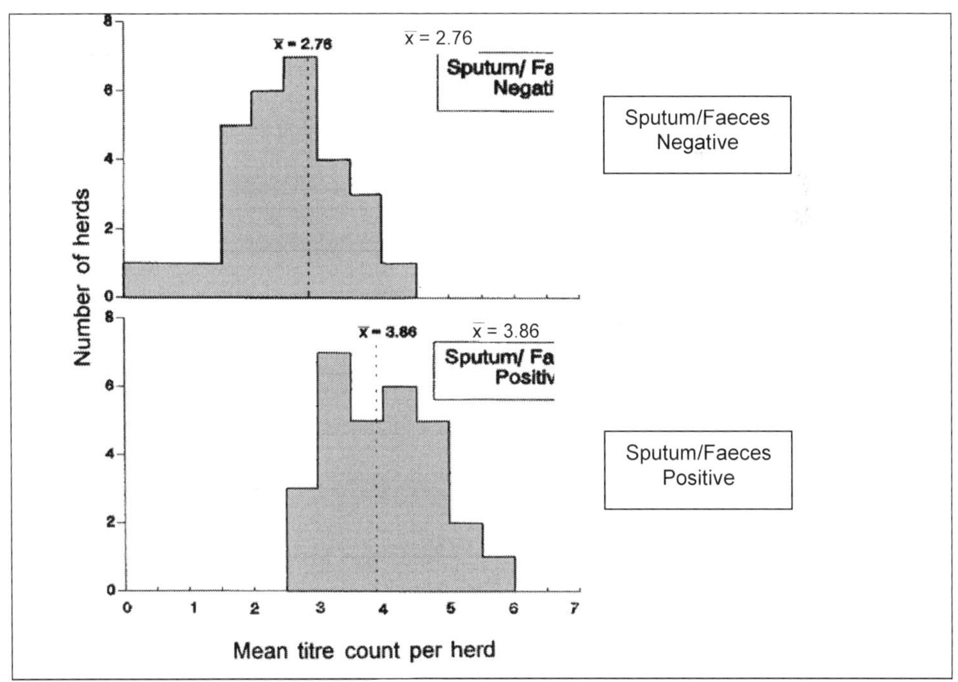

Figure 4.1. Distribution of mean titre count per herd for positive and negative herds (data from Boon *et al.*, 1982).[14]

[14] Reproduced with permission of the publisher

The difference of the average titre count of positive and negative herds is statistically significant. However, there is considerable overlap between negative herds with relative high titres and positive herds with relative low titres. If one wants to use the ELISA test as the only test to determine the presence of lungworm, one would have to adopt a cut-off (threshold) value. Herds with an average titre higher than this cut-off value will be regarded as positive, those with a lower average titre will be regarded as negative. The cut-off value, therefore, determines the sensitivity and the specificity. If a titre value of 4.5 is chosen as the cut-off value, then there will be no false-positives and the specificity would be 1.0. However, there will be a high number of positive farms that would be designated as negative. Thus, the number of false-negatives would be high, indicating that the sensitivity is very low. On the other hand, if one determines a titre value of 2.5 as the cut-off value, then no false-negatives will occur (SE = 1), but many false-positives will be present (low SP). This inverse relationship between SE and SP is presented in Figure 4.2.

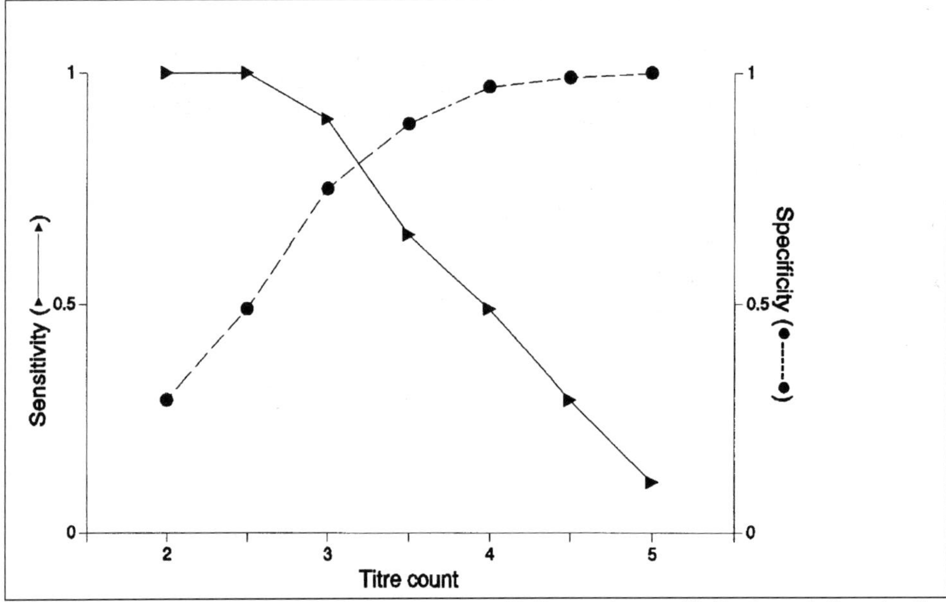

Figure 4.2. The relationship between sensitivity and specificity in relation to the chosen cut-off value (data from Boon *et al.*, 1982).[15]

The value actually chosen as cut-off value, will depend on the purpose of the test. In case of a serious threat for human health (zoonosis) or a very contagious disease that normally is absent, one would aim for a high SE to prevent or minimize the risk of assigning a truly diseased animal (or herd) as negative. If the prevalence of the disease is not high, one might consider slaughter of affected animals. In this case the specificity also would be important, because one would like to minimize the risk of slaughtering many false-positive animals (herds).

[15] Reproduced with permission of the publisher

Tests with high sensitivity are appropriate as tools for diagnosis:

- in early phases of pathogenesis when many aetiologic possibilities exist;
- in case no truly diseased individuals are allowed to escape detection (no false-negatives; e.g., severe zoonotic diseases);
- if the probability of disease is low.

Tests with high specificity are useful:

- to confirm diagnosis set earlier with other methods (if this test result is negative, then there is a high probability that the animal is truly negative);
- if false-positive results have large effects (for instance when positive animals must be slaughtered).

From the previous it is clear that the SE and SP are not fixed values but are determined by the chosen cut-off value. One way to get more insight in an optimal cut-off value is to calculate the SE and SP at several cut-off values. Next, the results can be plotted in a so-called ROC curve, where ROC stands for Receiver Operating Characteristic. In such a plot, the false-positive fraction (or 1-SP) is at the X-axis and the true positive fraction (or SE) on the Y axis. See Figure 4.3 for an example (data from Boon *et al.*, 1982). In such a curve, tests that plot in the left upper corner are best (high sensitivity and high specificity). The optimal cut-off value can then be chosen, depending on the purpose of the test. An alternative to this method is to calculate likelihood ratios (see also paragraph 3.3) at several cut-off values. This ratio is best obtained by determining specific areas or heights of the frequency distributions of the positive and negative populations at a specific cut-off value. A nice explanation of this method is in Gambino (1989).

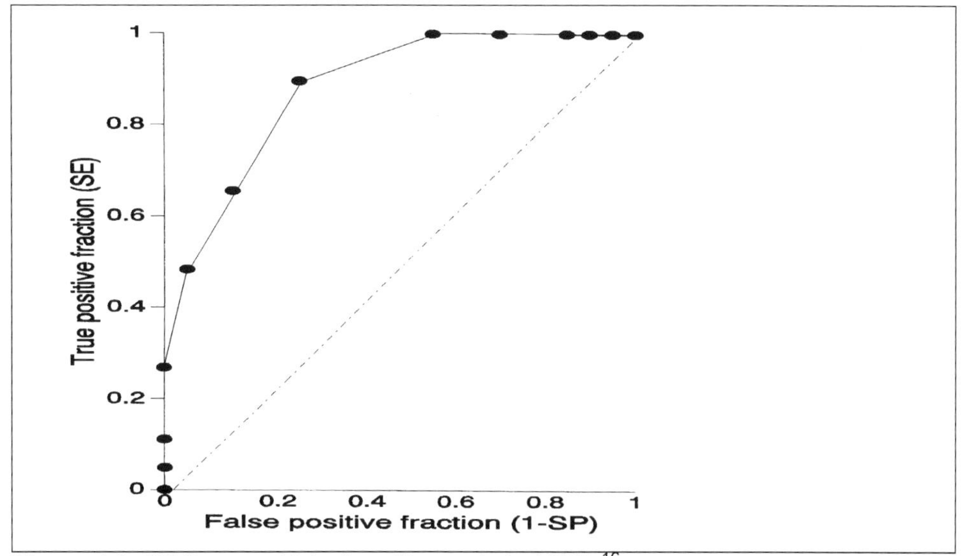

Figure 4.3. ROC curve (data from Boon *et al.*, 1982).[16]

[16] Reproduced with permission of the publisher

As for any proportion (Prop), the precision of the SE and SP can be obtained by calculating its confidence interval (CI). This interval is given by the formula:

$$Prop \pm z * \sqrt{\frac{(Prop * (1 - Prop)}{n}}$$

where z is the standardized Normal deviate and n is the sample size. E.g., if z is 1.96, then the formula determines a 95% confidence interval. The standard error of the proportion is given by $\sqrt{(Prop * (1 - Prop)/n)}$ which only depends on the magnitude of the proportion and the sample size n. The part after the ± sign is called the precision. The larger the sample size, the better the precision is which is intuitively correct: an SE based on a panel of 100 samples is better than an SE based on a panel of only 10 samples while both might produce an SE of say 80%. SE and SP, with their confidence intervals, are easily calculated using (WIN)EPISCOPE (Frankena *et al.*, 1990).

Given a desired precision and a pre-estimate of the proportion, the formula above can also be used to decide upon the size of the panel that is needed to evaluate the test (see Chapter III, paragraph 4.3).

3.2. Relation between SE, SP and prevalence

If one wants to know the prevalence of disease in a population, a number of individuals is sampled and tested as being diseased or non-diseased according to a test. It should be realized that the true prevalence does not equal the prevalence as measured in such a sample. The measured prevalence will depend on the sensitivity of the test, its specificity, and the true prevalence in the population. This can be deduced from Table 4.2. This table is easily constructed, starting with the probabilities in **bold**. With N equal to 1, the proportion of diseased is equal to P, the proportion that is truly diseased *and* tested positive is equal to SE*P and the proportion that is truly healthy *and* tested negative equals SP * (1 - P). The other proportions can be obtained by summation or subtraction.

Table 4.2. Relation between SE, SP and prevalence.

		Truly diseased		
		yes	no	Total
Test result	+	**SE * P**	(1-SP) * (1-P)	SE*P + (1-SP) * (1-P)
	-	(1-SE) * P	**SP * (1-P)**	(1-SE)*P + SP*(1-P)
Total		**P**	1-P	**1**

Example: Suppose that the true prevalence is 0.01 (1%), the SE and SP are both 0.90 (90%). What is the apparent prevalence? Assume that the population size is 1000 animals. The true prevalence is 1% and, therefore, 10 animals are truly diseased. This means that 990 animals are truly healthy. Because SE is 90%, 9 animals of the truly 10 diseased animals will be detected. Because SP is also 90%, 891 of the 990 truly healthy animals will be designated as healthy. The 2x2 table is:

		Truly diseased		
		yes	no	Total
Test result	+	9	99	108
	-	1	891	892
Total		10	990	1000

The apparent prevalence will be 10.8%, while the true prevalence is 1%. If SE and SP are both 99% and the true P=1%, then the apparent prevalence equals 1.98% (= (0.99 * 0.01 + (1 -0.99) * (1 - 0.01)) * 100%). If the SE and SP are both 90% and the true prevalence 10, 25 and 50% respectively, then the apparent prevalence will be 18, 30, and 50% respectively.

The Apparent (or measured) Prevalence, AP, is (a + b)/N (from Table 4.1) or SE∗P+(1-SP)∗(1-P) with P being the true prevalence.

If the SE and SP of a test are known and this test is used to estimate a prevalence, it is simple to correct this estimated prevalence for the imperfect SE and SP. Using the formula AP = SE∗P + (1-SP)∗(1-P), it shows that:

$$P = \frac{(AP + SP - 1)}{(SE + SP - 1)}$$

Theoretically it is not possible to obtain a negative value for P. However, practically it might occur, especially when values for SE and SP have been determined on a panel that is not representative for the population that is investigated. If the panel contains animals having maternal antibodies, then the SP is too low when the test is used in a population having no animals with maternal antibodies. Then either, the numerator or denominator might become negative! Secondly, the SE and SP are based on a sample, inducing sampling variation; this might lead to estimates for SE and SP that differ somewhat (depending on the sample size) from the true SE and SP.

Example: Suppose the SE and SP of a test for leptospirosis in cattle amount to 93 and 91%, respectively. The test is to be used to determine the true prevalence. Suppose AP is 25%. Then P will be 19%.

$$P = \frac{0.25 + 0.91 - 1}{0.93 + 0.91 - 1} = \frac{0.16}{0.84} = 0.19$$

3.3. Predictive values

The proportion of animals that tested positive while they are truly diseased is called the positive predictive value. Its value can be obtained from Table 4.1 or Table 4.2 as:

$$PV^{+} = \frac{a}{a+b} = \frac{P * SE}{P * SE + (1-P) * (1-SP)}$$

The negative predictive value indicating the proportion of animals that tested negative while they are truly non-diseased is calculated as:

$$PV^{-} = \frac{d}{c+d} = \frac{(1-P) * SP}{P * (1-SE) + (1-P) * SP}$$

A predictive value is a population characteristic because it depends on the prevalence of disease.

Example: Suppose there is a barn with 200 slaughter pigs, of which 50% suffer from disease Z. A company has developed a test with a 90% sensitivity and 90% specificity. They are proud of this and with the test kit comes a leaflet that says that the test is very suitable for use in practice. The 2x2 table for this example is:

		Disease Z		
		yes	no	Total
Test result	+	90 (a)	10 (b)	100
	-	10 (c)	90 (d)	100
Total		100	100	200

The predictive value of a positive test is a/(a+b)=0.9, which is high.
The farmers' neighbour is also a pig farmer (actually a better one) but still 10% of his 200 pigs have disease Z. If the procedure to construct the 2x2 table is repeated, it will show that the predictive value of the test is only 0.5, i.e., comparable to flipping a coin among the test-positive animals to decide which are truly diseased and which are not.

If a disease has a low prevalence, the positive predictive value will largely depend on the specificity (Table 4.1: if the prevalence decreases, 'a + c' will be small and 'b + d' will be high. Then, with constant SE and SP, 'a' will decrease and 'b' will increase, resulting in a low positive predictive value).

In the example above, the odds (diseased animals versus non-diseased ones) before the test were 100:100 or 1:1; the post-test odds being 90:10 or 9:1. Thus, the test increases the likelihood of a test positive animal 9 fold. This is called the *likelihood ratio* (ratio between true positives and true negatives) which can be calculated as well as SE/(1 - SP) = 0.9/(1 - 0.9) = 9. This is also a measure, and may be a better one than predictive values, of what a test can do in a specific situation (Gambino, 1989). Moreover, the likelihood ratio is independent from the prevalence. At the neighbours' farm the pre-test odds were 2:18, while the post-test odds were 18:18 (also a 9-fold increase). So, the likelihood ratio is constant across prevalences, but the predictive value, which is a probability, varies with the prevalence.

3.4. Diagnostic tests and their interpretation at the herd level

When individuals are tested to determine the health status of an aggregate of animals (e.g., a herd) the validity of a test should be evaluated at the aggregated level: herd-level sensitivity (HSE) and herd-level specificity (HSP). HSE is the probability of a truly infected herd to be classified as infected by the test. HSP is the probability of a truly non-infected herd to be classified as non-infected with the test.
HSE and HSP not only depend on the SE and SP of the test but also on the number of animals tested and the critical number of positives at which the herd is declared positive. Major goals of determining HSE and HSP is the assessment of the percentage of herds affected with the disease of interest, and to assess the probability that a herd is actually diseased, based on the test result of the individual animals.

Formulae to calculate the HSE and HSP are relatively simple if the critical number is set to 1. Then, the apparent prevalence AP can be used to calculate them (see Table 4.2: AP = SE ∗ P + (1 - SP) ∗ (1 - P)). Thus, an animal in a non-diseased herd (P = 0) has a probability of 1-SP to be tested (false-)positive and a probability of SP to be tested negative. This means that if the test specificity is not equal to 1, a negative animal might be declared (false-)positive and thus the herd is declared positive. Sampling n animals from a negative herd will decrease the herd specificity further, as:

$$HSP = SP^n$$

Thus, if the SP of a test is 0.90 then the probability that e.g., five animals all are negative, and thus the herd, is only $0.90^5 = 0.59$.

The formula for HSE is a bit more complicated. The herd is denoted as positive if at least one animal is tested positive. The formula for HSE with a critical number of 1 equals:

$$HSE = 1 - (1 - AP)^n$$

1 - AP is the probability of testing one animal as negative and $(1 - AP)^n$ is the probability of testing ***all*** n animals as negative. Thus $1 - (1 - AP)^n$ is the probability to test at least 1 animal out of n as positive.

Example: The table below contains results for a test with SE = 0.95 and SP = 0.99 and two levels of true prevalence. The results indicate that HSP decreases with increasing numbers of tested animals within a herd, whereas HSE increases. Herd sensitivity also increases with an increasing true prevalence, whereas herd specificity is, by definition, not influenced by prevalence.

Herd-level specificity (HSP) and sensitivity (HSE) by true prevalence (P) and number of animals tested per herd, given an individual animal test sensitivity of 95% and a specificity of 99% (modified from Martin et al. (1992).

number tested	HSP (%)	HSE (%)	
	P=0, 10, 30	P=10	P=30
1	99	10	28
2	98	20	48
5	95	42	81
10	90	66	96
30	74	96	100
60	55	100	100
100	37	100	100

If the critical number is set larger than 1, then the formulae for HSE and HSP become more complicated and it is better to use formulae derived from a binomial distribution. This more basic approach is well described by Martin *et al.* (1992) and Jordan (1996).

$$HSP = \sum_{i=0}^{c-1} \frac{n!}{i! * (n-i)!} * p_f^{\,i} * q_f^{\,n-i}$$

$$HSE = 1 - \sum_{i=0}^{c-1} \frac{n!}{i! * (n-i)!} * p_d^{\,i} * q_d^{\,n-i}$$

where:

- n = sample size
- c = critical number
- p_f = AP if the herd is truly free of the disease
- q_f = $1 - p_f$
- p_d = AP if the herd is truly positive
- q_d = $1 - p_d$

Fortunately, Jordan (1996) also describes a free domain computer programme (HERDACC to be downloaded from http://epiweb.massey.ac.nz) that makes quick calculations and produces nice tables on HSE and HSP.

In literature, it is common to find references stating that larger herds were more frequently affected with a specific disease. This association is important because if the relationship between herd size and health status truly exists, explanations for it should be sought. However, if in larger herds more samples are taken (often the sample size is related to herd size), truly negative herds will be classified disproportional as positive ones, due to decreasing HSP. Thus, in the analysis it looks like that larger herd size is positively associated to the disease. This should be realized when interpreting results of epidemiologic studies at the aggregate level.

3.5. Multiple testing

Diagnosis is seldom based on the outcome of a single test only. It is common to perform multiple testing. The interpretation of multiple test results depends on the sequence in which the tests are conducted and the way in which their results are integrated (Smith, 1991). Table 4.3 summarizes the factors to be considered.

Table 4.3. Effects of multiple test strategies (modified from Smith, 1991).

	Test Strategy	
Considerations	Parallel Testing	Serial Testing
Effect of test strategy	Increase sensitivity	Increase specificity
Greatest predictive value	Negative test result	Positive test result
Clinical use	Rule out a disease	Rule in a disease
Purpose; clinical seting	Rapid assessment of individual patients; vaccination, clinics, emergencies	Time not crucial; avoid excessive testing of groups of animals; test and removal programmes
Comments	Useful when there is an important penalty for missing disease, i.e., false-negative results	Useful when there is an important penalty for false-positive results

Parallel testing

In parallel testing two or more different tests are applied at the same time. Diagnostic tests are usually done in parallel when rapid assessment of the health status is necessary. The net effect of parallel testing is to prove that the animal is healthy (a high sensitivity causes a high negative predictive value)! Only animals that have negative results on all tests are considered to be free of disease (see Table 4.4 for an example). The sensitivity and specificity of a parallel test procedure equal:

$$SE_{par} = 1 - (1 - SE_1) * (1 - SE_2)$$

$$SP_{par} = SP_1 * SP_2$$

Serial testing

In serial testing only those animals that tested positive on an initial test are retested. The net effect is to prove that the animal is truly affected by the disease tested for. Serial testing maximizes specificity and the positive predictive value, but lowers sensitivity and the negative predictive value (Table 4.4). Because of the sequence in which serial testing is done, an animal is classified as affected only if it is positive on all tests. Serial testing might be used in eradication programmes. The sensitivity and specificity of a serial test procedure equal:

$$SE_{ser} = SE_1 * SE_2$$

$$SP_{ser} = 1 - (1 - SP_1) * (1 - SP_2)$$

When using multiple tests, it should be realized that it is assumed that all results are independent from each other. If this is not the case, the benefits from multiple testing will be overestimated.

Table 4.4. Predictive values for test T1, T2 and a combination of both (modified from Smith, 1991).

Test	Sensitivity (%)	Specificity (%)	Positive Predictive Value (%)[1]	Negative Predictive Value (%)[1]
T1	80	60	40	90
T2	90	90	75	96
T1 and T2 (parallel)	98	54	42	99
T1 and T2 (serial)	72	96	86	91

[1] For 25% prevalence.

3.6. Test agreement

Often the sensitivity and specificity of a test are unknown, because the true values are difficult or costly to establish, costly in terms of money or time. Hence, tests with unknown validity are used. When a new test is being developed, it is then compared to current tests. Also, when two clinicians undertake diagnoses, their results will differ to some degree. How can the agreement in results with different test(er)s be quantified? The relative quality can be quantified as the *kappa* value (Table 4.5).

Table 4.5. Contingency table to evaluate test agreement.

		Test 2/Clinician 2		
		+	-	Total
Test 1/Clinician 1	+	a	b	a + b
	-	c	d	c + d
	Total	a + c	b + d	N

The number of identical results amounts to *a + d*. The proportion of agreement equals *(a + d)/N*. However, this proportion of agreement includes agreement due to chance as well as underlying genuine agreement. The agreement due to chance can be calculated as: *(Ea + Ed)/N*. In this formula, *Ea* stands for the expected value of *a* when chance alone is at work; *Ea* equals *[(a + b) ∗ (a + c)]/N* and *Ed=[(c+d)∗(b+d)]/N*. The total agreement, i.e., including chance, can be 1.0 at maximum. This means that the total agreement due to comparability between tests beyond chance can be *1 - ((Ea + Ed)/N)* at maximum, with *[((a+d)/N) - ((Ea+Ed)/N)]* as indication of agreement beyond chance. Therefore, *kappa* equals:

$$\text{Kappa} = \frac{\frac{a+d}{N} - \frac{Ea+Ed}{N}}{1 - \left(\frac{Ea+Ed}{N}\right)} = \frac{a+d-Ea-Ed}{N-Ea-Ed}$$

If *kappa* = 0, then there is no agreement at all beyond chance. If *kappa* = 1, there is perfect agreement. Values of *kappa* between 0.4 to 0.5 indicate a very moderate level of agreement, those between 0.5 and 0.6 can be regarded as just sufficient (about the level expected when two clinicians diagnose the same case), those between 0.6 and 0.8 are good (about the level expected when the same clinician diagnoses the same case on a different occasion). It should be realized that a *kappa* value compares test results, and should not be used to state anything about the absolute value of the tests: tests can have a high *kappa* value, but still be equally wrong! *Kappa* values can easily be calculated and statistically evaluated using the computer programme (WIN)EPISCOPE (Frankena *et al.*, 1990 to be downloaded from http://www.zod.wau.nl/qve).

Test agreement can also be evaluated when the outcomes are not discrete events (like diseased yes or no), but are measured on a continuous scale (like optical densities in certain immuno-assays). It is then very tempting to evaluate the agreement by means of a correlation coefficient, but Bland and Altman (1986) give five reasons why this is inappropriate. They propose a graphical approach based on simple calculations as an alternative. The further interested reader is referred to this paper.

References

Bland, J,M.; Altman, D.G. (1986). Statistical methods for assessing agreement between two methods of clinical measurement. Lancet, 1, 307-310.

Boon, J.; Kloosterman, A.; Brink, R. van den (1982). The incidence of *Dictyocaulus viviparus* infections in cattle in The Netherlands. I. The Enzyme Linked Immunosorbent Assay as a diagnostic tool. Veterinary Quarterly, 4, 155-160.

Frankena, K.; Noordhuizen, J.P.; Willeberg, P.; Voorthuysen, P.F. van; Goelema, J.O. (1990). EPISCOPE: computer programs in veterinary epidemiology. Veterinary Record, 126, 573-576.

Gambino, R. (1989). The misuse of predictive value - or why you must consider the odds. Laboratory Report, 11, 65-72.

Jordan, D. (1996). Aggregate testing for the evaluation of Johne's disease herd status. Australian Veterinary Journal, 73, 16-19.

Martin, S.W.; Shoukri, M.; Thornburn, M.A. (1992). Evaluating the health status of herds based on tests applied to individuals. Preventive Veterinary Medicine, 14, 33-43.

Smith, R.D. (1991). Veterinary Clinical Epidemiology - A Problem-oriented Approach. Butterworth-Heinemann, Boston.

Thrusfield, M. (1995). Veterinary Epidemiology. 2nd edn. Blackwell Science, Oxford.

4. Exercises

4.1. Incidence

At a fur farm, newly bought minks are put in a special enclosure during a period of 3 weeks. Due to stress of transport, change of feeding and the new environment, lung infection and deaths might occur. The following table shows what happened in a four week period. At the first day, 112 animals were present.

Week no.	Number of minks added during the week	Number of new cases	Number of new cases that died
1	36	9	0
2	46	23	1
3	0	22	1
4	0	10	0

It is assumed that minks that recover have acquired immunity which protects against the disease at least for a period of 1 month.

Estimate for each of the 4 weeks the cumulative incidence and the true incidence rate.

4.2. Prevalence and Incidence

In a dairy herd of 30 cows, milk samples were collected for examination on subclinical mastitis at two dates: August 23, 1994 and September 22, 1994. At the first sampling date 10 cows were mastitic, at the second only 6. After a visit of the practitioner at August 31, 1994, cow 68, 30 and 33 were culled and one new cow (no. 398) was included in the herd. Results are in the tables below.

Results of mastitis test on samples of August 23, 1994.

Cow no.	RF quarter	LF quarter	RH quarter	LH quarter	Culled
23			+		
68		+	+	+	+
28	+				
30		+			+
33			+	+	+
35	+	+		+	
38				+	
335		+			
336				+	
339		+			

Results of mastitis test on samples of September 22, 1994.

Cow no.	RF quarter	LF quarter	RH quarter	LH quarter
12				+
43	+			
46		+		+
41		+		
335	+	+		
337			+	

Assume that cows marked as positive in the table of August 23, 1994 and that were not culled will, at average, recover in two weeks.

1. What are the prevalences of infection at the two dates of examination?
2. What is the incidence rate of subclinical mastitis in the period between both dates?
3. What is the risk that a cow will become subclinically infected in the course of a 10 months lactational period? What additional assumptions must be made in this calculation? Are these assumptions reasonable?

4.3. Diagnostic tests

Atrophic rhinitis (AR) is a disease that causes worldwide economic losses to the pig breeding industry. It is best diagnosed by visual inspection of the conchae. Prospective studies were done to detect AR in carcasses at the slaughterline. Longitudinal sections (LS) of nasal cavities, made and inspected at the slaughterline, were compared with transverse sections (TS) made at a later stage. Transverse sectioning is the recommended method, but this method is impossible to perform at high speed slaughterlines. The research was done in a large slaughterhouse. Three data sets were created:

1. Two hundred and forty eight randomly selected pig heads were taken from the slaughterline and inspected with respect to nasal cavity deviations using the LS and TS methods.
2. From 638 pig heads that passed the slaughterline within an hour, 107 heads were classified as abnormal using LS (under force of high speed!). Afterwards, without the demand/pressure of speed, the 107 heads were again classified with LS as well as TS.
3. Pigs (n = 385) from 6 herds with AR problems.

The results (in percentages) of the three groups are presented in the next tables (LS = longitudinal section; TS transverse section; N=normal conchae; CA = conchae atrophy) (Tielen *et al.* (1988). Tijdschrift voor Diergeneeskunde, 113, 1345-1355. (In Dutch)).

Results of group 1 (N = 248)

		LS		
		N	CA	Total
TS	N	89.7	0.5	90.2
	CA	6.6	3.2	9.8
	Total	96.3	3.7	100

Results of group 2 (N = 107)

		LS		
		N	CA	Total
TS	N	40.2	14.0	54.2
	CA	19.6	26.2	45.8
	Total	59.8	40.2	100

Results of group 3 (N = 385)

		LS		
		N	CA	Total
TS	N	49.8	9.2	59.0
	CA	20.1	20.9	41.0
	Total	69.9	30.1	100

Prevalence:

1. What is the prevalence of AR on pig farms based on TS with data of group 1. Do the same for LS. Calculate also the 95% confidence intervals for these prevalences.
2. Do the prevalences or their 95% confidence intervals change when using numbers instead of percentages? Calculate!
3. Using the data of group 2, that is from the 638 heads of which 107 were found to be positive, it can be deduced that the prevalence amounts to 107/638 = 16.8% using LS at high speed. What are the prevalences based on LS and TS when scored afterwards at quiet conditions, assuming that the initial 531 (= 638 - 107) indeed are negative?

Sensitivity, specificity and predictive values:

Suppose TS is the 100% reference method ("golden standard").

4. Calculate SE and SP of the LS method with data of group 1. Interpret the outcome in your own words. Calculate the 95% confidence intervals.
5. Calculate the predictive value for a positive score with LS. Calculate the predictive value for a negative score with LS. Interpret the outcome in your own words. Calculate the 95% confidence intervals.
6. Based on the low SE one is intended to conclude that LS is not a good method. However, both PV^+ and PV^- are high which might indicate that LS is good. How would you interpret this seemingly discrepancy?

Test agreement

7. Calculate *kappa* between LS and TS using the results of group 1.
8. Which method is best: LS or TS?
9. Does *kappa* change when we use numbers instead of percentages?
10. If *kappa* did not change in your answer to the previous question, do you have ideas what will be affected by using percentages instead of numbers?

Conclusions

11. Do you agree that LS is a good method to determine the prevalence of AR?
12. Might LS provide a tool to trace AR positive herds?

Further exercises on these data:

13. Calculate prevalences, sensitivities, specificities, predictive values and *kappa* values using data of group 2 and 3.

4.4. Diagnostic tests and cut-off value

A Veterinary Institute developed a diagnostic test for the infectious pig disease SMD (Swine Misery Disease). SMD becomes clinically manifest after an incubation period of 3 months and results in growth reduction in animals younger than 6 months old. SMD is without any symptoms in sows. The test, SMDETEC, is based on detection of antibodies in serum.

1. Mention some reasons why SMDETEC might give false-positives and false-negatives.
2. An evaluation of SMDETEC in a group of 100 infected (G1) and 100 non-infected (G2) animals shows the following frequency distribution:

Antibody-titre	Frequency in		Antibody-titre	Frequency in	
	G1	G2		G1	G2
0.0	0	41	2.5	10	2
0.5	0	25	3.0	26	2
1.0	1	17	3.5	34	1
1.5	3	7	4.0	16	1
2.0	7	4	4.5	3	0

Which titre value would you decide upon to be the cut-off value? Explain why you select that particular one. Also produce the ROC curve.
In the subsequent questions we assume that a titre larger than or equal to 3.0 denotes a positive animal.

3. Calculate the sensitivity and the specificity of SMDETEC and their 95% confidence intervals.
4. In a national survey using SMDETEC, it shows that 10% of all animals is positive. Calculate the true prevalence. Calculate also the negative and positive predictive values and interpret them. Mention the main reason why the predictive value of a negative test result is that high.
5. A pig multiplier with 250 sows is accused by the fatteners of delivering piglets which are affected with SMD. The multiplier phones the vet and all 250 sows are sampled. Ten (10) samples are indicated as positive to SMD. The fatteners think they now have the evidence that they can make a claim. However, the multiplier keeps denying that the disease is present. Who is right and why?

4.5. Predictive values

Suppose you are asked to advise a farmer who wants to buy 20 animals which are tested free of disease X with a diagnostic test Y. Nevertheless the farmer hesitates to buy the animals because they come from a country where disease X is present at a rather high level (prevalence = 55%) so he fears the risk for bringing disease X to his farm. In the documents you find that the SE of test Y was about 90.9% and the SP 100%.

1. According to the test results (all animals were tested negative): should the farmer buy these animals or not?
2. What is the predictive value of a positive test result? Why is it that high?

4.6. The impact of false-positives

The prevalence of para-tuberculosis has been determined by bacteriological techniques as being 5%. However, bacteriology with regard to this disease is cumbersome: culture is difficult, it takes a long time before results are available and last but not least it is expensive. So there is a big need for an alternative method. You developed a serological technique to detect antibodies. When compared to bacteriology it appears that the SE of your test is 95% and the SP 80%. The Veterinary Service in your country decides to use your test for eradication of the disease: animals tested positive are slaughtered. Each slaughtered animal causes an economic loss of 100 dollars.

1. When 1 million cows are tested what are the financial losses due to slaughter?
2. What is the extra loss due to inappropriateness of the test?
3. Due to the answer on the previous question, the Veterinary Service asks you to improve your test because too many animals are slaughtered. Should the SE or the SP of the test be increased to minimize the costs most effectively?

5. Answers

5.1. Incidence

On basis of the stated figures the following table can be drawn up (NAR is number at risk at first or last day of the week):

Week	NAR first day	Average NAR	Weeks at risk	Number affected	Incidence rate/week	Risk for the week
1	112	130	125.5	9	0.0717	0.0692
2	139	162	150.5	23	0.1528	0.1420
3	162	162	151	22	0.1457	0.1358
4	140	140	135	10	0.0741	0.0714

The number at risk for each period is calculated as all animals present at the beginning of the first period plus the animals added in the previous period(s) minus the animals that acquired immunity in the previous period(s). Thus, 139 is simply 112 + 36 - 9; and 162 equals 112 + 36 + 46 - 9 - 23. Note that animals that died are already included in the number of new cases.

The number of weeks at risk is determined by assuming that, at average, minks are added halfway the week and that, again at average, the infection will occur as well halfway the week. Thus, 125.5 = 112 + 36/2 - 9/2 which is also equal to (112 + 139)/2.

The incidence rate for week 1 is calculated as 9/125.5; the cumulative incidence after week 1 is 9/130.

5.2. Prevalence and Incidence

1. Prevalence rate_1 = 10/30 = 0.33
   Prevalence rate_2 = 6/28 = 0.21
   Both prevalences are at the cow level.

2. The period of risk can be calculated in several ways, differing in precision. Two methods are shown below:

   a. Most precise: Incidente rate= 5/85=0.0588 cases per cow-week

3 cows culled	3 * 0 weeks = 0 weeks
1 cow (no 335) mastitic the whole period	1 * 0 weeks = 0 weeks
6 cows recovered after 2 weeks	6 * 2 weeks = 12 weeks
5 cows with new onset regarded as mastitis-free for 2 weeks	5 * 2 weeks = 10 weeks
15 cows without mastitis in the whole period	15 * 4 weeks = 60 weeks
1 new cow without mastitis for three weeks	1 * 3 weeks = 3 weeks
	85 weeks

b. Less precise: Incidence rate=5/84=0.0595 cases per cow-week

Because 20 and 22 cows, respectively, are mastitis-free at the 1st and 2nd tests, the average number at risk is (20 + 22)/2 = 21 and the number of weeks at risk equals 21 ∗ 4 = 84 weeks.
As the observation period is 1 month (and assuming that 1 month is 4 weeks), the total risk period will be 21 cows ∗ 1 month = 21 cow-months. Seeing that there are 5 new cases (no. 335 is assumed to have had mastitis throughout the period), the incidence rate is calculated as: 5/21 cases per cow-month = 0.238 per cow-month.

3. The risk that a cow gets mastitis in a 10 month lactation period may be calculated in two ways:

either:
Incidence rate (10 months) = 2.38 cases per 10 cow-months. Then, the risk for an individual cow to get subclinical mastitis during its 10 months of lactation can be estimated from the incidence rate as $1 - e^{-2.38} = 0.91$

or:
The risk during the month of observation can be calculated directly as:

$$R_1 = \frac{5 \text{ cases}}{20 \text{ cows at risk at the beginning of the period}} = 0.25$$

as the risk can only be calculated directly on the basis of the number of animals at risk from the beginning of the period. The risk of NOT getting mastitis is 0.75 and thus the risk of NOT getting mastitis in a 10 month period is $0.75^{10} = 0.056$. The risk of getting mastitis in a 10 month period is then 1-0.056 = 0.944.

Intrinsic to the extrapolation of the observations made in a 4 week period to a whole lactation, is the assumption that the mastitis incidence is evenly distributed over the year. It is hence also assumed that all factors influencing mastitis incidence are equal for all months. Such an assumption is most likely unrealistic under practical conditions.

5.3. Diagnostic tests

1. Prevalence with LS = 3.7%; prevalence with TS = 9.8%.
The large difference occurs because LS classifies 6.6% untruly as normal, thereby underestimating the prevalence of CA with a factor 3.
The 95% CI is given by:

$$P \pm 1.96 * \sqrt{\frac{P*(1-P)}{N}}$$

with:

P = prevalence,
√ = square root and
N = total number of heads.

P according to TS amounts to 9.8%, so the 95% CI is:

$$0.098 \pm 1.96 * \sqrt{\frac{0.098 * 0.902}{100}} = [0.040; 0.074]$$

In analogy, the 95% CI using LS:

$$0.037 \pm 1.96 * \sqrt{\frac{0.037 * 0.963}{100}} = [0.000; 0.074]$$

2. The frequencies are given below:

Results of group 1 (N = 248)

		LS		
		N	CA	Total
TS	N	223	1	224
	CA	16	8	24
	Total	239	9	248

prevalence using TS = 24/248 = 9.7%
prevalence using LS = 9/248 = 3.6%

Thus, prevalences do not change when using numbers! The CI, however, does change when using n = 248.

95% CI using TS: [0.061; 0.135]
95% CI using LS: [0.014; 0.060]

The confidence intervals are smaller with a multiplication factor of: √248/√100 = 1.57. **Use numbers when calculating a CI!**

3. Of the 107 heads scored as CA positive in a hurry, ultimately 43 have CA when judged at more quiet conditions (40.2% of 107). So, prevalence with LS amounts to 43/638 = 6.7% Prevalence with TS is: 49/638 = 7.7%. This is much lower than the original 107/638 = 16.8% based on judgement along the slaughterline and lower than the prevalence of 9.8% (see question 2).

4. SE = (248∗0.032) / (248∗0.098) = 0.327 or 32.7%.

SP = (248∗0.897) / (248∗0.902) = 0.994 or 99.4%.
The SE is very low, only 1/3 of all real positive heads are being scored as such. The SP is very high, nearly all normal heads are scored as such.

For SE:
95% CI: 0.327 ± 1.96∗√(0.327∗0.673/24) = [0.139; 0.515]
with n = number of CA positive heads.

For SP:
95% CI: 0.994 ± 1.96∗√(0.994∗0.006/224) = [0.984; 1.000]
with n = number of normal heads.

5. PV^+ = (248∗0.032) / (248∗0.037) = 0.865 or 86.5%. In 86.5% of the cases a head scored as CA with LS really is CA.

   PV^- = (248∗0.897) / (248∗0.963) = 0.931 or 93.1%. Thus, in 93.1% of the cases a head scored as normal, indeed is normal.

   For PV^+:
   95% CI: 0.865 ± 1.96∗√(0.865∗0.135/9) = [0.642; 1.000].

   For PV^-:
   95% CI: 0.931 ± 1.96∗√(0.931∗0.069/239) = [0.899; 0.963].

6. Predictive values not only depend on SE and SP, but also on ..... the prevalence! If the prevalence was 50%, then we would have obtained the following 2x2 table:

		LS		
		N	CA	Total
TS	N	49.7	0.3	50
	CA	33.7	16.3	50
	Total	83.4	16.6	100

   PV^+ = 16.3/16.6 = 0.982 or 98.2%.
   PV^- = 49.7/83.4 = 0.596 or 59.6%.

   So, PV^+ remains high, because SP is high and the number of false-positives is low. PV^- decreases, because SE is low and the number of false-negatives high.

7. a. proportion agreement = (89.7 + 3.2)/100 = 0.929
   b. expected agreement due to chance alone

$$\frac{\left(\frac{90.2*96.3}{100}+\frac{3.7*9.8}{100}\right)}{100}=0.872$$

c. maximal proportion agreement beyond chance: 1 - 0.872 = 0.128
d. realized proportion agreement beyond chance: 0.929 - 0.872 = 0.057
e. *kappa* = 0.057/0.128 = 0.45, very moderate agreement

8. It is not possible to conclude about the absolute value of the tests. *Kappa* only quantifies the degree of agreement beyond chance. It might be that both tests are equally wrong.

9. See at answer 2 for the exact frequencies.
The outcome now is:
a. (223 + 8)/248 = 0.931
b.

$$\frac{\left(\frac{224*239}{248}+\frac{24*9}{248}\right)}{248}=0.874$$

c. 1 - 0.874 = 0.126
d. 0.931 - 0.874 = 0.057
e. 0.057/0.126 = 0.45 = *kappa*
So, *kappa* does not change! (the small deviations are caused by rounding errors).

10. What does change, however, is the width of the confidence interval. When using percentages, one actually increases or decreases the number of sampling units to 100 thereby manipulating the standard error of the mean. Calculation of the confidence interval (CI) for *kappa* is too complex to perform on a small calculator, therefore they will be given (CI's for *kappa* are given by WINEPISCOPE):

95% CI using percentages:	0.45 ± 1.96∗0.17 [= 0.12; 0.78]
95% CI using numbers:	0.45 ± 1.96∗0.11 [= 0.23; 0.67]

11. LS is not a good instrument to determine the prevalence of AR. The AR prevalence is underestimated by a factor 3, that is, about 2/3 of truly positive heads are diagnosed as normal, even at quiet conditions.

12. If a large number of heads per herd is tested, especially when the prevalence within a herd is low, this might be a good method. Diagnosing one CA would classify the herd as CA. There is hardly any danger for diagnosing a truly negative herd as positive, because SP is high.

13. Results for group 2:

Parameter	Results (%)	95%CI
P (TS)	45.8	36.4 to 55.2
P (LS)	40.2	30.9 to 49.5
SE	57.2	42.3 to 71.0
SP	74.2	62.9 to 85.4
PV^+	65.2	50.9 to 79.4
PV-	67.2	55.7 to 78.7

Based on 107 heads, *kappa* = 0.32

Results for group 3:

Parameter	Results (%)	95%CI
P (TS)	40.8	35.9 to 45.7
P (LS)	29.9	25.4 to 34.4
SE	51.0	43.1 to 58.8
SP	84.7	80.0 to 89.3
PV^+	69.6	61.2 to 78.0
PV^-	71.5	66.1 to 76.9

Based on 385 heads, *kappa* = 0.37

5.4. Diagnostic tests and cut-off value

1. False-positives: cross reactions, earlier infection, vaccination, laboratory errors
   False-negatives: time-lag between infection and immune response, tolerance inappropriate test, immunosuppression, laboratory errors

2.

Cut-off value	SE	SP	LR
0	100	0	1
0.5	100	41	1.7
1.0	100	66	2.9
1.5	99	83	5.8
2.0	96	90	9.6
2.5	89	94	14.8
3.0	79	96	19.8
3.5	53	98	26.5
4.0	19	99	19.0
4.5	3	100	--

It depends on the use of the test whether a high SE or a high SP is wanted!

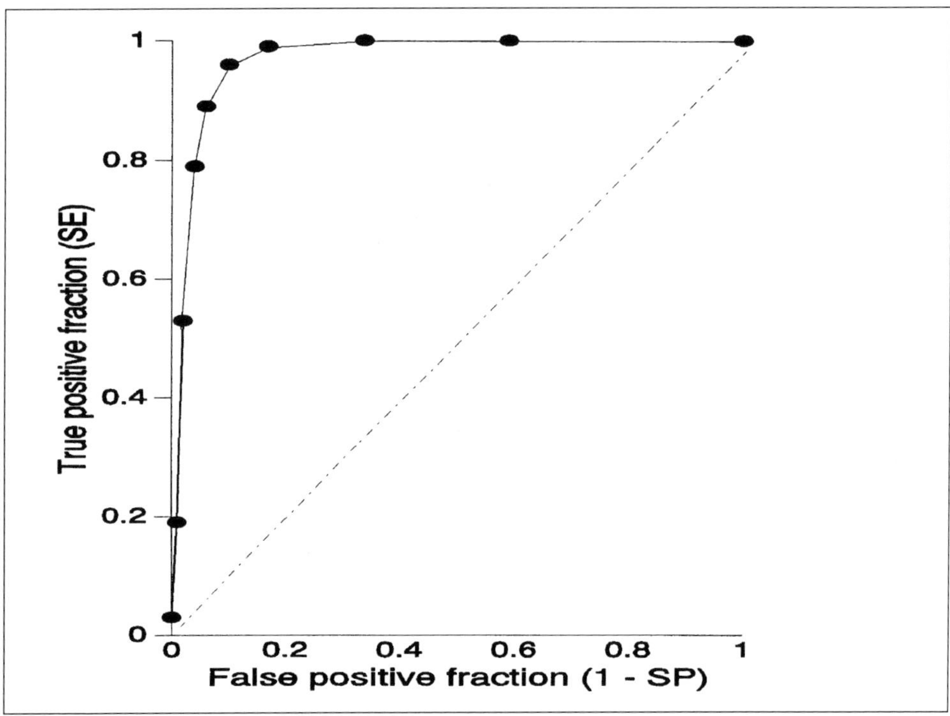

Figure 4.4. ROC curve of SMDETEC.

3. Create a 2x2 table:

		True status		
		G1 pos.	G2 neg.	Total
Test	Pos.	79	4	83
	Neg.	21	96	117
	Total	100	100	200

SE =	79/100 = 79%; SP = 96/100 = 96%
95% CI for SE =	SE ± 1.96 ∗ Standard Error
Standard error =	√(SE ∗ (100 - SE)/n)
n =	is corresponding marginal which is 100 for both
Standard error SE =	√(79 ∗ (100 - 79)/100) = 4.07
95% CI for SE =	79 ± 1.96 ∗ 4.07 = [71; 87]
Standard error SP =	√(96 ∗ (100 - 96)/100) = 1.96
95% CI for SP =	96 ± 1.96 ∗ 1.96 = [92; 100]

4. AP = 0.10

$$P = \frac{0.10 + 0.96 - 1}{0.79 + 0.96 - 1} = \frac{0.06}{0.75} = 0.08 = 8\%$$

$$PV+ = \frac{0.08 * 0.79}{(0.08 * 0.79) + (1 - 0.08)(1 - 0.96)} = 0.632$$

$$PV- = \frac{(1 - 0.08) * 0.96}{0.08 * (1 - 0.79) + (1 - 0.08) * 0.96} = 0.981$$

The predictive value of a negative test result of 98% means that 98% of the negative tested animals are truly negative. This is due to the low prevalence and high specificity.

5. AP = 10/250 = 0.04

$$\Rightarrow P = \frac{0.04 + 0.96 - 1}{0.79 + 0.96 - 1} = \frac{0}{0.75} = 0$$

Both might be correct, but 'at average' the multiplier is correct! If you just calculate the true prevalence from the AP and sensitivity and specificity then p = 0! Thus, most likely no animals are truly infected.

The PV^+ = 0%. So, this means that at average 0% of the positively tested animals are truly positive.
The PV^- = 100%. This means that all negative tested animals are truly negative. Hence, if fatteners might say that there may be some false negatives then the multiplier can state that negatively tested animals are most likely to be truly negative.

5.5. Predictive values

1. The parameter you need must express 'the possibility of being not diseased when the test is negative'. This is, of course, the PV^-.

2x2 table:

		INFECTED		
		Y	N	
TEST	+	50	0	50
	-	5	45	50
		55	45	100

The PV- = 45/50 = 90%. So, 90% of all animals tested free from the disease are really free. The other 10% is positive. So from the 20 animals, at average, 18 are negative and 2 are positive. The farmer should not buy these animals!!

2. The PV^+ = 100%, because there are no false-positives (SP = 100%). So when a test result is positive the animal is indeed infected.

5.6. The impact of false-positives

1. The results (in percentages) are as follows:

		INFECTED		
		Y	N	
TEST	+	4.75	19	23.75
	-	0.25	76	76.25
		5	95	100

Of the 1 million cows 23.75% (237,500) is tested positive. This would result in a financial loss of 237,500 ∗ 100 dollar = 23.75 million dollar

2. The extra loss amounts to 190,000∗100 dollar = 19 million dollar. This is 19/23.75 = 80% of the total costs!

3. The extra loss is caused by animals that are slaughtered but are not infected (false-positives = 19%). So, the SP should be increased.

Chapter V

Basics of Observational Studies

K. Frankena
Wageningen University & Research Centre
Department of Animal Sciences
Quantitative Veterinary Epidemiology Group
The Netherlands

M.V. Thrusfield
University of Edinburgh
Department of Veterinary Clinical Studies
United Kingdom

1. Introduction

Epidemiological research is conducted at the level of the ***population***, whatever the units of the population may be (animals, herds, farms, regions, countries). Essentially, there are two reasons why an epidemiologist performs population-level research (mostly by looking at a sample of a population). First, he might want to quantify a characteristic of that population, for instance, the prevalence of a disease. This type of research is called 'descriptive research' and is often undertaken using surveys (e.g., by blood sampling). Secondly, the epidemiologist may wish to test an association between a disease and exposure to a suspected causal factor. The main focus of such research is to test an hypothesis. This research is called 'analytical research'. Both types are observational, because the researcher observes events, without intervention/experimentation. Because of this non-intervention, observational epidemiology is different from experimental epidemiology in which the epidemiologist is interested in the effect of an intervention, be it a single exposure like vaccination or therapy, or a whole farm advisory program. Figure 5.1 shows an overview of the several components of veterinary epidemiology, in which descriptive research (surveys) and analytical research (observational studies) are put in the wider epidemiological context.

Since the main focus of analytical research is to test the association between disease and exposure to a suspected causal factor in the population, ***measures of association***, expressing the ***absolute or relative change in risk due to exposure***, are central. In general terms, risk is defined as the probability of hazard, bad consequences, loss, etc.... (Brown, 1993).

Whatever the type of observational research, the population is usually too large to allow observation of all units. Moreover, estimates of association often can obtained to an acceptable degree of precision by selection a number of animals smaller than the population size. Thus, ***samples*** of units are observed. Three basic types of sampling protocol are used in observational analytical research, producing three main study designs:

1. cross-sectional: in which units (individuals or herds) are sampled without considering health and exposure status beforehand;
2. case-control: where units are intentionally chosen for their health status;
3. cohort: where units are intentionally chosen for their exposure status.

The techniques of sampling were discussed earlier (see Chapter III). The 2x2 table below illustrates the differences between the three types:

		Disease		
		+	-	
Factor	+	A	B	A + B
	-	C	D	C + D
		A + C	B + D	N

This table can be generated in three ways, according to the method of sampling:

- random sampling of N units, without selection according to either disease or exposure status (cross-sectional studies);
- sampling according to disease status, involving selection of A + C (diseased) and B + D (healthy) (case-control studies);
- sampling according to factor status, involving selection of A+B (exposed) and C + D (unexposed) individuals (cohort studies).

2. Types of Study and Measures of Association

In this paragraph, three types of study will be discussed. The following example will be used for illustration.

	Diseased	Healthy	Total
Exposed	600	400	1,000
Unexposed	400	1,600	2,000
Total	1,000	2,000	3,000

Thus, the population consists of 3,000 animals, of which 1,000 are exposed. Of the 1,000 exposed animals, 600 develop disease X and 400 remain free of this disease. Of the 2,000 unexposed animals, 400 develop the disease and 1,600 remain free.

2.1. Cross-sectional studies

In a cross-sectional study, individuals are tested for the presence of the disease under study and for the exposure status at the same time. Cross-sectional studies therefore take a 'snapshot' of the situation at a specific moment.

The measure of association that can be calculated with this type of study is the prevalence ratio (PR) which is the ratio of the fraction diseased among the exposed and the fraction diseased among the unexposed:

$$PR = \frac{\frac{A}{A+B}}{\frac{C}{C+D}}$$

If the prevalence ratio equals 1.0, then there is no association; if the measure is greater than 1.0, then exposure might be a risk factor; if the measure is less than 1.0, then exposure might be a preventive factor.

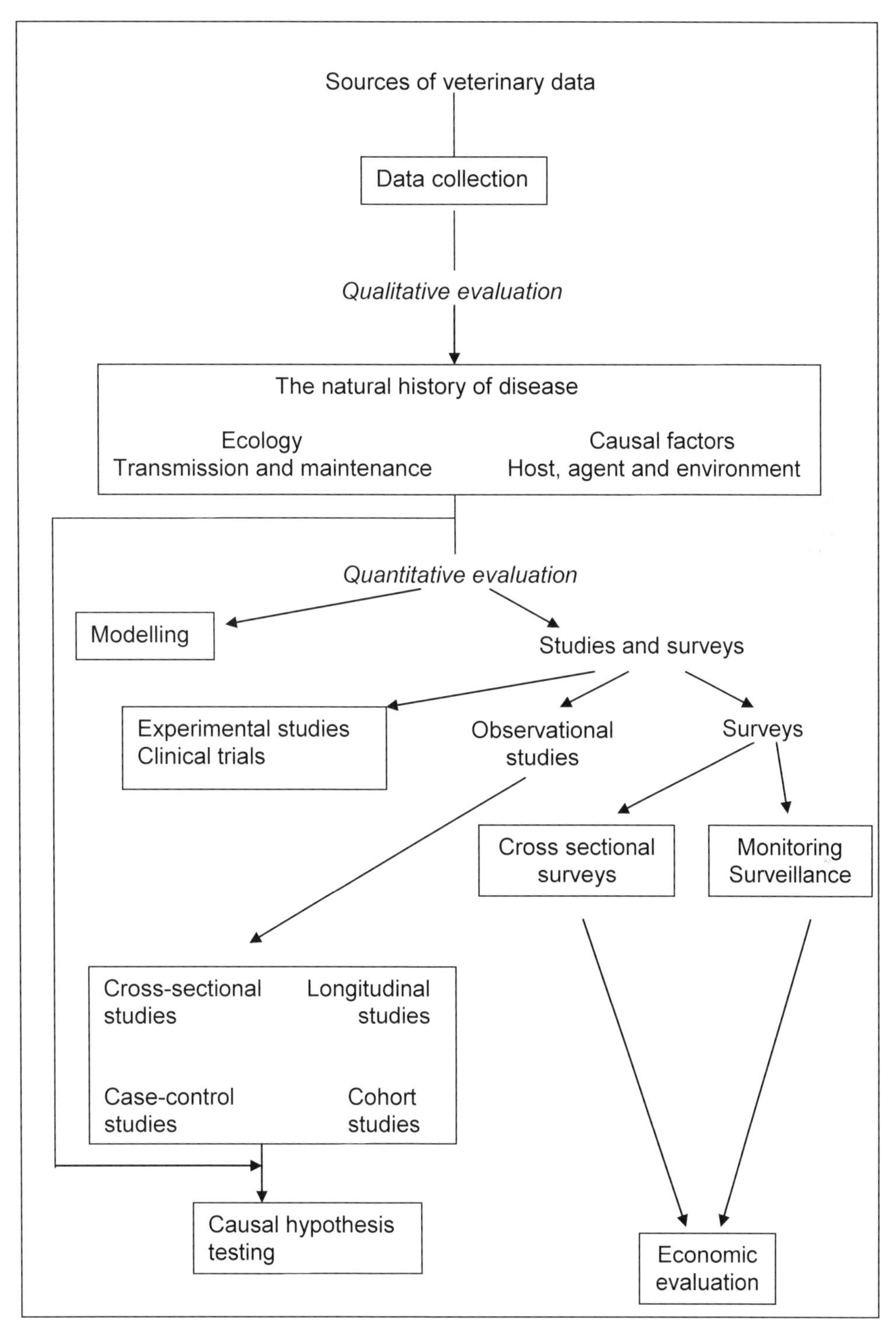

Figure 5.1. Components of veterinary epidemiology (from Thrusfield, 1997).

If a cross-sectional study is performed on a random sample of 300 animals out of the population serving as an example, the 2x2 table would most likely be as follows:

	Disease X	No disease X	Total
Exposed	60	40	100
Unexposed	40	160	200
Total	100	200	300

The prevalence ratio is (60/100) / (40/200) = 3.0. This figure indicates that the prevalence in exposed animals is three times higher than in unexposed animals.

Cross-sectional studies are less suitable for identifying relationships between *variable* or *transient* exposures and the disease of interest, because the current exposure information might be too recent to be etiologically meaningful. For exposures that are constant throughout the individual's life (like blood group, breed, sex and sometimes housing system), cross-sectional studies can be useful. Conclusions about causality therefore cannot be drawn, except for those factors that do not change over time. A second disadvantage of cross-sectional studies is that diseases with low incidence or short duration (fast recovery) will lead to a small number of cases (low prevalence). This can be deduced from the following relation that is valid for stable endemic diseases:

$$P = I * D$$

P = prevalence, i.e., the ratio of the number of cases at a certain time to the total number of animals at risk in the population (which is also the probability that an animal at risk suffers from that disease at a specific time);

I = incidence rate (incidence density), i.e., the number of new cases per time unit that are arising;

D = duration of disease, i.e., the length of the period after contracting the disease during which an animal would be designated as having the disease.

For analyses, a certain number of cases will be required. To meet this, diseases with low I or short meaningful D will require large scale studies, i.e., high N.

2.2. Case-control studies

In a case-control study, diseased (A + C) and non-diseased (B + D) animals are intentionally chosen as the units to be sampled (Schlesselman, 1982).

To measure whether or not exposure is more common in the diseased group than in the control group, the (exposure) odds ratio (OR) is the measure of association that indicates the relative change in risk. The OR is calculated as:

$$OR_{exp} = \frac{\frac{A}{C}}{\frac{B}{D}} = \frac{A * D}{B * C}$$

The numerical value of the odds ratio is interpreted in the same way as that of the prevalence ratio.

If a case-control study was performed with 150 individuals in each of the two health status groups, then the frequencies in our example would be close to:

	Diseased	Healthy
Exposed	90	30
Unexposed	60	120
Total	150	150

Note that the relative frequencies of exposure within the diseased and healthy group are equal to those in the original population. The OR equals (90/60) / (30/120) = 6.0. This figure means that exposure is six times more common in cases than in controls.

One cannot estimate the prevalence of disease in the population from which the cases or controls are taken because the case-control ratio (as determined by the investigator) is usually not the same as that in the population. Because the groups to be sampled are based on health status, this type of study is suitable for diseases with low incidence or of short duration. When cases and controls are known, the factor status can be assessed in retrospect. The objective is to investigate whether or not a possible risk factor occurs more frequently in the diseased than in the control group. Since the factor status is often assessed in retrospect, bias can occur, especially when this is done from memory (recall bias).

Case-control and cross-sectional studies are especially suited to screen for potential risk factors. The proof of causality is best left to cohort studies, starting with healthy individuals that are either exposed or unexposed to the factor of interest.

2.3. Cohort studies

In epidemiology, 'cohort' is reserved for a group of individuals that either do, or do not, possess a factor that may influence the occurrence of disease or other health-related event. A group possessing the factor (the exposed group) is then followed over time with respect to change in health status. A reference group, comprising individuals that do not possess that specific characteristic but are otherwise similar (the unexposed group), is also selected and similarly followed. This type of study follows, in chronological order, the effect of exposure and the change from the healthy to the diseased state.

Two types of cohort study can be distinguished: retrospective and prospective. In a retrospective study, the allocation of individuals to the cohorts is based on exposure experience in the past. Subsequently, the occurrence of disease can be in the past (but after the start of the moment of exposure) or at present/in future (if the study still has not finished). In a prospective study, the allocation to cohorts is based on current exposure and one has to 'sit and wait' for the development of disease in both cohorts.

The frequency of exposure in the population cannot be estimated in cohort studies (c.f., case-control studies in which the frequency of disease in the population cannot be computed). To estimate the relative change in risk, the cumulative incidence ratio (CIR) can be calculated, the incidence being the number of animals that developed the disease during the study divided by the total number of animals that were at risk at the start of the study. Synonyms for the CIR are the risk ratio and the relative risk (RR), although the latter sometimes is used as a general indicator for all types of relative measures of association. As a formula:

$$CIR = \frac{\frac{A}{A+B}}{\frac{C}{C+D}}$$

The numerical value of the CIR is interpreted in the same way as those of the prevalence ratio and odds ratio. The (disease) odds ratio can also be calculated:

$$OR_{dis} = \frac{\frac{A}{B}}{\frac{C}{D}} = \frac{A*D}{B*C}$$

A cohort study with 150 individuals per cohort in the example would yield:

	Disease X	No disease X	Total
Exposed	90	60	150
Unexposed	30	120	150

The CIR equals (90/150) / (30/150) = 3.0 and the OR = (90/60) / (30/120) = 6.0.
In cohort studies one can take into account the individual time at risk for each animal (see Chapter IV) as well. The number of cases and the number of time units an animal has not shown the event of interest are counted per cohort and next the ***incidence rate ratio*** (IRR, synonym rate ratio incidence density ratio, relative risk) is calculated as:

$$IRR = \frac{\frac{A}{T_1}}{\frac{C}{T_0}}$$

where A and C denote the number of cases in the exposed group (group 1) and the unexposed group (group 0). T_1 and T_0 indicate the total time at risk in each group. The use of the incidence rate ratio is recommended if populations are dynamic, when animals are commonly lost during follow-up, or new animals enter the cohorts after the initial observations have started. In the numerical example below the IRR equals (50/500) / (25/400) = 1.6.

	Exposure		
	+	-	
Number of cases	50	25	75
Time at risk	500	400	900

2.4. Summarizing study types

In Tables 5.1 and 5.2, the temporal setting and the advantages and disadvantages (according to Thrusfield, 1997) of the three types of study are summarized:

Table 5.1. Overview of the three basic types of observational study.

Type	Past	Present	Future
Cross-sectional		Disease Exposure	
Case-control	Exposure	Disease	
Retrospective cohort	Exposure/Disease	Disease	Disease
Prospective cohort		Exposure	Disease

Table 5.2. Advantages and disadvantages of the three types of observational studies.

	Cross-sectional	Case-control	Cohort
Advantages	- When a random sample of the target population is selected, proportions exposed and unexposed in the target population can be estimated - Relatively quick to mount and conduct - Relatively inexpensive - Require comparatively few subjects (unless disease is rare) - Current records occasionally can be used - No risk to subjects - Allow study of multiple potential causes of disease	- Well-suited to the study of rare diseases or of those with long incubation periods - Relatively quick to mount and conduct - Relatively inexpensive - Require comparatively few subjects - Existing records occasionally can be used - No risk to subjects - Allow study of multiple potential causes of a disease	- Incidence in exposed and unexposed proportion can be calculated - Permit flexibility in choosing variables to be systematically recorded
Disadvantages	- Moderate sample sizes are required to study rare diseases - Control of extraneous variables may be incomplete - Incidence in exposed and unexposed individuals cannot be estimated	- Exposed and unexposed proportion in target population cannot be estimated - Rely on recall or records for information on past exposures - Validation of information is difficult or sometimes impossible - Control of extraneous variables may be incomplete - Selection of an appropriate comparison group may be difficult - Incidence in exposed and unexposed individuals can be estimated	- Exposed and unexposed proportion in target population cannot be estimated - Large numbers of subjects are required to study rare diseases - Potentially long duration for follow-up - Relatively expensive to conduct - Maintaining follow-up is difficult - Control of extraneous variables may be incomplete

Table 5.3 summarizes the calculated measures of association. It can be seen that the OR overestimates the effect of a risk factor. This means that the OR is larger than the CIR (or PR) if the CIR (or PR) is greater than 1.0 and that the OR is smaller than the CIR (or PR) when the CIR (or PR) is less than 1.0 (overestimation of preventive effect). The CIR (or PR) and OR are equal in case A/(A + B) equals (A/B) and C/(C + D) equals (C/D). This is true if both A and C are equal to 0 (or: there are no diseased animals). If A and C are relatively small (prevalence or incidence is low) then the CIR an OR are about equal. Therefore, in follow-up studies preference should be given to the CIR and in cross-sectional studies to the PR (see also Nurminen, 1995).

Table 5.3. Measures of association using the frequency tables of paragraphs 2.1, 2.2 and 2.3 (n.a. = not allowed).

	Prevalence ratio	Cumulative incidence ratio	Odds ratio
Cross-sectional study	3.0	n.a.	6.0
Case-control study	n.a.	n.a.	6.0
Cohort study	n.a.	3.0	6.0

2.5. Measures of effect

In addition to the relative measures of association (OR, CIR and PR), measures of ***effect*** can be calculated. A measure of effect indicates to what extent the event can be prevented if the risk factor is neutralized, removed or avoided.
As an example: a cohort study of the effect of exposure to disease X gave the following results:

		Disease X	
		Yes	No
Exposure	Yes	15	45
	No	8	72

The CIR equals (15/60) / (8/80) = 2.5 and the OR = (15/45) / (8/72) = 3.0.

A simple measure of effect is the ***attributable risk*** (AR). As disease might occur in the unexposed group as well, only part of the disease in the exposed group can be attributed to the exposure. It is calculated as the risk of disease in the exposed group minus the risk of disease in the unexposed group. Hence, this measure cannot be calculated in case-control studies. A logical synonym is ***risk difference***. In the cohort example above the AR equals 15/60 - 8/80 = 0.15. This means that the risk in the exposed group, associated exclusively with exposure, is 0.15.

A second measure of effect is the ***population attributable risk (PAR)***. This is the incidence in the population minus the incidence in the unexposed group. It can therefore only be calculated when the population incidence is known. This can only be determined in cohort studies if exposed and unexposed groups are selected in the same proportion as they occur in the population from which they are selected. Thus, if in the example above, the numbers exposed and unexposed reflect the proportion exposed and unexposed in the population from which they are drawn, the PAR equals (23/140) - (8/80) = 0.064. This means that the incidence of disease in the population associated with the factor is 0.064. A PAR based on prevalence can be estimated directly in a cross-sectional study.

The ***attributable fraction*** (AF, also termed the aetiological fraction or attributable proportion) is the attributable risk divided by the risk of disease in the exposed group. In the example above this is 0.15 / (15/60) = 0.60. This figure is the proportion of exposed cases that could have been prevented if the exposure had not been present. This can be made more clear by calculating the number of expected cases if the exposure had no effect. The proportion of cases in the unexposed group is 8/80 = 0.10 and this proportion is then also expected in the unexposed group, being 0.10∗60 = 6 cases. However, 15 cases were diagnosed and that is 9 more than expected if there was no relation between the disease and the exposure. Thus 9 cases could have been saved by removing the exposure, which is equal to 9/15 = 0.60 (or 60%) of all exposed cases. A shorthand formula giving the same result is (CIR - 1)/CIR = (2.5 -1) /2.5 = 0.60. The AF can be estimated using odds ratios, thus: (OR - 1)/OR = (3 -1)/3 = 0.67.

A last measure of effect, closely related to the attributable fraction, is the ***population attributable fraction*** (PAF), which expresses the proportion of **all** cases that could have been prevented if the exposure had not been present. It is most easily calculated as the number of excess cases divided by the total number of cases, that is: 9/23 = 0.39 (or 39%). In the example, it is equal to the AF times the proportion of cases that is exposed (0.60 ∗ 15/23 = 0.39).

It should be noted that the AF and PAF will give negative values if the CIR (or OR) is smaller than 1.0. Then, the AF should be calculated as 1 - CIR or 1 - OR (Rothman, 1986). Suppose the OR in a study involving vaccination is 0.6, with vaccination being preventive. Then the AF will be 1 - 0.6 = 0.4, this is the proportion of potential cases that would be prevented by vaccination, in comparison with the total number of cases that would occur if vaccination was not implemented. One could also say that the OR for non-vaccination is 1/0.6 = 1.67 and then the AF = (1.67 - 1)/1.67 = 0.40 (or 40% of the cases in the non-vaccinated group can be prevented by vaccination).

The calculation of epidemiological parameters and their interpretation is summarized in the text below.

$$CIR = \frac{\left(\frac{15}{60}\right)}{\left(\frac{8}{80}\right)} = 2.5$$

The incidence of disease in exposed animals is 2.5 times higher than in animals not exposed (or: exposure increases the risk developing disease 2.5-fold compared with unexposed animals).

$$OR = \frac{(15 * 72)}{(8 * 45)} = 3.0$$

The odds of disease in exposed animals is 3 times the odds of disease in unexposed animals (NB: 1: in a case-control study, the odds ratio is interpreted as the odds of exposure in cases *vs.* controls; 2: in a cross-sectional study, the odds ratio can be interpreted in relation to both disease odds and exposure odds, based on prevalence - hence the synonym 'prevalence odds ratio').

$$AR = \left(\frac{15}{60}\right) - \left(\frac{8}{80}\right) = 0.15$$

The incidence of disease in exposed animals that is associated with exposure is 0.15 (15 per 100).

$$AF = \frac{(2.5 - 1)}{2.5} = 0.60$$

60% of exposed cases is associated with exposure.

$$PAF = \frac{(2.5 - 1)}{2.5} * \frac{15}{(15 + 8)} = 0.391$$

39.1% of all cases in the population is associated with exposure.

$$PAR = \left(\frac{23}{140}\right) - \left(\frac{8}{80}\right) = 0.064$$

The incidence of disease in the population associated with exposure is 64 per 1000. This can only be computed when the population incidence is known. However, it can be derived in cross-sectional studies, where it is based on prevalence, rather than on incidence.

For the parameters mentioned above, confidence intervals (CI) can be calculated. A confidence interval indicates the precision of the estimated parameter. The CI gives, with a defined probability (commonly 0.95, and often expressed as a percentage: 95%), the range (a lower and an upper value) in which the value of the measure will be in the population from which the study sample was drawn. For the most frequently used parameters (CIR, OR and IRR), interval calculations will be shown later (paragraph 3.9). In Rothman (1986), calculation of CI's for the AR (and some other parameters, not mentioned here) are described as well.

3. Design and Analysis of a Study

The general procedure that should be adopted is:

1. definition of objectives of the study;
2. description of target population;
3. calculation of sample size and choice of sampling method;
4. measurement of disease;
5. measurement of exposure;
6. bias;

7. data validation and editing;
8. descriptive results;
9. data analysis (testing for associations);
10. report the results.

3.1. Objectives of the study

It is essential that the objectives of the study are clearly defined. Hypotheses can then be generated; these will determine which factors require scrutiny so that an appropriate study design can be formulated.

3.2. Description of target population

A study is invariably conducted on a sample of a larger population to which the results of the study are to be extrapolated (the target population). This may for example, be all intensively-reared dairy herds, or all dogs, in a country. Therefore, one should take care to maintain representativeness, although there are often restrictions because of organisational problems or financial limitations. In all cases, however, the target population should be unambiguously defined.

3.3. Sample size and sampling method

The formulae for calculation of sample sizes in observational studies have been dealt with in Chapter III. Besides an adequate number of samples, the samples should be representative. In the first instance, it is tempting to select controls that are representative of the total non-diseased population. However, Rothman (1986) states that this is invalid: controls should be representative of the group from which the members automatically would be diagnosed as cases after developing the disease. Suppose you have a list with all herds in a region (the sampling frame). Some herds use herd health programmes and you select case herds (e.g., those with a high incidence of cystic ovarian disease: COD) from databases of practitioners that are involved in these herd health programmes. However, controls should not be selected from the complete sampling frame. They should be selected from those herds that have a low COD incidence and that also participate in a herd health programme. Thus the sampling frame consists not of all herds in the region, but of all herds using a herd health programme.

3.4. Measurement of disease status

Sometimes the disease that is being studied is not identified unambiguously either by clinical examination or by the use of auxiliary diagnostic tests; that is, the diagnostic methods do not have a diagnostic sensitivity and diagnostic specificity of 100% (Chapter IV). The net result is that animals may be misclassified as either affected or unaffected (see paragraph 3.6).

3.5. Measurement of exposure

In cohort and cross-sectional studies, the actual exposure can be recorded and sometimes measured quantitatively. In case-control studies the information on exposure may have to be recalled from memory by the owner of the animal. This might easily lead to recall bias. Only in very few instances (e.g., feeding, medication) this information is stored in on-farm databases.

A popular way of assessing information on exposure, especially for diseases with a multifactorial aetiology, is the questionnaire. A considerable literature exists on how to correctly design questionnaires (e.g., Dillman, 1978), and this should be consulted if a questionnaire-based study is to be undertaken. A danger of measuring exposure in this way is that one is not always certain whether or not the exposure preceded the onset of disease. Secondly, real measurements (e.g., about the size of the barn, the percentage of slatted area, the quality of hygienic measures) are not carried out, but are estimated. Another danger is that so much data are collected that the statistical analysis becomes unfeasible. When collecting exposure data, one should avoid missing values, because subjects with missing data will be excluded from the analysis. For situations with a low expected response rate, the original sample size should be increased by, say, a factor of 2 or 3. As sample size calculations are difficult to perform in a multivariate setting, one should try to balance the number of questions and the number of responders. About 4 to 5 responders for each factor are recommended (Greenland, 1985). Thus, if the questionnaire has 50 questions, one needs at least 200 responders. Questionnaire design is further addressed in Chapter XII, part 4.

3.6. Bias

Bias is a systematic error in the design, performance, or analysis of a study, that makes the results invalid. This contrasts with random error. There are several sources of bias. The most common are:

a. selection bias;
b. misclassification;
c. information bias;
d. confounding.

a. The essential feature of an epidemiological study is a comparison of groups with respect to disease or exposure frequency. Selection bias results in a distortion of the measured effect in the study from the true effect in the entire population because the units included in the study are not representative of the population from which they were selected. Cases and controls should therefore be comparable. So, if hospital cases are used, controls can be individuals that entered the hospital for other reasons or they should be selected among the whole population.

b. Bias due to misclassification occurs when cases are not recognized as such and might be selected as controls, and *vice versa*. These mistakes occur when the sensitivity and specificity of diagnostic methods are not 100%. This results in misclassification with respect to disease status. Exposure status, similarly, may be misclassified. This is a particular danger when exposure factors are transient or variable (e.g., drug use and dose levels). Both disease and exposure misclassification can distort the measures of association (odds ratio and relative risk). The extent of this distortion varies, but can render a computed measure insignificant (i.e., not significantly different from 1: see Thrusfield (1997) for a graphical representation of this effect). A strategy for decreasing the effect of misclassification of disease status is to choose a diagnostic method (including the cut-off point if the method is based on a continuous variable) that keeps the number of false-positives low. The risk estimate will then be on the 'safe side' (i.e., the estimate will be conservative).

c. If questionnaires are used and the respondent knows the reason for performing the study, he or she might subconsciously favour certain answers. Also, the information may need to be recalled from memory. This has a high chance of introducing errors (recall bias). If the interviewer is not trained, he or she might subconsciously direct the respondent's answers (interviewer bias).

d. Confounding relates to the fact that effects of factors cannot be directly estimated without bias when the numbers/classes of one factor are not equally distributed among the numbers/classes of another factor. This can again cause the estimates of odds ratios and relative risks to diverge from their true values. Further explanation will be given in paragraph 3.9 of this chapter.

3.7. Data validation and editing

The validity of the results of the study not only depends on the amount of bias but also on the percentage of errors in the initial data. Therefore, the data set should be checked for missing values and typing errors. Missing values should be coded in a unique way (e.g., -1 if the milk production of a cow is not known), so that the software is able to recognize it as such. Some typing errors can be detected by descriptive calculations (minima, maxima, frequencies). However, this method does not detect typing errors that result in a value that is permissible. Thus, suppose, a parameter can be coded as either 1, 2 or 3 and the actual value equals 2. If the value 3 is recorded either on paper or via the keyboard, this error will not be detected. Data validation and editing is an essential step. The validity of the results is directly related to the number of errors in the data ('garbage in = garbage out'!).

3.8. Descriptive results

Before starting the statistical analysis, the investigator has to describe the contents of the data set in terms of means and frequency distributions. It will give a direct insight into the number of typing errors, but he or she also gets a 'feeling' for the data. Some examples might be: number of animals, number of herds, general location of herds, overall prevalence, prevalence per herd (between-herd variation), mean age and breed of the animals, and the number of animals deleted from the data set with reasons for their deletion.

3.9. Data analysis

The strategy for analysis of the data should be defined before the study is undertaken. This, and the study's objectives, should then be included in a research proposal. Thus, a clear idea of how the data will be analyzed is required *before* the study is conducted. In order to estimate how much data should be collected, one must make assumptions about a most likely range of outcomes of the study because the sample size calculation needs this as input. In this section the analysis of the relationship between disease and a single factor (often termed 'crude' analysis), including calculation of confidence intervals, is discussed first. This is called univariate analysis and can easily be done by hand. However, unlike experimental settings, observational studies may need to reckon with the effects of various factors at the same time. Therefore, these factors should be analyzed simultaneously. In the second and third parts of this section, two features of multivariate analysis will be discussed: confounding and interaction (effect modification). If confounding is present, the estimate of the measure of association is biased. Interaction indicates that the effect of the factor depends on the level of another factor (hence, 'effect modification'). Reference will be made to the Mantel-Haenszel technique. More sophisticated methods for multivariate analysis are dealt with in Chapters VI and VII.

Crude analysis

The objective of the data analysis is to support or refute hypotheses of association between two or more features, specifically whether there is an increased (or decreased) risk of disease associated with specific factors. Apart from the sample estimate of the measure of association, the latter's confidence interval should be known. If the value 1.0 is ***not*** included in the confidence interval, then the measure deviates significantly from 1.0 at the level of significance corresponding to that interval, (the 10% level of significance for a 90% interval, the 5% level of significance for a 95% interval and the 1% level of significance for a 99% interval).

Several methods are available for obtaining confidence intervals. Some methods involve exact estimation of the intervals, other use approximations which are valid if the expected cell frequencies exceed a minimum. Here an overview of the estimation methods (and a reference where the method is explained) is given:

- Mid-p exact limits (Rothman, 1986)
- Fisher exact limits (Rothman, 1986)
- Test based limits (Rothman, 1986)
- Taylor series limits (Kleinbaum *et al.*, 1982)
- Cornfield limits (Kleinbaum *et al.*, 1982)

A comprehensive critique of the various methods of confidence interval estimation is provided by Sahai and Khurshid (1995). The most simple and most frequently used method will be shown in its full form for the OR. It is a method based on the so-called first-order Taylor series, which is an 'asymptotic' method. This means that the approximation is reasonable if 'large' sample sizes are used. As a rule of thumb, the ***expected*** cell frequencies in a 2x2 table should be at least 5 to have accurate interval estimation. If one of these expected frequencies is less than 5, exact methods must be used (e.g., within EPI-INFO). The procedure to calculate a CI for the CIR is almost identical.

The OR is not Normally distributed. Values will be concentrated somewhat around 1.0 with the minimum value at least greater than zero and a maximum value theoretically as high as infinity. The way of calculation of the confidence interval, specifically the use of the significance thresholds (Z-values), assumes Normality. Therefore, the data are first transformed to attain Normality. Transformation by taking the natural logarithm (ln) is best suited when the distribution is skewed to the right (i.e., the peak of the curve is to the left of centre). Then, after transformation, the confidence interval of the transformed OR can be calculated:

lower border: $\ln(OR) - Z_\alpha * \sqrt{}$ (variance $\ln(OR)$)
higher border: $\ln(OR) + Z_\alpha * \sqrt{}$ (variance $\ln(OR)$)

By transforming back via:

$$e^{\text{lower border}} \quad \text{and} \quad e^{\text{higher border}},$$

the interpretable lower and higher border values of the confidence interval of the untransformed OR are obtained. It should be realized that these borders are not symmetrical around the calculated OR. The value of Z_α in the above formula can be set as desired, for instance 1.96 for a confidence level of 95%, and 2.58 for a confidence level of 99%. The variance of the ln of the OR can be calculated from a 2x2 table as:

$$\text{var}\left(\ln(OR)\right) = \left(\frac{1}{A}\right) + \left(\frac{1}{B}\right) + \left(\frac{1}{C}\right) + \left(\frac{1}{D}\right)$$

The calculation of the CI for the CIR differs in the way the variance of ln(CIR) is calculated:

$$\text{var}\left(\ln(CIR)\right) = \frac{\frac{B}{A}}{A+B} + \frac{\frac{D}{C}}{C+D}$$

(This formulation can also be used for prevalence data in the calculation of confidence intervals for prevalence ratios.)

For incidence rate data:

$$\text{var}\left(\ln(IRR)\right) = \left(\frac{1}{A}\right) + \left(\frac{1}{B}\right)$$

The results of a hypothetical case-control study may be used as an example:

		Diseased	
		+	-
Factor	+	115	67
	-	16	64

OR = (115 ∗ 64) / (16 ∗ 67) = 6.87
The OR transformed = ln (6.87) = 1.93
The variance of ln(OR) = 1/115 + 1/67 + 1/16 + 1/64 = 0.10
The confidence is set at 95%, i.e., Z_α = 1.96.
The upper border: 1.93 + 1.96 ∗ √(0.10) = 2.55
The lower border: 1.93 - 1.96 ∗ √(0.10) = 1.31
The 95% confidence interval for the OR:

$$\text{from } e^{1.31} \text{ to } e^{2.55} \text{ (= from 3.71 to 12.81)}$$

This confidence interval does not include 1.0. Thus, it can be concluded that the factor is positively associated with disease occurrence. At 99% confidence (Z_α = 2.58) the interval ranges from 3.0 to 15.6. This larger confidence interval is intuitively correct: if one wants to be more confident, one needs to pay something; in this case one has less precision.

Confounding

Suppose one has a set of data relating to the occurrence of milk fever (hypocalcaemia) after calving in relation to body condition in the dry period:

		Milk Fever	
		Yes	No
Condition	Fat	50	150
	Normal	30	170

The OR = 1.89 (95% CI = 1.14 - 3.12). This would mean that cows that score as being fat in the dry period have an increased risk of milk fever after subsequent calving. However, parity also may be important in this respect. Therefore, the researcher also scored this characteristic.

		Parity			
		1 or 2		3 or higher	
		MF	no MF	MF	no MF
Condition	Fat	5	45	45	105
	Normal	15	135	15	35

The OR for young (first and second parity) cows is 1.0 and the OR for higher parity cows is also 1.0. So, within each parity class, condition certainly has no effect. How can it be that, in the overall analysis, fat condition was a risk factor? The reason is that apparently parity is a risk factor, i.e., higher parity cows have a higher risk of getting milk fever (OR = 3.86, within each condition class as well as overall). The parity 1, 2 cows had an odds of fat to normal condition of 1:3 while the higher parity cows showed an odds of 3:1 (OR = 9 indicating that higher parity cows have a 9 times higher risk than young cow as being scored as fat).

Graphically:

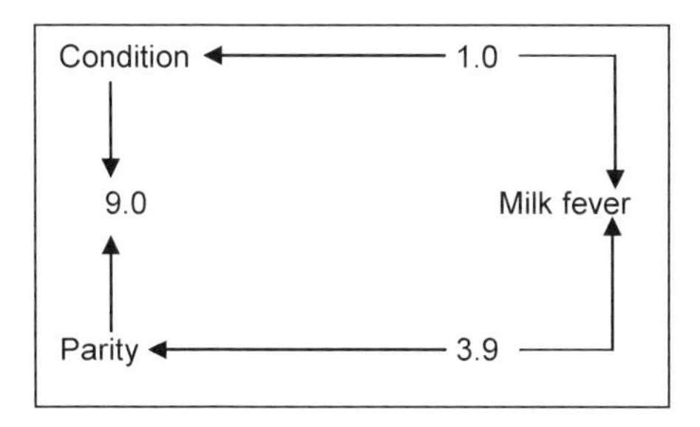

Thus, the unbiased effect of condition could only be estimated when corrected for parity. There may have been more confounders at work, such as breed or season, but they were not measured in this study. One should always be aware of the fact that relationships may be caused by confounding with other factors!

In the above example, an unbiased estimate of the effect of condition can be directly obtained by calculating the Mantel-Haenszel OR via:

$$OR_{M-H} = \frac{\frac{A_1 D_1}{N_1} + \ldots + \frac{A_k D_k}{N_k}}{\frac{B_1 C_1}{N_1} + \ldots + \frac{B_k C_k}{N_k}} = \frac{\sum \frac{A_i D_i}{N_i}}{\sum \frac{B_i C_i}{N_i}}$$

Substituting the data:

$$OR_{M-H} = \frac{\left(\frac{5 * 135}{200} + \frac{45 * 35}{200}\right)}{\left(\frac{15 * 45}{200} + \frac{15 * 105}{200}\right)} = 1$$

The OR_{M-H} gives a direct estimate that is weighted for differences in distribution of numbers among classes.

Factors are called confounders when they are:

- related to the disease;
- related to the exposure factor(s) under studie;
- not a necessary intermediate step between the factor and the disease.

In the above example, parity is a confounder for condition, but condition is not a confounder for parity because adjusted and non-adjusted OR's for parity are equal (OR = 3.86; OR_{M-H} = 3.86).

Assessment of confounding includes the following steps:

1. calculate the crude OR (this is the univariate OR)
2. calculate the adjusted OR (this is the multivariate OR)
3. decide on whether the difference between 1 and 2 is 'big' (arbitrary decision), if the answer is yes, then there is confounding and the adjusted OR should be presented if there is no interaction.
4. calculate whether the stratum specific OR's are homogeneously distributed across strata. If not, there is interaction (see later).

There are three ways of dealing with confounding. The first way was discussed above: to ***control*** for it during the statistical analysis. The second and most simple way is by ***exclusion***, that is, include only one stratum in your study. This strategy is undesirable because much information is lost. The third way is to use ***matching***. Two main types of matching exist: individual and frequency matching. Individual matching is the coupling of one or more controls to each case by selecting the cases and controls that are similar with respect to potential confounders; for instance, choosing the same breed for a case and a control. If frequency matching is applied, the *distribution* of matching variables in the comparison groups is forced to be similar. The objective of matching is the elimination of bias due to confounding by selecting a 'balanced' group of cases and controls. The whole idea is to get an unbiased estimate of the effect of the factor of interest. It should, however, be realized that the relation between the matching variable and the disease cannot be studied in itself because these OR's are by definition 1.0 as their frequency in cases and controls have become identical. Matching is especially applied when the number of observations is relatively low. Then, one cannot be sure beforehand that analytical control will be possible. Typical matching variables in veterinary epidemiology are: herd, breed, litter, parity and lactational stage.

In the following two situations matching (or analytical control) is required:

→ = causal relation
↕ = non-causal relation
F = factor of interest
M = matching factor (potential confounder)
D = disease

a.

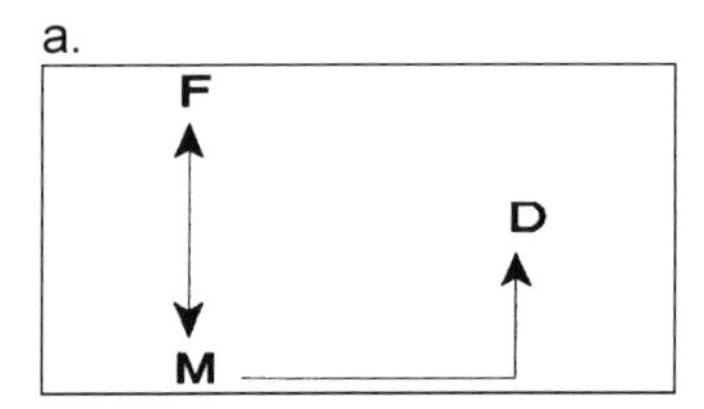

b.

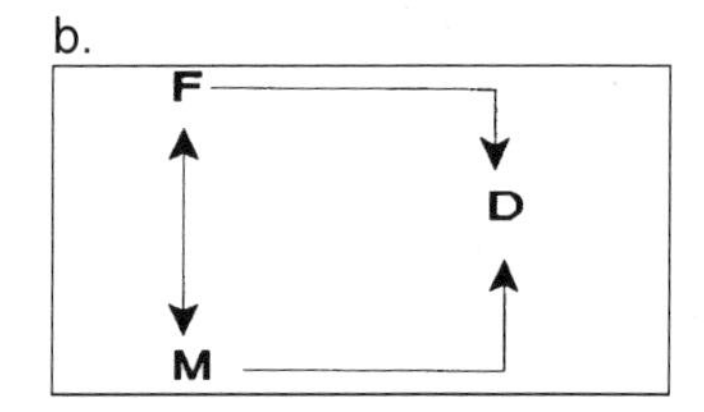

a. Indirect association between exposure to the factor of interest and disease due to the fact that the factor is related to another factor that really is a risk factor. Remember the example of condition (F), parity (M) and milk fever (D) where analytical control was used.

b. F and M are both separate risk factors, but they are also related to each other. For instance, age (F) as well as milk production level (M) are risk factors for mastitis (D). Also age and milk production level are associated indicating that, without matching for level of milk production, the effect of age will be overestimated.

In the next two cases matching is not necessary:

c.

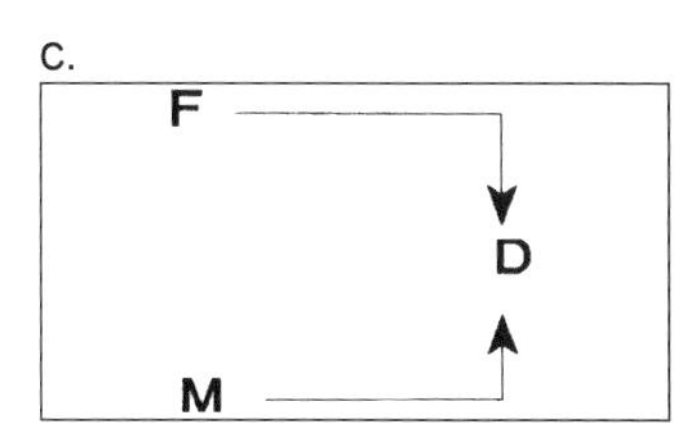

d.

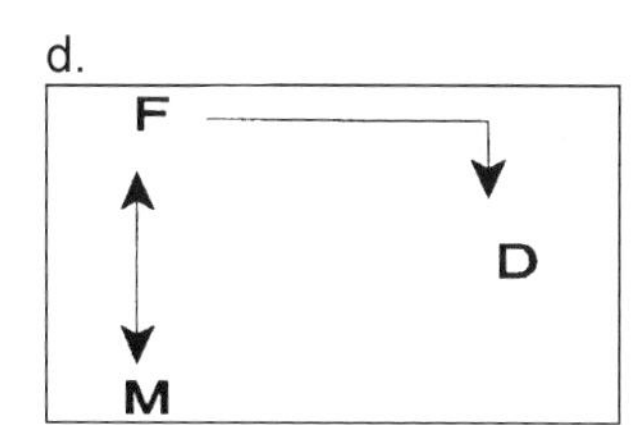

c. F and M are not associated, indicating that the effect of F can be estimated unbiased without matching for M. For instance, in a case-control study into the effect of age and sex on disease X, it is not necessary to match one for the other.

d. Although M is associated with F, it is not a risk factor for D, and there is no need to control for M.

Interaction

Controlling for confounding is necessary to have unbiased estimates for the measure of association. These estimates can be obtained by specific formulae (e.g., Mantel-Haenszel) and, in fact, these formulae calculate one value for the measure of association from 2 (or more) 2x2 tables. Hence, the term 'pooled estimate' is often used. However, there is one important condition determining whether or not this pooling is allowed: the measures should be homogeneously distributed across the 2x2 tables, i.e., there should not be large differences between the stratum-specific measures. If not, it is said that interaction (synonym effect modification) exists or, in other words, that the effect of exposure is different on the several levels of the second factor (the effect is modified by the second factor). Fortunately, interaction can be evaluated statistically. One such statistic is the Breslow-Day statistic, which has a Chi-square distribution. No elaboration will be made on computational details (they are rather lengthy). If this statistic has a 'significant' value (it exceeds 'the' critical value), then interaction is present. The Breslow-Day statistic is illustrated with an hypothetical example concerning culling and mastitis. Note: culling is the 'disease' and mastitis is the 'exposure'!

Parity 1: 25 culled cows from which 5 showed mastitis
42 cows not culled from which 7 showed mastitis
Parity 2: 11 culled cows from which 6 showed mastitis
15 cows not culled from which 4 showed mastitis
Parity 3: 23 culled cows from which 19 showed mastitis
73 cows not culled from which 33 showed mastitis

If parity is disregarded, the OR equals 2.02. Parity-specific ORs are 1.25, 3.30 and 5.76. The Mantel-Haenszel OR equals 3.09. Is confounding present? If you think that the difference between 3.09 and 2.02 is important, then the answer is yes.

Is interaction present? It means: are the parity-specific ORs homogeneous? The Breslow-Day statistic can be calculated as 3.13. As we have 3 strata, the number of degrees of freedom equals 2. In the Chi-square table it can be found that the critical value at the 5% level and 2 *df* equals 5.99. Thus, the parity specific ORs are (statistically) homogeneous and interaction is not significantly present (3.13 is less than 5.99). Below is part of the output of the SAS software package (SAS, 1989).

Estimates of the Common relative risk (Row1/Row2)

Type of Study	Method	Value	95% Confidence Bounds	
Case-Control	Mantel-Haenszel	3.086	1.502	6.340

The confidence bounds for the M-H estimates are test-based.

Breslow-Day Test for Homogeneity of the Odds Ratios

Chi-Square = 3.126 DF = 2 Prob = 0.210

Total Sample Size = 189

Recall that the result of a statistical test heavily depends on the number of observations. Now, if the number of animals in the example above is multiplied by a factor 2 (50 culled cows from which 10 showed mastitis, etc.), recalculation of all ORs gives exactly the same results. However, the Breslow-Day statistic is now 6.25 (this is above 5.99) and it is concluded that interaction is present!

Estimates of the Common Relative Risk (Row1/Row2)

Type of Study	Method	Value	95% Confidence Bounds	
Case-Control	Mantel-Haenszel	3.086	1.502	6.340

The confidence bounds for the M-H estimates are test-based.

Breslow-Day Test for Homogeneity of the odds Ratios

Chi-Square = 6.252 DF = 2 Prob = 0.044

Total Sample Size = 378

Confounding is a bias that should be prevented or removed from the data. However, interaction is a description of a real effect and should therefore be reported. Much emphasis should be put on the (bio)logical interpretation of the interaction. In the example above it is logical that the OR increases with parity because older animals are already more likely to be culled because of their age. If, besides that, a disease (like mastitis) becomes evident, the farmer will be more prone to replace these animals with young, healthy heifers.

3.10. Report the results

The results of a study should be brought to the broader public, (i.e., scientists, policy-makers, farmers, consumers etc). Those who made a significant contribution to the study, (e.g., by filling in a questionnaire or by giving access to the farm to collect data), especially, should be given feed back in order to maintain or increase their willingness to participate in further studies.

References

Brown, L. (1993). The New Shorter Oxford English Dictionary on Historical Principles. 2 vols. Oxford University Press, Oxford.

Dillman, D.A. (1978). Mail and Telephone Surveys: the Total Design Method. John Wiley and Sons, New York.

Greenland, S. (1985). Power, sample size and smallest detectable effect determination for multivariate studies. Statistics in Medicine, 4, 117-127.

Kleinbaum, D.G.; Kupper, L.L; Morgenstern, H. (1982). Epidemiologic Research. Van Nostrand Reinhold Company, New York.

Martin, S.W.; Meek, A.H.; Willeberg, P. (1987). Veterinary Epidemiology: Principles and Methods. Iowa State University Press, Ames, Iowa.

Nurminen, M. (1995). To use or not to use the odds ratio in epidemiologic analyses? European Journal of Epidemiology, 11, 365-371.

Rothman, K.J. (1986). Modern Epidemiology. Little, Brown and Company, Boston/Toronto.

Sahai, H.; Khurshid, A. (1995). Statistics in Epidemiology: Methods, Techniques and Applications. CEC Press, Boca Raton.

SAS Institute Inc. (1989). SAS/STAT® Users Guide. SAS Institute Inc., Cary, NC.

Schlesselman, J.J. (1982). Monographs in Epidemiology and Biostatistics - Volume 3: Case-Control Studies: Design, Conduct, Analysis. Oxford University Press, New York/Oxford.

Thrusfield, M. (1997). Veterinary Epidemiology. Revised 2nd edn. Blackwell Science, Oxford.

4. Exercises

4.1. Coccidiosis

Suppose a case-control study was performed into the effect of lighting regime on the presence of intestinal lesions due to coccidiosis in broilers. In total, data from birds of 208 flocks were obtained. Coccidiosis lesions were found in broilers in 99 flocks. Nearly 50% of the positive (= with lesions) flocks were reared under an intermittent lighting regime, while this figure was 28.4% for the negative flocks.

Calculate the OR and its 95% confidence interval for exposure to intermittent lighting regime. Also calculate the AF and PAF. Give an interpretation of the outcomes in your own words.

4.2. Salmonellosis in poultry

Introduction

Salmonellosis is the disease complex caused by *Salmonella spp.* bacteria. Salmonellosis is a zoonosis, that is, the disease can spread from animals to humans (and *vice versa*). Salmonellosis in poultry has been the subject of investigation for many years. Currently, problems are arising with the great number of more facultatively pathogenic *Salmonella* species, not because of an adverse effect on the technical results of poultry production, but because of the increasing awareness of the hazard to human health. Since the outbreak of *S. enteritidis* in man in the United Kingdom in 1989 the relevance has been increased further. The infection can spread easily and effectively in the production chain and then to food products for man. Various aspects of *Salmnella* infections in poultry have been studied. These include vertical (transovarial) and/or horizontal transmission, effects of feeding, housing, disinfection, colonization-resistance, vaccination, importance of wild birds, rodents, surface water, transportation and cross-contamination in slaughterhouses. However, an integrated and quantitative epidemiological approach to the salmonellosis problem, studying more than one factor simultaneously, has not been made until now. The study described in this section is a quantitative analysis of risk factors for salmonellosis in poultry (in (Great) Grand Parent Stock) by means of a retrospective study. The objective was to determine risk factors by estimating the odds ratio from pre-existing data. However, one must take into account that the initial sampling of data was not done primarily to undertake an epidemiological study with respect to salmonellosis in poultry.

Materials and methods

The study covered a 5-year period (1984-1989). In total, 111 flocks on 32 farms were involved. Flocks were divided into a *Salmonella*-positive or *Salmonella*-negative group, based on bacterial culture and serological typing. A flock was considered positive when there was at least one positive finding. In total, 86 flocks were diagnosed *Salmonella*-positive and 25 as *Salmonella*-negative. Additional information was obtained by means of a questionnaire survey. The procedure of allocation of flocks to a group defines this study as a case-control study. A listing of the major variables with the percentage of exposure among *Salmonella*-positive (case) and *Salmonella*-negative (control) flocks is presented in Table 5.4.

Table 5.4. Listing of the major variables, with percentage of exposure among cases and controls.

Variable	% exposure in cases	% exposure in controls
Feedmill (small *vs.* large)	55.8	16.0
Geographic region (north *vs.* south)	52.3	24.0
Ventilation (natural *vs.* mechanical)	53.5	44.0
Other poultry within 1 km (no *vs.* yes)	43.0	40.0
Other species on farm (no *vs.* yes)	34.9	32.0
Flock size (> 15000 *vs.* ≤ 15000)	36.0	12.0
# Buildings (> 1 *vs.* 1)	66.3	20.0
# Egg collection (1/day *vs.* freq.)	26.2	22.7
Hygiene barriers (poor *vs.* good)	52.4	28.0
Disinfection tub present (no *vs.* yes)	80.0	68.2
Farm type (litter *vs.* battery)	94.2	80.0

Univariate analysis

1a. Calculate with data from the table above, the odds ratios with their 95% confidence interval for the first two variables.

1b. We know that many northern farms obtain their feed from small feedmills. Therefore, confounding might be present. Data on stratification according to feedmill are given below.

Stratum 1: feedmill large

	Region		
	North	South	Total
Case	9	29	38
Control	4	17	21
Total	13	46	59

Stratum 2: feedmill small

	Region		
	North	South	Total
Case	36	12	48
Control	2	2	4
Total	38	14	52

Calculate the OR of the variable region after stratification according to feedmill (use the Mantel-Haenszel technique).

1c. What is your conclusion after answering 1b?

1d. The estimate of the adjusted OR is only valid in a certain situation. What situation?

4.3. Swine enzootic pneumonia (SEP

Reference:
P. Willeberg (1980). The analysis and interpretation of epidemiological data. In: Geering, W.A.; Roe, R.T. and Chapman, L.A. (Editors); Proceedings of the Second International Symposium on Veterinary Epidemiology and Economics, Canberra, Australia, 7-11 May 1979. Australian Government Publishing Service, Canberra; pp. 185-198.

Introduction

In Denmark, pig producers are well organised and supportive of their cooperatively managed slaughterhouses. This has made it possible to introduce a national swine herd health programme to deal with current health problems in the pig population.

Disease problems in intensive swine production are mainly multifactorial. These disorders affect primarily the respiratory and the intestinal tracts. The aim of the national health programme is to minimize the negative effects associated with such multifactorial diseases. These negative effects include economic losses, decreased quality of the products, and increased use of antibiotics with associated expenses and risks of tissue residues.

Use of post-mortem observations obtained by routine meat inspection at the slaughterhouse is considered useful to farm management practices. Health surveillance at the herd level will benefit from an immediate feedback of slaughterhouse information. More detailed information will be available with application of individual animal identification. Then, the health implications of various medications, feeding, genetic constitution, etc. can be evaluated by comparing prevalence values at slaughter among simultaneously raised groups of swine. However, in this case there has to be a complete history of each animal. In the following study, findings at meat inspection were matched with the individual pig's record. The total file contained 4576 pigs. One of the epidemiological analyses concerned the associations between clinical disease (as established on farm and subsequently treated) and swine enzootic pneumonia (SEP) at slaughter (properly speaking: a retrospective cohort). Some of the results are shown in the Table 5.5. Since all clinical cases were treated, it was not possible to evaluate the efficacy of treatment versus no treatment. However, it is possible to compare the results of treatment with 100% successful prevention, e.g., based on a Specified Pathogen Free (SPF) programme.

Exercises

1a. What is the recovery rate of treated pigs?
1b. Supposing that a 100% effective treatment exists, how many animals would have been saved from dying and from chronic SEP lesions?
1c. Supposing that an SPF programme prevents the occurrence of SEP, how many pigs would have been saved from dying and from chronic lesions?
1d. Willeberg claims that the routine diagnostic data are valid, because lesions have been detected in 26.9% of prior clinical cases compared with 7.8% among clinically normal pigs (see Table 5.5). What do you think of this statement?

Table 5.5. Occurrence of swine enzootic pneumonia (SEP) in Denmark.

Disease outcome	CLINICALLY DISEASED			CLINICALLY HEALTHY			TOTAL	
	# cases	% of total # cases	% of all pigs	# cases	% of total # cases	% of all pigs	# cases	% of all pigs
Mortality due to SEP	30	7.5	0.7	33	0.8	0.7	63	1.4
SEP lesions at slaughter	107	26.9	2.3	324	7.8	7.1	431	9.4
No lesions[1]	261	65.6	5.7	3821	91.5	83.5	4082	89.2
Total	398	100.0	8.7	4178	100.0	91.3	4576	100.0

[1] includes slaughtered pigs without SEP as well as pigs dying from other diseases.

Based on slaughterhouse records and findings, problem herds and a series of non-problem herds were identified. They were compared with respect to the presence of causal or disease-enhancing factors. A questionnaire survey was undertaken in the herd. The objective was to determine if certain housing or management factors were associated with a high prevalence of SEP at slaughter. Case herds were defined as having a three-year average SEP rate of 5% or more, control herds were herds with prevalence values lower than 5%. Examples of the data and results are shown in Table 5.6.

Table 5.6. Analysis of determinants of swine enzootic pneumonia in herds from a Danish slaughterhouse.

Variable	Case	Control	OR	95% CI	$OR_{M\text{-}H}$
Herd size					
< 400 pigs slaughtered/yr	49	111	1		-
≥ 400 pigs slaughtered/yr	67	22	6.9	3.8-12.4	-
Mechanical ventilation					
no	25	60	1		1
yes	91	73	3.0	1.7-5.2	1.8
Replacement					
on-farm weaning	12	61	1		1
purchase of weanlings	104	72	7.3	3.7-14.6	5.1
Diarrhoea					
not infectious	56	86	1		1
infectious	60	47	2.0	1.2-3.3	1.5
Freq. of other diseases					
prevalence <3% at slaughter	55	85	1		1
prevalence ≥3% at slaughter	61	48	2.0	1.3-3.3	1.9
Total number of herds	116	133			

2a. How is the OR and the 95% confidence interval of the variables HERD SIZE and VENTILATION calculated? Calculate also the 99% CI.

2b. In Table 5.7, data on the variable VENTILATION, stratified to HERD SIZE, is shown. Calculate the OR for the use of mechanical ventilation adjusted for herd size, and the OR of large herd size adjusted for ventilation with the Mantel-Haenszel technique.

2c. In the last column of Table 5.6, the ORs adjusted for herd size are given. Was it necessary to make these adjustments? Why did the investigators not adjust for the variable VENTILATION? Explain your answer.

Table 5.7. Number of cases and controls with and without mechanical ventilation, stratified to herd size.

Herd size	With ventilation		Without ventilation	
	Case	Control	Case	Control
< 400	30	56	19	55
≥ 400	61	17	6	5

The investigators were not satisfied with the rough division into herds larger than 400 and smaller than 400 pigs so they made a more detailed division. The results are shown in Table 5.8.

Table 5.8. Number of cases and controls in herds with and without mechanical ventilation, stratified to herd size and the results.

INPUT OF DATA (A,B,C,D for each stratum)					
herd size (stratum)	Cases		Controls		EXP=ventilation N.EXP = without ventilation
	EXP (A)	N.EXP (B)	EXP (C)	N.EXP (D)	Total
1 < 200	2	4	7	27	40
2 200 - 300	15	8	30	18	71
3 300 - 400	13	7	19	10	49
4 400 - 500	7	2	5	4	18
5 > 500	54	4	12	1	71
Total	91	25	73	60	249

RESULTS: CRUDE AND ADJUSTED (pooled) ESTIMATES

Desired level of confidence (90, 95, 97.5, 99, 99.5): 95.00
Number of strata: 5

	OR	CI LIMITS Log. approx. Lower	Upper	CI LIMITS Chi-sq. approx Lower	Upper	Chi
Crude	2.99	1.71	5.23	1.73	5.19	3.90
Pooled (direct)	1.26	.66	2.43			
Pooled (Mantel-H)	1.26	.66	2.42	.66	2.42	.70

Breslow-Day test for homogeneity of OR's across strata using MH-OR:

Q (BD) = 1.02 with 4 *df*: see Chi-sq. table for p-value

2d. Show the calculation of the adjusted OR (Mantel-Haenszel) of the variable VENTILATION. Is calculation of a pooled OR allowed?

2e. What is your conclusion, after all your calculations, with respect to ventilation?

Subsequently, all data were analyzed for the different effects that may occur when several determinants are present in varying combinations among the herds. Table 5.9 contains the number of cases and controls with SEP problems among herds which are simultaneously exposed to some of the three factors given in Table 5.6.

Table 5.9. Multiple disease determinants for swine enzootic pneumonia.

	Mechanical ventilation	Purchase of pigs	≥3% of other diseases	No. cases	No. controls
1	no	no	no	1	14
2	no	no	yes	2	11
3	no	yes	no	13	27
4	no	yes	yes	9	8
5	yes	no	no	3	19
6	yes	no	yes	6	17
7	yes	yes	no	38	25
8	yes	yes	yes	44	12

3. How do you calculate a risk for combinations of factors? Show this for the combination of 5 and 8.

5. Answers

5.1. Coccidiosis

The cell frequencies of the 2x2 table should first be calculated:

	Coccidiosis		Total
	Yes	No	
Intermittent	49	31	80
Not intermittent	50	78	128
Total	99	109	208

Nearly 50% of 99 positive flocks (49) are exposed.

Also:

$$OR = \frac{49/31}{50/78} = 2.47$$

Exact interpretation: the odds of exposure (to intermittent lighting regime) is about 2.5 times greater in the coccidiosis positive flocks than in the negative flocks.

Common interpretation: the risk of having a coccidiosis positive flock is 2.5 times greater when an intermittent lighting regime is used compared with a constant lighting regime.

95% CI for the OR:

ln(OR) = 0.90; var (ln (OR)) = 1/49 + 1/31 + 1/50 + 1/78 = 0.09

Z_α = 1.96 and the 95% CI for the ln(OR) is: 0.90 ± 1.96 ∗ √(0.09) = [0.31; 1.49]

The 95% CI for the OR is: [$e^{0.31}$; $e^{1.49}$] = [1.36; 4.44], which means that the true OR is, with probability 0.95, between 1.4 and 4.4. As 1.0 is excluded from this interval, we might say that there is a significant ($P < 0.05$) positive association between intermittent lighting regime and coccidiosis.

Attributable Fraction:

$$AF = \frac{OR - 1}{OR} = \frac{1.47}{2.47} = 0.60$$

Sixty per cent of the exposed cases can be prevented by changing the intermittent lighting regime to a constant lighting regime.

$$PAF = AF * \frac{49}{49 + 50} = 0.29$$

Twenty-nine per cent of all cases can be prevented by changing the intermittent lighting regime to a constant lighting regime.

5.2. Salmonellosis in poultry

1a. The cell frequencies of the 2x2 table should first be calculated.

	Salmonellosis	
	Yes	No
Small feedmill	48	4
Large feedmill	38	21
	86	25

There are 86 positive flocks and 25 negative flocks; 55.8% of the 86 positive flocks obtained feed from a small feedmill (A = 48), while it was 16% of the negative flocks (B = 4).

OR = (48 ∗ 21)/(38 ∗ 4) = 6.6 95% CI = [2.1; 21.0]

For REGION the OR = 3.5 with a 95% CI of [1.3; 9.6]

1b. **Mantel-Haenszel:**

$$OR = \frac{\frac{9 * 17}{59} + \frac{36 * 2}{52}}{\frac{4 * 29}{59} + \frac{2 * 12}{52}} = 1.64$$

1c. We may assess confounding. If it is thought that the difference between 3.5 and 1.6 is large then confounding is defined to be present.

1d. Presenting an adjusted OR is only correct if the odds ratios are homogenous over strata, which means that interaction should not exist.
The stratum specific ORs are 1.3 and 3.0, respectively. Though these 2 ORs differ considerably, the Breslow-Day Chi-square yields 0.44 with 1 *df* and, because this is much lower than the critical value of 3.84 (at $P < 0.05$), this is far from significant ($P = 0.51$). The 0.44 was calculated using computer software. The insignificance is due to the rather small numbers in some cells of the 2x2 tables.

5.3. Swine enzootic pneumonia (SEP)

1a. This question concerns all clinical cases that were treated but that showed no lesions at slaughter. Thus the clinical recovery rate equals: 261/398 = 65.6%

1b. Only clinically diseased pigs will be treated and thus 30 (0.7%) animals would have been saved from dying and 107 (2.3%) from chronic lesions.

1c. If SEP were totally absent, 63 (1.4%) animals would have been saved from dying and 431 (9.4%) from chronic lesions.

1d. The cell frequencies of the 2x2 table are:

	SEP	
	Yes	No
Lesions at slaughter	107	324
No lesions at slaughter	261	3821
	368	4145

From this table the value of KAPPA can be calculated (see Chapter IV), indicating agreement between diagnosis of SEP and findings at slaughter. KAPPA equals 0.19 which indicates a poor agreement.

2a. OR = (67/22) / (49 /111) = 6.9; ln(OR) = 1.93
var(ln(OR) = 1/49 + 1/22 + 1/67 + 1/111 = 0.09

$Z_{(0.05)} = 1.96$;

lower border: $e^{1.93 - 1.96 * \sqrt{(0.09)}} = 3.8$
upper border: $e^{1.93 + 1.96 * \sqrt{(0.09)}} = 12.4$

$Z_{(0.01)} = 2.58$
lower border: $e^{1.93 - 2.58 * \sqrt{(0.09)}} = 3.2$
upper border: $e^{1.93 + 2.58 * \sqrt{(0.09)}} = 14.9$

A similar procedure can be followed for the variable VENTILATION, resulting in the values mentioned in Table 5.6. The 99% CI equals [1.4; 6.2].

2b. Crude OR for VENTILATION equals {(30+61)/(56+17)} / {(19+6)/(55+5)}=3.0

Herd size adjusted OR for VENTILATION:

2x2 table for herds < 400 (≥ 400):

	Case	Control
MV+	30 (61)	56 (17)
MV-	19 (6)	55 (5)

$$OR_{M-H} = \frac{\left(\frac{30 * 55}{160}\right) + \left(\frac{61 * 55}{89}\right)}{\left(\frac{56 * 19}{160}\right) + \left(\frac{6 * 17}{89}\right)} = 1.8$$

Crude OR for HERD SIZE equals {(61+6)/(17+5)} / {(30+19)/(56+55)} = 6.9

VENTILATION adjusted OR for HERD SIZE:

$$OR_{M-H} = \frac{\left(\frac{56 * 61}{164}\right) + \left(\frac{6 * 55}{84}\right)}{\left(\frac{30 * 17}{164}\right) + \left(\frac{19 * 5}{84}\right)} = 5.8$$

2c. If the crude and adjusted ORs differ 'considerably' then there is confounding. Herd size is considered as a potential confounder and indeed some ORs change considerably. The ORs for the other risk factors are unlikely to change much when adjusted for ventilation type. In 2b, a change from 6.9 to 5.8 was calculated.

2d. Use the Mantel-Haenszel formula with 5 strata:

$$OR_{M-H} = \frac{\left(\frac{2 * 27}{40} + \ldots + \frac{54 * 1}{71}\right)}{\left(\frac{4 * 7}{40} + \ldots + \frac{4 * 12}{71}\right)} = 1.3$$

This is insignificant at the 0.05 level because 1.0 is included in the 95% confidence interval (see Table 5.8). This adjusted OR can be used, because the Breslow-Day statistic is (far) less than 9.5, being the critical value of Chi-square with 4 *df* at the 0.05 significance level. Thus, the stratum-specific ORs are assumed to be homogenous.

2e. In first instance, the OR for the use of mechanical ventilation was 3.0 (significantly larger than 1.0). After adjusting for herd size (2 classes), the OR decreased to 1.8, and after a further refinement (5 classes) its value was 1.3. Thus, the effect of type of ventilation is not significantly associated with SEP in this data set.

3. If combination 1 (all variables 'no') is selected as a reference then the OR of mechanical ventilation in the absence of purchase and high levels of other disease is: (3/1) / (19/14) = 2.2
   If all variables have the opposite value of the reference (meaning that piglets are purchased, other diseases are present and ventilation is mechanical), then the OR is:
   (44/1) / (12/14) = 51.3.
   All combinations and their respective relative risks R (the odds ratio approximations) can be put in a Venn diagram (Figure 5.2).

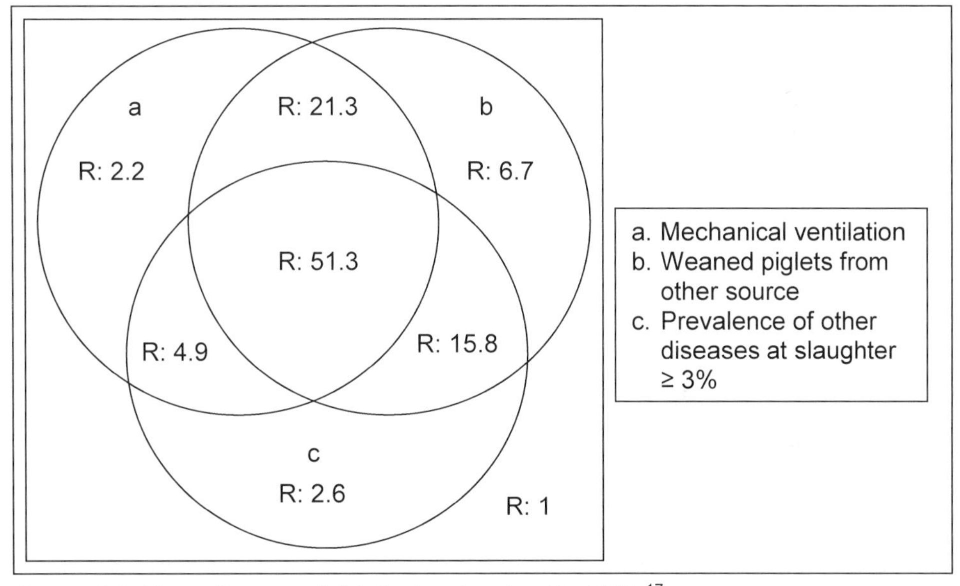

Figure 5.2. Venn diagram of risk factors involved in SEP.[17]

[17] From Willeberg, 1980. 2nd Symposium ISVEE, Canberra, Australia, Commonwealth of Australia Copyright, reproduced by permission.

Chapter VI

Multivariate Analysis: Logistic Regression

K. Frankena
Wageningen University & Research Centre
Department of Animal Sciences
Quantitative Veterinary Epidemiology Group
The Netherlands

E.A.M. Graat
Wageningen University & Research Centre
Department of Animal Sciences
Quantitative Veterinary Epidemiology Group
The Netherlands

1. Introduction

As shown at the end of Chapter V, univariate analyses might not always give the correct risk estimates, due to confounding and/or interaction. In observational studies we generally deal with many potential risk factors and interaction and/or confounding will often be present.

The existence of interaction is evaluated by statistical analysis. The Breslow-Day statistic has been introduced in Chapter V as a measure to indicate whether or not interaction is statistically present.

To account for confounding, 2 approaches are available:

1. use a matched design (if you know beforehand that confounding will occur);
2. correct for it in the statistical analysis.

The principle of matching has been dealt with in Chapter V. A statistical technique that adjusts for confounding (Mantel-Haenszel) has been shown briefly. The Mantel-Haenszel technique is suitable for (even large) data sets with a limited number of factor classes (strata). However, its use is limited when large numbers of 2 by 2 tables need to be interpreted. What about data from a 2-year study in which you want to adjust for the effect of herd (10 herds), breed (6 breeds) and month (24 months) ending up in $10*6*24 = 1440$ strata? Also, how are parameters handled that are measured on a continuous scale (growth, milk production, distances between farms, etc.)?

An attractive alternative is regression using the logistic function. Although other types of functions might be suitable as well, we restrict discussion to the logistic one because:

a. its interpretation is simple as the result equals the logarithm of the *odds ratio*;
b. it is suitable for analyzing data that are collected retrospectively.

If the data include time at risk parameters, Cox proportional hazard regression (survival analysis) might be an attractive alternative (Chapter VII). The principle of logistic regression is quite similar to linear regression. A disadvantage is that primarily odds ratios can be evaluated, while in some studies relative risks are more appropriate, although with additional calculations the cumulative incidence ratio can be obtained.

In this chapter the following will be discussed:

- introduction into the need for logistic regression
- significance testing
- extension to polytomous and continuous predictor variables
- how to check whether or not confounding does occur
- how to check whether interaction is present
- model-building strategy
- goodness-of-fit
- logistic regression on ordinal response variables

Only the most important aspects of logistic regression will be dealt with. A more complete elaboration of logistic regression and related matters easily could cover an entire book (see e.g., 'Applied Logistic Regression' by Hosmer and Lemeshow, 1989). It is intended that the reader will see the necessity of multivariate analysis, will pick up the principle of logistic regression and will be able to read and interpret the output of the logistic calculations. For a better theoretical background the books in the reference list are recommended.

2. Introduction to the Theory of Logistic Regression

The objective of an analysis using logistic regression is the same as that of any analysis using linear regression. First of all, it describes the relationship between an outcome variable (synonyms dependent or response variable) and one or more predictor (synonyms independent or explanatory) variables. Secondly, it tries to find the best estimation in a biologically plausible model, where model stands for a number (1 to n) of predictor variables. The predictor variables are often called covariates. The most common example of modelling is the ordinary linear regression model in which the outcome variable generally is continuous. The difference between logistic regression and linear regression is in the nature of the outcome variables. In logistic regression the outcome variable is binary (e.g., diseased/non diseased, dead/alive).

When the observation period is equal for all experimental units and the outcome is binary, logistic regression is a powerful statistical method for estimating odds ratios with the possibility of controlling for confounding and to estimate effect modification (i.e., interaction). The methods applied in logistic regression follow the same general principles as those used in linear regression.

A linear regression equation is represented by: $E(Y|X) = \beta_0 + \beta_1 * x_1 + ... + \beta_n * x_n$, where X stands for $x_1 ...... x_n$. $E(Y|X)$ is the ***expected*** outcome of an observation given the values of the predictor variables (in statistical language: $E(Y|X)$ is the conditional mean). The β's are the 'weights' that are put on each predictor variable. These β's are estimated by statistical techniques available in statistical software and a subsequent statistical test might be to check whether or not the calculated β's differ 'significantly' from 0. The formula of $E(Y|X)$ indicates that it can take any value when X ranges between $-\infty$ and $+\infty$. However, with binary data, $E(Y|X)$ ranges between 0 and 1, while Y is equal to 0 or 1.

A simple numerical example: you have investigated 200 relatively young cows regarding clinical lameness and recorded also the age of the animal as parity 1 or parity 2. The summarized data set is in the next table.

		PARITY		
		1	2	Total
LAME	yes	10	30	40
	no	65	95	160
	Total	75	125	200

In this case, LAME is the outcome variable (Y) and PARITY the predictor variable (x_1). Using linear regression in STATISTIX[18], the following output will be obtained (x_1 was coded as 0 when PARITY was 1 and x_1 was coded as 1 when parity was 2):

STATISTIX 4.0

UNWEIGHTED LEAST SQUARES LINEAR REGRESSION OF LAME

PREDICTOR VARIABLES	COEFFICIENT	STD ERROR	STUDENT'S T	P
CONSTANT	0.13333	0.04603	2.90	0.0042
PARITY	0.10667	0.05823	1.83	0.0685

R-SQUARED	0.0167	RESID. MEAN SQUARE (MSE)	0.15892
ADJUSTED R-SQUARED	0.0117	STANDARD DEVIATION	0.39865

SOURCE	DF	SS	MS	F	P
REGRESSION	1	0.53333	0.53333	3.36	0.0685
RESIDUAL	198	31.4667	0.15892		
TOTAL	199	32.0000			

CASES INCLUDED 200 MISSING CASES 0

We learn from this that there is a positive association between Y and X (COEFFICIENT for PARITY is positive), that is almost significant at the 0.05 level (*P* = 0.0685). Also, Y increases with 0.107 when x_1 increases with 1 unit.

Thus, $E(Y|x_1=0) = 0.133+0.107*0 = 0.13$ and
$E(Y|x_1=1) = 0.133+0.107*1 = 0.24$

And indeed 10/75 = 0.13 and 30/125 = 0.24. The probability of being lame is higher for animals of parity 2.
Theoretically, $E(Y|X)$ might range from $-\infty$ en $+\infty$, if X varies from $-\infty$ en $+\infty$. E.g., if in the example above x_1 is equal to 10 (of course, this is an extrapolation), then $E(Y|X)$ equals $0.133 + 0.107 * 10 = 1.203$. Thus, the expected probability of an animal being lame when it is of parity 10, has a value larger than 1! However, if this value of x_1 had been in the data set the analysis was applied on, the β's might have had other values and $E(Y|X)$ might have been between 0 and 1. But even without extrapolation seemingly illogical expected outcomes may occur when using linear regression. This problem is definitely not present when logistic regression is used.

To simplify the formulae, $\pi(X)$ will be used instead of $E(Y|X)$, the conditional mean of Y given X. First, some (known) calculation rules which are needed to manipulate expressions used in logistic regression will be addressed.

[18] STATISTIX 4.0, Analytical Software (1992), 1958 Eldridge Avenue, St. Paul MN55113, USA.

1. $\ln(a/b) = \ln a - \ln b$
2. $\ln(a*b) = \ln a + \ln b$
3. $e^{(a+b)} = e^a * e^b$
4. $e^{(a-b)} = e^a / e^b$
5. $e^{-a} = 1/e^a$
6. $e^{\ln a} = a$
7. $\ln(e^a) = a$

Logistic regression uses a log linear model in which the ***risk of developing disease*** is defined as the following function of predictive variables:

Probability of disease:

$$P(Y=1 \mid X) = \pi(X) = \frac{e^{\beta_0 + \beta_1 * x_1}}{1 + e^{\beta_0 + \beta_1 * x_1}} \quad \text{(sigmoid curve)} \mathbf{(6.1)}$$

By dividing numerator and denominator by $e^{\beta 0 + \beta 1 * x1}$ in (1) and then applying rule 5, it follows that:

$$\pi(X) = \frac{1}{1 + e^{-(\beta_0 + \beta_1 * x_1)}} \quad \mathbf{(6.1a)}$$

From expression (6.1a) it can be deduced that if X goes to infinity, $\pi(X)$ goes either to 1 (if β_1 is positive) or to 0 (if β_1 is negative). Also, if X goes to minus infinity, $\pi(X)$ goes either to 0 (if β_1 is positive) or to 1 (if β_1 is negative). In other words: $E(Y \mid X)$ will always be between 0 and 1, which is theoretically correct. In Figure 6.1 this is shown graphically. A continuous variable called TRAIT is at the horizontal axis while the variable EVENT (yes = 1, no = 0) is at the vertical axis. It shows that at the highest values of TRAIT, the EVENT occurs more frequently. Fitting a linear regression to these data gives the straight line in Figure 6.1 (note that the predicted value exceeds 1.0 at the highest levels of TRAIT). The sigmoid curve results from a logistic regression. In a very large data set, there will be many observations at each value of TRAIT. Some of those observations will have an outcome of 1 and others of 0. Thus, for each value of TRAIT, the proportion of observations showing the EVENT can be calculated and this proportion is equal to the probability of having an outcome of 1 given the value of TRAIT. This is shown in Figure 6.2 where TRAIT is categorized into 10 classes in order get a substantial number of observations for each X-value. From this figure we see even better that logistic regression predicts the actual probability better than linear regression and that the logistic prediction is restricted to values between 0 and 1.

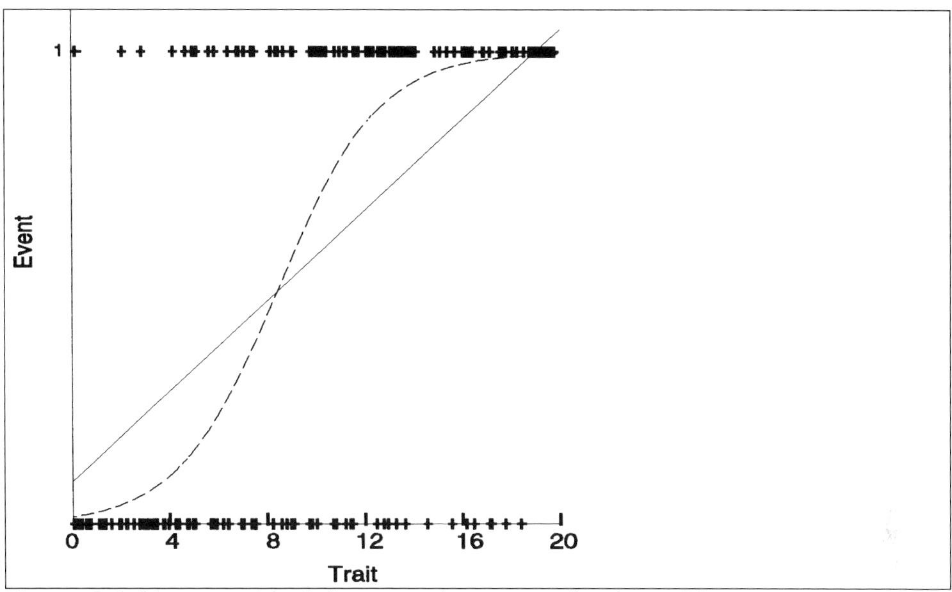

Figure 6.1. Linear and logistic regression curves fitted to a binary outcome variable and a continuous predictor variable.

Based on formula (6.1) the following 2x2 table can be constructed:

OUTCOME VARIABLE		PREDICTOR VARIABLE	
		x_1=1 (exposed)	x_1=0 (non-exposed)
	y=1 (diseased)	$\Pi(1) = \frac{e^{\beta_0 + \beta_1}}{1 + e^{\beta_0 + \beta_1}}$	$\Pi(0) = \frac{e^{\beta_0}}{1 + e^{\beta_0}}$
	y=0 (healthy)	$1 - \Pi(1) = \frac{1}{1 + e^{\beta_0 + \beta_1}}$	$1 - \Pi(0) = \frac{1}{1 + e^{\beta_0}}$

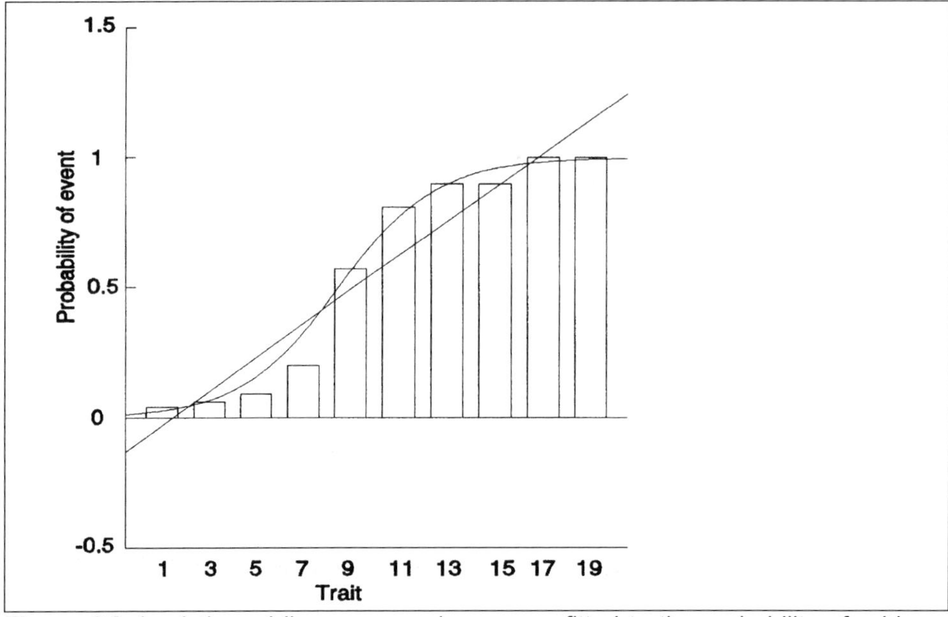

Figure 6.2. Logistic and linear regression curves fitted to the probability of a binary outcome using a categorized predictor variable.

The odds of being diseased among exposed ones (x_1=1) is: $\pi(1)/(1-\pi(1))$

The odds of being diseased among non-exposed ones (x_1=0) is: $\pi(0)/(1-\pi(0))$

The odds ratio is defined as the odds for exposed ones to the odds for non-exposed ones (Chapter V):

$$OR = \frac{\frac{\pi(1)}{1-\pi(1)}}{\frac{\pi(0)}{1-\pi(0)}}$$

Using the expressions from the Table above (and calculation rule 4), the odds ratio is (note that in the odds the denominators cancel out!):

$$OR = \frac{\frac{e^{\beta_0+\beta_1}}{1}}{\frac{e^{\beta_0}}{1}} = e^{\beta_1}$$

Taking the natural log of the odds ratio yields:

$\ln(OR) = \ln(e^{\beta 1}) = \beta_1$, which is the estimate obtained from logistic regression.

Just as in linear regression, β_0 and β_1 are parameters that need to be estimated from the data. It looks rather complicated to solve the β's from formula (6.1), and only in simple cases it can be done by a simple calculation (see Appendix 1). In general, the solution of the β's requires special algorithms. These algorithms are *iterative* and have been implemented in software like SAS, GLIM, GENSTAT, STATA, BMDP, STATISTIX and EGRET. The first step in solving the β's concerns the ***logit transformation*** of $\pi(X)$. This transformation involves the natural log and is central to logistic regression. This transformation is defined, in terms of $\pi(X)$, as:

$$\text{logit}(\pi) = \ln(\frac{\pi}{1-\pi}) = \ln(e^{\beta_0 + \beta_1 * x_1}) = \beta_0 + \beta_1 * x_1 \qquad \text{(linear)}$$

The logit function "links" the probabilities π (expectations of observations Y) to a "linear predictor", $\beta_0 + \beta_1 x_1$. Note that in the ordinary linear regression model the link function is the identity function. Although logit π is a non-linear function of π, its outcome in terms of β_0 en β_1 is linear. The logit can range from $-\infty$ en $+\infty$, depending on the range of explanatory variables in X.

The β's are solved by the software and then OR's are calculated easily by exponentiation (some software packages give β's and OR's). The interpretation of coefficients is similar for both cohort and case-control studies, except for β_0 (see Hosmer and Lemeshow, (1989), page 181). To compute OR's, β_0 is not necessary and so the interpretation of remaining parameters is identical. The estimated coefficient of the predictor variable states the degree of change in the outcome variable per unit of change in the predictor variable. However, if the odds ratio is interpreted as (an estimator of) the cumulative incidence ratio (relative risk) one always should remember that this interpretation is only sound when the event is relatively rare. Hence, at high incidences it is better to model to 'no occurrence'; i.e., if the event did not occur (which then is rare), the outcome variable should have the value 1 and if the event did occur the outcome variable should have the value 0. Another 'escape' is to interpret the odds ratio in its original meaning: the ratio of two odds. One should speak about odds being increased OR-fold due to exposure. Below is the output of the logistic analysis of the lameness example, where β_0 and β_1 are in the column 'COEFFICIENT'.

UNWEIGHTED LOGISTIC REGRESSION OF LAME

PREDICTOR VARIABLES	COEFFICIENT	STD ERROR	COEF/SE	P
CONSTANT	-1.87180	0.33834	-5.52	0.0000
PARITY	0.71912	0.39866	1.80	0.0713
DEVIANCE		196.67		
P-VALUE		0.5133		
DEGREES OF FREEDOM		198		
CASES INCLUDED 200		MISSING CASES 0		

The odds ratio for parity 2 (x_1=1) is $e^{0.72}$ = 2.05. The standard error of β_1 equals 0.40. The 95% confidence interval, based on the Normal approximation, (Z_α = 1.96) for β_1 is 0.72 ± 1.96∗0.40 = [-0.06; 1.50] and thus the 95% confidence interval of the OR equals:

$$e^{0.72 \pm 1.96*0.40} = [e^{-0.06}; e^{1.50}] = [0.94; 4.48]$$

As 1.0 is just not excluded from the interval, it can be concluded that the relation is not significant at the 5% level. We can also read the *P*-value from the output, being 0.07.

Direct calculation of the OR from the 2x2 table shows that the OR equals (30/95)/(10/65) = 2.05 (!). The variance of the ln(OR) is estimated as 1/A+1/B+1/C+1/D (Taylor series - see Chapter V). The standard error in this particular case is √(1/30+1/65+1/10+1/95) = 0.40, identical to the standard error of β for PARITY.

As mentioned before $E(Y = 1|x_1 = 1) = \pi(1)$ equals $1/[1+e^{-(\beta 0+\beta 1*1)}]$ and $E(Y=1|x_1=0)=\pi(0)$ equals $1/[1+e^{-(\beta 0 + \beta 1*0)}]$. Knowing β_0 and β_1 from the output above, one can calculate these probabilities as being:

$$\pi(1) = 1/(1+e^{-(-1.8718+0.7191*1)}) = 0.24$$
$$\pi(0) = 1/(1+e^{-(-1.8718+0.7191*0)}) = 0.13$$

Thus, the E(Y|X) is identical if we compare linear (see page 141) and logistic regression! Also, the test of significance of the coefficient yields about the same result.

So, why the need of logistic regression instead of linear regression? First of all, the theoretical range of E(Y|X) in ordinary linear regression is from -∞ to +∞, while in real life it is a probability if the outcome is binary. Secondly, one of the assumptions underlying the estimation method used in linear regression is violated. This assumption concerns a Normal distribution N(0,σ) of the residuals (errors). The residuals result from the discrepancy between the actual value of the outcome (y) and its expected value (E(Y|X).

In formula: $y = E(Y|X) + e$, or equivalently: $e = y-E(Y|X)$

The residual e is the difference between the observed and the predicted value of y. In linear regression, e should follow a Normal distribution with mean 0 and a variance that is constant at all levels of the predictor variable. This is not true in case of a binary outcome variable. Then, y = π(X) + e and e can have at most 2 values. If y = 1 then e = 1-π(X) and if y = 0 then e = -π(X). Thus, the distribution of the error follows a Binomial distribution. In particular, this implies that var(e) = var(y) = π(1-π) which depends on X through π and thus this variance is not constant. Standard software for logistic regression is based on the Binomial distribution and takes differences between variances into account.

Other link functions than the logistic link are capable of handling Binomially distributed data in an appropriate way. General preference for the logistic function arises from the fact that it gives a meaningful parameter (the odds ratio) and that it is an easily used function.

In summary, logistic regression analysis with a binary outcome variable employs:

1. a (conditional) mean of the regression equation between 0 and 1;
2. a Binomial distribution of the errors, not a Normal distribution;
3. a linear combination of explanatory x-variables, e.g. $\beta_0 + \beta_1 x_1$ for the logit of the (conditional) means.

3. Significance Testing

After the coefficients have been estimated, one wants to know whether or not the predictor variables are significantly associated with the outcome variable. Equivalently one could ask whether or not the inclusion of the predictor variable improves the model (and thus the prediction) significantly. A comparison of observed values of the outcome variable to predicted values obtained from logistic regression models with and without the predictor variable, can be made with the **log likelihood function**. To clarify the use of the likelihood a bit, assume that a full model (e.g., a regression line through two data points) exists. For the current model which will generally be more parsimonious than the full model, the deviance D is defined as:

$$D = -2\ln\left[\frac{\text{likelihood current model}}{\text{likelihood full model}}\right]$$

May be you are wondering why D is defined in such a complicated way by referring to a full model. This is because the full model corresponds to the maximal achievable likelihood. It offers a baseline for measuring the goodness of fit of the current model when binary data are grouped and entered into the analysis as counts y out of total n (see paragraph 8). The quantity inside [ ] is the ***likelihood ratio***. The use of -2ln (likelihood ratio) follows from statistical theory about hypothesis testing. For assessment of the significance of a predictor variable, two values of D need to be obtained: one for the model with and one for the model without the predictor variable. The change in D (deviance difference) due to including the predictor variable in the model is calculated as:

$$G = D\ (\text{model without } x_1) - D\ (\text{model with } x_1)$$

Since the likelihood of the parsimonious model appears in both values of D, it cancels out and G can also be computed as:

$$G = -2\ [(\text{log likelihood without } x_1) - (\text{log likelihood with } x_1)]$$

Calculation of the likelihood, the log likelihood and/or the -2 log likelihood ratio test are standard features in the majority of statistical packages.

If the predictor variable is dichotomous or continuous, the significance of a variable can also be derived from its regression coefficient and its standard error (se), by use of an approximation with the Normal distribution. A confidence interval is calculated and a check is made whether 0 is in the interval. Such an interval is given by:

$$\beta \pm Z_\alpha * se(\beta)$$

When the lower limit limit of this interval is larger than 0:

$$\beta - Z_\alpha * se(\beta) > 0 \text{ or } \beta > Z_\alpha * se(\beta),$$

we conclude that β differs significantly from 0 and is valued positively.

When the upper limit of this interval is below 0:

$$\beta + Z_\alpha * se(\beta) < 0 \text{ or } \beta < -Z_\alpha * se(\beta),$$

β differs significantly from 0 and is valued negatively.

Squaring both equations, yields:

$$\beta^2 > Z_\alpha{}^2 * se(\beta)^2$$

which is equivalent to:

$$W > Z_\alpha{}^2$$

where W is the Wald statistic (or Wald Chi-square):

$$W = \left[\frac{\beta}{se(\beta)} \right]^2$$

For $P < 0.05$, Z_α at 1 degree of freedom (*df*) = 1.96 and thus W should exceed 1.96^2 = 3.84 to have a significant regression coefficient. However, various studies suggest that the likelihood ratio test may be more powerful then the Wald test (Hosmer and Lemeshow, 1989). As an example of the Wald statistic (W) and the deviance difference (G), we present the SAS output of an analysis of the factor AGEGROUP and RED DISCOLORATION (RD). See Appendix 2a, b and c for more information.

variable	coefficient	stand. error	Wald
constant(β_0)	-1.1688	0.0993	138.6097
AGEGROUP(β_1)	1.1431	0.1275	80.3335
Model	-2 log likelihood	G	
Intercept only	1564.416		
Intercept+AGEGROUP	1479.450	84.966 with 1 df (p = 0.0001)	

The β_1 indicates that the risk of showing RD is $e^{1.1431}$ = 3.1-fold increased when x_1 = 1 (is AGEGROUP = 1). The Wald statistic equals 80.335 which shows a probability of less than 0.0001. The Chi-square for G is somewhat larger than the one for the Wald.

4. Extension to Polytomous and Continuous Predictor Variables

In paragraph 2 and 3 of this chapter, predictor variables that had only 2 classes were discussed. In logistic regression it is also possible to handle predictor variables that have more than two classes (polytomous) or that are continuous. We will first discuss polytomous predictor variables.

Suppose, a predictor variable has more than two categories (k>2). Then, a set of (k-1) ***dummy variables*** (or design variables) needs to be created. The choice of a particular method to create dummy variables (reference cell coding or mean coding) depends to some extent on the goals of the analysis. The next table shows hypothetical data for 360 individuals and a predictor variable with 4 classes:

	Age class 1	2	3	4
diseased	20	40	60	80
healthy	40	40	40	40
total	60	80	100	120
OR	1.0	2.0	3.0	4.0
95% CI		[1.0; 4.0]	[1.5; 5.9]	[2.1; 7.7]
β = ln(OR)	0.0	0.69	1.10	1.39

In the table above, the odds ratio is calculated for each category in the situation with age class 1 as a ***reference***. Thus, the OR of 2.0 results from (40/40) / (20/40) = 1600/800.

The same estimates of the odds ratios are obtained from a logistic regression with an appropriate choice of dummy variables. The method for specifying the dummy variables, arbitrarily (but logical) named D2 to D4, is shown below.

	dummy variable		
class	D2	D3	D4
1	0	0	0
2	1	0	0
3	0	1	0
4	0	0	1

For age class 1, the reference group, all the dummies have the value 0. For the other classes one and only one of the dummies has value 1. This method is called "reference cell coding" or "corner stone condition". These 3 dummy variables fully specify all 4 classes. That is also the reason that in case of a dichotomous variable no dummy variables need to be created. The dichotomous variable already specifies both classes e.g., coded as 0 and 1. Logistic regression on these coded variables yields the following results:

Analysis of Maximum Likelihood Estimates				
Variable	Parameter Estimate	Standard Error	Wald Chi-Square	PR > Chi-Square
INTERCPT	β_0 = -0.6931	0.2739	6.4061	0.0114
D2	β_{12} = 0.6931	0.3536	3.8437	0.0499
D3	β_{13} = 1.0986	0.3416	10.3454	0.0013
D4	β_{14} = 1.3863	0.3354	17.0831	0.0001

The β's, and thus the odds ratios, are identical to the ones calculated before. Comparison of classes cna be made using the logit difference. For example, comparison of age class 2 to class 1 is as follows:

$$\ln[OR(\text{class } 2, \text{class } 1) = \text{logit}(\text{class } 2) - \text{logit}(\text{class } 1) =$$
$$[\beta_0 + \beta_{12}*1 + \beta_{13}*0 + \beta_{14}*0] - [\beta_0 + \beta_{12}*0 + \beta_{13}*0 + \beta_{14}*0] = \beta_{12} = 0.6931$$

Confidence intervals are obtained in a way similar to binary predictor variables. Also the deviance difference (G, the -2log likelihood of the model without the variable minus the -2log likelihood of the model with the variable) can be calculated:

Model	- 2 log likelihood	G
Intercept only	494.612	
Intercept + dummies	474.651	19.961 with 3 df (P=0.0002)

Note that the G statistic now has 3 degrees of freedom. The model with the 3 dummies fits significantly better than the model without the dummy variables (P = 0.0002). In case of a polytomous predictor variable one cannot conclude anything about the significance of the specific β's using the G statistic, for that purpose we need to rely on the Wald statistic. This statistic shows that class 2 to 4 all significantly differ from class 1. **Be aware**: none of the dummy variables might be significant while the G is significant. In this case you probably have chosen a reference class which has an intermediate risk compared to the other classes (some dummies have negative β's other positive β's, none of them being significantly differing from 0, while the most negative β's and the most positive ones might differ significantly from each other!). In general, one can state that if the G statistic is significant, at least two classes differ significantly, although this might not be deduced from the Wald statistics directly, due to the choice of the reference category.

Whether or not class 4 differs significantly from class 2, cannot be deduced from the output directly, although we see that this specific OR will be 2.0 (using class 1 as reference, the OR for class 4 is **twice** the OR for class 2). In order to calculate the standard error of this ln(OR), we need to have the variance/covariance matrix. Another way is to run the model for a second time, re-specifying the dummies in such a way that class 2 is now the reference.

The ln(OR) of class 4 (D4) versus class 2 (D2) equals:

$\beta_{14} - \beta_{12} = 1.3863\text{-}0.6931 = 0.6932$ and the OR equals: $e^{0.6932} = 2.0$.

The covariance matrix yields:

Variable	INTERCPT	D2	D3	D4
INTERCPT	0.075	-0.075	-0.075	-0.075
D2	-0.075	0.125	0.075	0.075
D3	-0.075	0.075	0.117	0.075
D4	-0.075	0.075	0.075	0.1125

The variances of the estimated beta's are on the diagonal. Covariances are off-diagonal elements, e.g., $cov(\beta_{12},\beta_{14}) = 0.075$. Now, the variance of the ln(OR) of class 4 (D4) versus class 2 (D2) equals:

$$var(\beta_{14} - \beta_{12}) = var(\beta_{12}) + var(\beta_{14}) - 2cov(\beta_{12},\beta_{14}) = (0.125 + 0.1125 - 2*0.075) = 0.0875.$$

Then, the standard error of the ln(OR) is $\sqrt{(0.0875)} = 0.2958$

Based on the β and its standard error we calculate the 95% confidence interval of the OR as $[e^{0.69 \pm 1.96*0.30}] = [1.1; 3.6]$. As 1.0 is not included in this interval, the association is significant at the 0.05 level.

The second run of the model, re-specifying class 2 as reference, shows the following output (D1=1 if class is 1, D3=1 if class is 3 and D4=1 if class is 4):

Model		- 2 log likelihood	G	
Intercept only		494.612		
Intercept + dummies		474.651	19.961 with 3 df (P=0.0002)	

Variable	Parameter Estimate	Standard Error	Wald Chi-Square	PR > Chi-Square
INTERCPT	2.95E-16	0.2236	0.0000	1.0000
D1	-0.6931	0.3536	3.8437	0.0499
D3	0.4055	0.3028	1.7935	0.1805
D4	0.6931	0.2958	5.4909	0.0191

Indeed, $e^{0.6931}$ = 2.0 and the standard error equals 0.2958. Note also that the -2 log likelihood has not changed!

In Appendix 2b, the polytomous situation is adapted to the RD example, using 10 classes (30 day intervals) for age where the eldest group is taken as reference.

When the predictor variable is continuous, the regression coefficient indicates the change in the log odds for an increase of one unit in the predictor variable. Predictor variables that are typically continuous are weight, growth, milk production, age, etc. Returning to our RD example, we might include AGE as a continuous variable into our model. Appendix 2c then gives the output. As age is measured in days, the β_1 tells us that the risk of showing RD increases with $e^{0.00825}$ ***per day***. As it is not really realistic to calculate this figure per day, one might multiply it by, for example, 28 to get the increase per 4 weeks (also the standard errors should be multiplied by 28 then, all other parameters remain the same), which equals 1.26. As the data cover an age range of about 300 days, the highest OR that can be calculated is $e^{300*0.00825}$ = 11.9. Thus, animals of one year old have an 11.9 times higher probability of having RD than animals that are 10 weeks old. Although the β_1 is very small (due to the time unit of only one day), it is very significant. The Wald statistic equals 98.766, having a probability of less than 0.0001. It is advised to run the analyses with variables already in the proper units, because a too small unit might result in very small coefficients, printed by the software for example as 0.0000. Then, multiplication to get the estimate for the desired larger units is useless.

To treat a predictor variable as continuous, the assumption that the logits are linear needs to be fulfilled. Robustly, this can be done by breaking the range of the predictor variable into groups, creating dummy variables, performing the logistic regression analysis using the lowest group as a reference and plotting the midpoint of the group (x-axis) versus the respective regression coefficients (the β of the reference group being 0). From such a plot the most logical shape (linear, quadratic, binary) can be derived. This robust eye-ball method is accurate enough for most applications (Hosmer and Lemeshow, 1989).

Returning to the RD example, one can deduce linearity from the output in Appendix 2b, because there, AGE was treated as a polytomous variable (10 groups), using the youngest group as a reference. Plotting the β's against age group results in Figure 6.3. It looks good enough to treat AGE as linear. A higher order term (e.g., quadratic)

for the explanatory variable aspect is in paragraph 8 of this Chapter.can also be included and a subsequent test might be whether the log likelihood ratio test indicates a significantly better fit. A more thorough elaboration on this

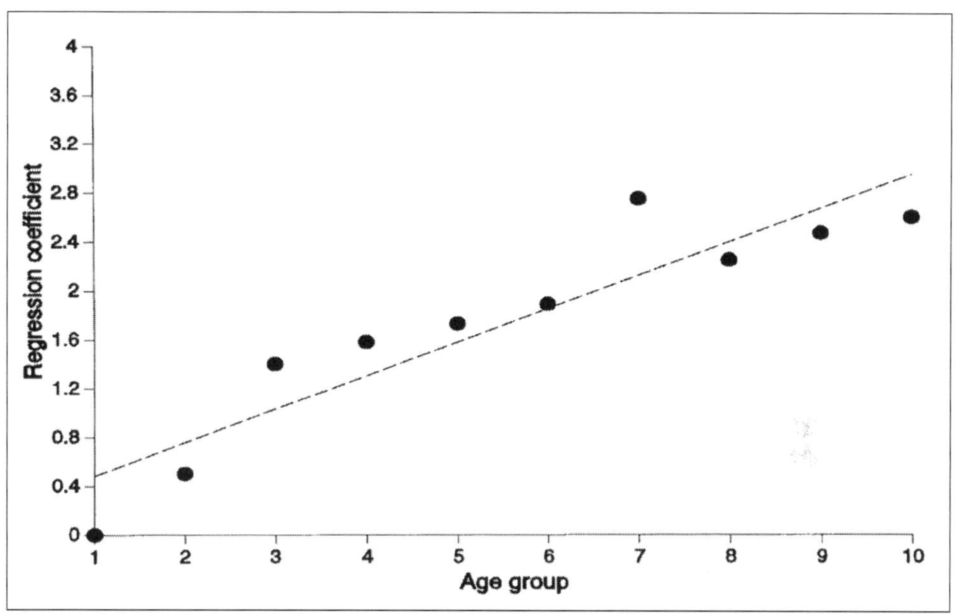

Figure 6.3. Logistic regression coefficients for each age group, using group 1 as reference group ($\beta = 0$).

5. Confounding

As mentioned in Chapter V, to be a confounder a parameter has to meet 3 conditions:

1. it is related to the outcome variable;
2. it is related to the exposure (predictor) variable;
3. it is not an intermediate step in the causal path between the exposure and the disease.

Now let us return to the milk fever/condition/parity example of Chapter V. Parity was related to milk fever, older cows having an increased risk of milk fever. Parity was also related to condition, older cows being in better condition than younger ones, and, thirdly, being of higher parity is not a pre-requisite to get milk fever.

The crude OR for condition was 1.89, while the parity-adjusted OR equalled 1.0. The same results can be obtained with logistic regression. For that purpose, two models needed to be evaluated. The first is a univariate model with condition as predictor variable and the second is a multivariate model containing condition and parity as predictors. The output is shown on the next page:

MODEL: MF = CONDITION

UNWEIGHTED LOGISTIC REGRESSION OF MF

PREDICTOR VARIABLES	COEFFICIENT	STD ERROR	COEF/SE	P
CONSTANT	-1.73460	0.19800	-8.76	0.0000
CONDITION	0.63599	0.25656	2.48	0.0132

DEVIANCE 394.02
P-VALUE 0.5470
DEGREES OF FREEDOM 398

CASES INCLUDED 400 MISSING CASES 0

MODEL: MF = PARITY+ CONDITION

UNWEIGHTED LOGISTIC REGRESSION OF MF

PREDICTOR VARIABLES	COEFFICIENT	STD ERROR	COEF/SE	P
CONSTANT	-2.19702	0.24510	-8.96	0.0000
PARITY	1.34972	0.31687	4.26	0.0000
CONDITION	1.458E-14	0.29718	0.00	1.0000

DEVIANCE 394.02
P-VALUE 0.5470
DEGREES OF FREEDOM 397

CASES INCLUDED 400 MISSING CASES 0

Exponentiation of the coefficient of CONDITION in the univariate model results in an OR of 1.89, while it approaches 1 (e^0 as 1.458E-14 is a short notation for $1.458 * 10^{-14}$) in the second model, including PARITY.

When comparing results of model 1 to the results of model 2 in order to check for confounding, it might be that estimates of the variable(s) change (as in the example above). Also standard error(s) might change and in consequence of this, the Wald statistic. How large changes in estimates must be for a variable to be defined as a confounding variable, is a decision made by the investigator. It is also important whether this change is defined in a relative or in an absolute sense. For example, a β of 0.03 that changes to 0.01 has a large relative change (67%) but a very small absolute change (0.02). Therefore, a combination might be chosen as well, say to be defined as a confounder, the relative change must be equal to at least 25% when the β is larger than 0.40 (or smaller than -0.40) and at least 0.1 absolute if it is between -0.40 and 0.40. Thus in the example above, PARITY should be considered as a confounder for CONDITION as the regression coefficient of the latter changes from 0.64 to 0.00.

If it is known (from literature or other studies) that some parameters (like age or breed) are confounding variables for other predictor variables, it might be decided to force those variables in the model, even if they are not confounders in the particular data set.

In practice: when adding/removing a variable to/from a model induces an 'important' difference in the estimate of the predictor variable of interest, then the added/removed variable should stay in the model, even if the variable itself does not show a significant association with the disease in the multivariate model.

6. Presence of Interaction and its Consequences

In this paragraph, it will be described how to account for interaction using the logistic regression model. Interaction can take many different forms. We begin by describing the situation when it is absent. For example, the model with a binary exposure variable (factor present/absent) and a second binary coded covariate. If the association between the exposure factor and the outcome variable is the same within each level of the covariate, then there is no interaction between the covariate and the exposure factor. Graphically, the absence of interaction yields a model with parallel lines (using the logistic scale), one for each level of the risk factor variable. When interaction is present, the association between the exposure factor and the outcome variable differs between, or depends in some way on, the level of the covariate. That is, the covariate modifies the effect of the risk factor. Epidemiologists often use the term ***effect modifier*** to describe a variable that interacts with an exposure factor.

A significance test, indicating whether or not the interaction is statistically significant, is based on the likelihood ratio test. The difference in deviance (G) between a model without the interaction terms and a model with these terms, follows a Chi-square distribution. The outcome of G will be almost identical to the Breslow-Day statistic that was mentioned in Chapter V, paragraph 3.9. This will be shown in the example at the end of this paragraph.

If effect modification exists, one needs to present several odds ratios for the exposure factor, namely an OR for each level of the covariate, or, if the covariate is continuous, one might calculate several odds ratios at specific levels of that covariate (e.g., if the covariate is milk production per lactation, one can show the OR for the exposure factor at 6,000 kg, at 8,000 kg and 10,000 kg). To calculate the odds ratio in presence of interaction, consider a model including a binary (0,1 coded) exposure factor F, a binary (also 0,1 coded) covariate X and their interaction is then defined as $F*X$. The latter has a value of 0 if F or X (or both) has a value of 0 and it has a value of 1 if both F and X have the value 1.

Thus, if X = 0 then the OR for F equals $e^{\beta(F)}$ and if X = 1, this OR will be $e^{\beta(F) + \beta(X)}$.

In a formal way this is shown by the logit formula:

$$g(F,X) = \beta_0 + \beta_1 F + \beta_2 X + \beta_3 FX$$

If X = 0:

$$g(F{=}1,X{=}0) = \beta_0 + \beta_1*1 + \beta_2*0 + \beta_3*1*0 = \beta_0 + \beta_1$$
$$g(F{=}0,X{=}0) = \beta_0 + \beta_1*0 + \beta_2*0 + \beta_3*0*0 = \beta_0$$

Then the log-odds equals g(F=1,X=0) - g(F=0,X=0) = β_1, and the OR is e^{β_1}.

If X = 1:

$$g(F{=}1,X{=}1) = \beta_0 + \beta_1*1 + \beta_2*1 + \beta_3*1*1 = \beta_0 + \beta_1 + \beta_2 + \beta_3$$
$$g(F{=}0,X{=}1) = \beta_0 + \beta_1*0 + \beta_2*1 + \beta_3*0*1 = \beta_0 + \beta_2$$

The log-odds equals g(F=1, X=1) - g(F=0, X=1) = $\beta_1 + \beta_3$ and the OR is $e^{\beta_1+\beta_3}$. To calculate a confidence interval for this OR, one needs the standard error of the ln(OR). The variance of $\beta_1 + \beta_3$ = var(β_1) + var(β_3) + 2 cov(β_1,β_3) and the standard error is the square root of the variance. Note that the variance / covariance matrix is needed to obtain the covariances. In general the variance is calculated as:

$$\text{var}\,[\ln(OR)] = (\delta F)^2*\text{var}(\beta_1) + (\delta F*X)^2*\text{var}(\beta_3) + 2*X*(\delta F)^2*\text{cov}(\beta_1,\beta_3),$$

where δF represents the difference in exposure level and x the value of the covariate. It is advised to use 0,1 coding whenever possible because this simplifies the calculation, while the OR and its variance are not affected.

Let us return to the example in Chapter V, concerning a binary exposure factor (mastitis) in relation to culling (yes/no) adjusting for the covariate parity having 3 levels. In logistic regression, one needs to create two dummies for the covariate: e.g., D2 and D3, assuming that parity 1 is the reference. This also implies that there are 2 interaction terms:

INT2 = D2*MASTITIS and INT3 = D3*MASTITIS

The output of the model without interaction:

MODEL: CULLING = MASTITIS + PARITY

UNWEIGHTED LOGISTIC REGRESSION OF MF

PREDICTOR VARIABLES	COEFFICIENT	STD ERROR	COEF/SE	P
CONSTANT	-0.73198	0.26825	-2.73	0.0064
MASTITIS	1.11600	0.36919	3.02	0.0025
D2	-0.02447	0.49273	-0.05	0.9604
D3	-1.10856	0.40026	-2.77	0.0056

DEVIANCE	219.97
P-VALUE	0.0401
DEGREES OF FREEDOM	185

CASES INCLUDED 189 MISSING CASES 0

The output of the model with interaction:

MODEL: CULLING = MASTITIS + PARITY + MASTITIS*PARITY

UNWEIGHTED LOGISTIC REGRESSION OF MF

PREDICTOR VARIABLES	COEFFICIENT	STD ERROR	COEF/SE	P
CONSTANT	-0.55962	0.28031	-2.00	0.0459
MASTITIS	0.22314	0.64918	0.34	0.7310
D2	-0.22884	0.60785	-0.38	0.7066
D3	-1.74297	0.59452	-2.93	0.0034
INT2	0.97078	1.06255	0.91	0.3609
INT3	1.52737	0.88275	1.73	0.0836

DEVIANCE	216.82
P-VALUE	0.0442
DEGREES OF FREEDOM	183

CASES INCLUDED 189 MISSING CASES 0

From this output it is concluded that:

1. The interaction does not significantly contribute to the model, because the G statistic equals 219.97 - 216.82 = 3.13 with 2 *df* (the critical value being 5.99). Thus the 3 odds ratios, being 1.25, 3.30 and 5.76, might be considered as homogeneous. However, it should also be noticed that the cell frequencies show low numbers and that the power of this analysis is low.
2. MASTITIS is significantly related to the disease, the OR being $e^{1.12}$ = 3.06 (assuming that the investigator decides that the PARITY indeed is a confounder).

Note that the deviance difference is almost identical to the value of the Breslow-Day statistic as calculated in Chapter V. In Chapter V we also showed an analysis in which the numbers were doubled. Doing the same using logistic regression, it shows (see output below) that the deviance difference equals 439.95 - 433.64 = 6.31 which is larger than the 0.05 critical value of 5.99 (derived from the Chi-square distribution at 2 *df*). Now we have to conclude that the 3 odds ratios of 1.25, 3.30 and 5.76 are not homogeneous. Remember that significance highly depends on numbers! Of course, we should not conclude from the first analysis that interaction does not exist, but that the data was too sparse to make definite conclusions about it. Note again that the deviance difference and the Breslow-Day statistic (6.25) are similar.

MODEL: CULLING = MASTITIS + PARITY

UNWEIGHTED LOGISTIC REGRESSION OF MF

PREDICTOR VARIABLES	COEFFICIENT	STD ERROR	COEF/SE	P
CONSTANT	-0.73198	0.18968	-3.86	0.0001
MASTITIS	1.11600	0.26106	4.27	0.0000
D2	-0.02447	0.34841	-0.07	0.9440
D3	-1.10856	0.28302	-3.92	0.0001

DEVIANCE 439.95
P-VALUE 0.0105
DEGREES OF FREEDOM 374

CASES INCLUDED 378 MISSING CASES 0

MODEL: CULLING = MASTITIS + PARITY + MASTITIS*PARITY

UNWEIGHTED LOGISTIC REGRESSION OF MF

PREDICTOR VARIABLES	COEFFICIENT	STD ERROR	COEF/SE	P
CONSTANT	-0.55962	0.19816	-2.82	0.0047
MASTITIS	0.22314	0.45900	0.49	0.6269
D2	-0.22884	0.42959	-0.53	0.5942
D3	-1.74247	0.41578	-4.19	0.0000
INT2	0.97078	0.75118	1.29	0.1962
INT3	1.52687	0.62108	2.46	0.0140

DEVIANCE 433.64
P-VALUE 0.0150
DEGREES OF FREEDOM 372

CASES INCLUDED 378 MISSING CASES 0

VARIANCE-COVARIANCE MATRIX FOR COEFFICIENTS

	CONSTANT	MASTITIS	D2	D3	INT2	INT3
CONSTANT	0.03929					
MASTITIS	-0.03927	0.21068				
D2	-0.03927	0.03927	0.18455			
D3	-0.03927	0.03927	0.03927	0.17287		
INT2	0.03927	-0.21068	-0.18455	-0.03927	0.56427	
INT3	0.03927	-0.21068	-0.03927	-0.17287	0.21068	0.38574

As interaction is now significant, 3 OR's should be calculated for MASTITIS, one for each level of the covariate. These are the parity-specific OR's and these need to be presented because PARITY significantly modifies the effect of MASTITIS on culling.

The OR's can be calculated directly from the parameter estimates and for the respective confidence intervals we need the variance\covariance matrix.

Parity	OR	variance of ln(OR)	95% CI OR
1	$e^{0.22} = 1.25$	0.21 = 0.21	$e^{0.22\pm1.96*\sqrt{0.21}}$ = [0.5; 3.1]
2	$e^{0.22+0.97} = 3.29$	0.21+0.56+2∗(-0.21) = 0.35	$e^{1.19\pm1.96*\sqrt{0.35}}$ = [1.0; 10.5]
3	$e^{0.22+1.53} = 5.75$	0.21+0.39+2∗(-0.21) = 0.18	$e^{1.75\pm1.96*\sqrt{0.18}}$ = [2.5; 13.2]

Note: in the output of the single data set and the double data set, the β's are identical. However, the variances in the second analysis have been reduced by a magnitude of 2 and thus the standard errors by a magnitude of $\sqrt{2}$.

When many exposure variables are potentially present, many interactions (also three-way and higher order interactions) might exist. It is tempting to screen all interaction terms on significance and this in fact guarantees that you will find some significant interactions: due to random error, 1 out of 20 interaction terms tested will be significant if 0.05 is used as threshold *P*-value. Moreover, what is the use of interactions you cannot explain in a biological perspective? Therefore, only biologically meaningful interactions should be tested (although this depends on (your) current knowledge of the biology of the disease).

7. Model Building Strategy

An ideal situation is to start the analysis with a full model containing all predictor variables and subsequently use a careful backward deletion procedure. However, in observational studies many potential risk factors and confounders might be screened. This might lead to problems during the analysis because too many information has been collected in relation to the number of observations. Then, one should attempt to reduce the number of variables before performing a multivariate analysis or to create summary variables and use those in the analysis (like in factor analysis). Hosmer and Lemeshow (1989) proposed a 4 step procedure in variable selection for a logistic regression model.

1. The analysis procedure should start with a univariate analysis of each predictor variable and potential confounder, preferentially using 2x2 tables (this will give you more 'feeling' with the data than using logistic regression in which you will not see any cell frequency). If a polytomous predictor variable is analyzed, all the design variables should be in the model! Special attention should be paid to erroneous looking odds ratios or confidence intervals (or regression coefficients and standard errors). This might indicate that there is at least one cell with a zero frequency. This will result in an OR of zero or infinity. Including such a variable in the logistic regression model will yield undesirable outcomes. It is best to recode such a zero cell by joining categories of the predictor variable in such a way that the zero cell disappears. Another way of accounting for this problem is to add 0.5 to each cell. All variables showing a *P*-value less than 0.25 (arbitrary threshold!) are selected for the next step. A disadvantage of the univariate analysis is that a set of variables, of which each is weakly associated with the outcome, can become important predictors when they are taken together. To prevent this, one should choose a significance level that is relatively safe (e.g., $P < 0.25$).

2. All selected variables and potential confounders from step 1 should be put together in one logistic model. This is only possible if the number of observations (sample size) is large enough when compared to the number of predictor variables in the model. When the data are (still) inadequate, one may exclude variables that have missing values for a relatively large number of observations. Also, if 2 variables are highly correlated (again an arbitrary threshold might be used, e.g., 0.6) one of them can be omitted from the model. If necessary, the next step might be to create several subsets of variables and reduce the number of variables per subset (as in step 3).

3. When the multivariate model of step 2 has been fitted, each variable should be examined on its significancy and on the change of the regression coefficient compared to the univariate analysis. Next, the least significant variable (highest *P*-value based on the deviance difference) is deleted from the model. Be aware: it is not allowed to delete a single dummy variable from the model, they should all stay in the model or they should all be left out! The model is fitted again, and the regression coefficients of this new model are compared to those of the old model and if any coefficient has changed 'considerably' (arbitrary threshold), it should be put back in the model as being a confounder. This process of ***deleting, refitting and verifying*** continues until all variables in the model exceed a pre-defined *P*-value (mostly 0.05) or act as confounders.

4. The next step concerns the inclusion of interaction terms. As expressed before, only biologically meaningful interactions should be evaluated.

This 4 step procedure should be used with utmost care, because weak relations of predictor variables with the outcome variable in the univariate step might become of larger importance when these variables are forced together in one model. Also interactions of variables that are not significant in the univariate step or deleted during step 3, will go undetected. Dohoo *et al.* (1997) give an overview of several techniques that can be used when many predictor variables need to be evaluated.

8. Goodness-Of-Fit (GOF) in Logistic Regression: Basic Ideas

GOF can be addressed in 2 ways:

1. relative
2. absolute

Relative GOF can be described as: does a model with variable x_1 tell us more than a model without variable x_1? It is based on the -2 log likelihood ratio test (deviance difference) as discussed in paragraph 3. However, the difference in -2 Log L does not indicate **how well** the model fits, which is: how close do the predicted values, based on the coefficients in the model, agree to the observed values. For that we need to assess the absolute GOF. An overall method to look at this is described by Hosmer and Lemeshow (1989). Their method is based on comparing observed and predicted numbers of individuals within each 'decile of risk'. In the first decile, the 10% of individuals with the lowest **estimated probability** of the event are grouped, the last decile contains 10% of the individuals with the highest estimated probability of the event. Subsequently, the observed and predicted numbers are statistically evaluated using a parameter C which is Chi-square distributed with 8 *df*. C is often called, the Hosmer-Lemeshow statistic. If this C has a significant value, it is concluded that the differences between observed and predicted values are not due to random error and that the model does not fit well enough.

A disadvantage of C is that quite large numbers are needed to calculate it (remember that the expected frequency should be at least 4 in each class to use the Chi-square approximation). Also, it is not calculated in case one of the deciles has a predicted number of 0. By comparing observed and predicted numbers within each decile, it can be seen which deciles are badly predicted, **but** it cannot be seen which individuals are really mispredicted.

STATISTIX also calculates a second statistic (H), which is based on **fixed** cutpoints (all animals with a predicted probability less than 0.10 are in group 1 etc.). Then, in each group an unequal number of animals will be present and hence it has been shown that the C statistic should be preferred to the H statistic. Below the output of STATISTIX is shown for the data in Appendix 2c (age as a continuous predictor for RD).

HOSMER-LEMESHOW GOODNESS-OF-FIT TESTS FOR RED

		Decile of Risk										
		1	2	3	4	5	6	7	8	9	10	
RED		0.18	0.21	0.25	0.32	0.38	0.43	0.48	0.52	0.58	0.64	Total
1	OBS	11	20	32	36	45	51	68	56	59	63	441
	EXP	18.6	23.5	28.3	33.8	41.0	47.6	53.5	59.3	63.6	71.7	441
0	OBS	103	100	90	83	73	68	50	62	57	58	744
	EXP	95.4	96.5	93.7	85.2	77.0	71.4	64.5	58.7	52.4	49.3	744
	Total	114	120	122	119	118	119	118	118	116	121	1185

HOSMER-LEMESHOW STATISTIC (C) 17.03; P-VALUE 0.0298; DEGREES OF FREEDOM: 8

		Decile of Risk										
		1	2	3	4	5	6	7	8	9	10	
RED		0.10	0.20	0.30	0.40	0.50	0.60	0.70	0.80	0.90	1.00	Total
1	OBS	0	20	72	74	117	137	21	0	0	0	441
	EXP	0.0	32.4	63.5	73.4	99.7	149.2	22.9	0.0	0.0	0.0	441
0	OBS	0	167	189	133	104	135	16	0	0	0	744
	EXP	0.0	154.6	197.5	133.6	121.3	122.8	14.1	0.0	0.0	0.0	744
Total		0	187	261	207	221	272	37	0	0	0	1185

NOTE:The Hosmer-Lemeshow statistic (H) has not been computed because some columns in the table have zero observed values.

It shows that the C statistic is significant and that the model does not fit well enough. The number of misfits are especially in deciles 1, 7 and 10 (which is also obvious from Figure 6.3).

It is also important to evaluate which individuals do not fit well. In fact, one should not speak of individuals but of 'covariate patterns' because individuals might have exactly the same values for all predictor variables. Test statistics commonly used for this are:

a. the Pearson Chi-square, being the sum of the squared Pearson residuals for covariate pattern x_1 to x_j: Σr_j^2;
b. the deviance Chi-square, being the sum of the squared deviance residuals for covariate pattern x_1 to x_j: Σd_j^2.

These statistics are based on comparing the difference between observed and predicted values per covariate pattern. In case the discrepancy is large for some patterns, one should think about the reasons **why** they fit badly and **how** they influence the Pearson Chi-square and/or the deviance Chi-square and the regression coefficients. This can be done by running the programme for a second time, without the specific covariate pattern and comparing the overall measure of fit (Pearson or deviance) and regression coefficients (β's). However, to evaluate all covariate patterns in this way would take many runs! Fortunately, these figures can be obtained directly from a single run, if the 'leverage' (h) for each covariate pattern j (h_j) is calculated. The leverage can be looked upon as the distance between x_j and the average of the data.

It can be shown that:

$$\delta X_j^2 = \frac{r_j^2}{1 - h_j}$$

$$\delta D_j^2 = d_j^2 + \frac{r_j^2 * h_j}{1 - h_j} = d_j^2 + \delta X_j^2 * h_j$$

$$\delta \beta_1 = \frac{r_j^2 * h_j}{1 - r_j^2} = \frac{\delta X_j^2 * h_j}{1 - h_j}$$

δX_j^2 = change in Pearson Chi-square after deleting a specific covariate pattern
δD_j^2 = change in deviance Chi-square after deleting a specific covariate pattern
$\delta \beta_j$ = influence of one covariate pattern on regression estimates

From these test statistics, influential covariate patterns can be detected. Deletion of any individual or covariate pattern from the data should be described, including the arguments why that deletion was performed.

It is strongly advised to read Chapter V of Hosmer and Lemeshow (1989) for a more detailed description of how the fit of a logistic model can be assessed.

9. Multilevel Data

In veterinary epidemiology it is very common to have data obtained from several levels. For example, recorded data at the animal level concern breed, sex, production and disease status while herd level data are related to management, housing type and several parameters related to feed. Then, a 'herd effect' (more generally, 'cluster effect') might be present which should be taken into account in the model. Where does the herd effect come from? Animals within a herd are more similar to each other when compared to animals from another herd, due to similar exposures (in statistical language: the observations are not independent). Some of these factors might have been measured. However, there may be many factors which are not measured in the screening but that do have an effect on the occurrence of disease.

On this basis it is presumed that animals within a herd are more similar (with respect to exposure) than animals from different herds. So, the variation of the standard error might be larger than can be expected on the basis of binomial variation that is expected to occur in the model. The variance of the estimated parameter will be too small, resulting in a too small confidence interval. Then, the variable might be declared as significant while it is not significant in reality. Of course, this is an undesirable situation. There are two ways to account for this problem. First, one may return to the herds to obtain extra information (if we have any idea about the information needed). This is rarely done (in general we have retrospective data). Second, one can try to account for it in the analysis. Different approaches exist (Curtis *et al.*, 1988):

1. to disregard the herd effect. This assumes homogeneity of risk across all groups and this is often not the case;
2. be more restrictive with the significance level (e.g., lower it to 0.01);
3. inclusion of the herd effect in the model as a ***fixed*** effect: a disadvantage is that the risk is fixed for a particular herd and that N-1 dummy variables are needed for N herds (thus statistically unattractive). If interactions occur with these dummy variables interpretation will be difficult;
4. include the herd effect in the model as a ***random*** effect.

A fifth alternative is to calculate a so-called 'variance inflation factor', based on the variance between clusters and within clusters. The variance is then multiplied by this factor, resulting in increased standard errors and thus in decreased significancies. It has been shown that a random effect model is the best way to deal with the cluster effect, resulting in an increase of the standard errors of the coefficients **and** also the regression coefficients might change considerably. Software that can handle random effect logistic models is commercially available (among others: STATA 6.0, GENSTAT, SAS - requires a GLIMMIX macro -, EGRET, MLn) although the size of the data set and/or the model might be a limiting factor. Also the amount of computer time needed might be considerable when evaluating these models, especially when more levels of random effects are fitted.

Besides the herd effect, other dependencies might occur, e.g., animals within litters, lactations within cows, milking quarters within cows etc. Also second or higher levels of dependency might occur. For example, if the unit of observation is the piglet (more than one piglet per litter), and several litters per sow exist and several sows per herd are present then 3 levels of dependency are potentially present (a litter effect, a sow effect and a herd effect). In statistics it is often said that a **nested** or **hierarchical structure** is underlying these data and that a **multilevel analysis** is most appropriate.

10. Ordinal Outcome Variables

Logistic regression can also be applied to ordinal and nominal outcome variables. The most basic theory can be found in McCullagh and Nelder (1989). Only ordinal responses will be discussed here, because those are more common in veterinary epidemiology than nominal responses. The effect of two antibiotics on demeanour scores will be used as an illustration.

Ordinal responses, like a demeanour score (1 = alert, 2 = apathy, 3 = marked depression and 4 = moribund), have no exact quantitative meaning. However, it is very tempting to perform a straightforward analysis of variance to these data, but for that the distances between scores need to be equal; i.e., the difference between alert and apathy should be the same as the difference between marked depression and moribund; equal to the difference between 1 and 2 kg is the same as the difference between 99 and 100 kg. If not, the interpretation of the outcomes might be biased. Logistic regression can be used to approach ordinal scores in a more justified way. This is done by using cumulative probabilities, also referred to as a 'threshold-model' (see later). In formula:

$$\Pr(\text{outcome}_j \geq i) = \frac{1}{1 + e^{-\beta_{0i} - \beta_j * x_j}}$$

From this formula the probabilities of each outcome can be derived. What is different compared to binary logistic regression is that k-1 intercepts are calculated where k is the number of possible outcomes. Thus, in the demeanour score example, 3 intercepts will be calculated (if all scores occur in the data set). The meaning of these intercepts is identical to that in binary logistic regression, they can be used to recalculate the probabilities for each outcome.

In ordinal logistic regression, k-1 regressions are performed simultaneously. In the first regression, the lowest score is compared to all the higher scores (2 to k). In the second, the scores 1 and 2 are compared to score 3 to k, etc. The fact that the regressions are performed simultaneously results in the same regression coefficients for the predictor variables in all regressions. One can also say that k-1 parallel logit functions are fitted simultaneously and that the parallelism derives from the uniform regression coefficients.

Exponentiation of these regression coefficients gives the odds ratios. The interpretation of an odds ratio larger than 1.0 is that the probability of ***higher*** scores is larger if the value of the predictor variable increases. One basic assumption is that the regression coefficients in all regressions are statistically equal. For that e.g., SAS calculates a Chi-square statistic to test whether this proportional odds assumption is true. If significant, the proportional odds assumption does not hold and the regression outcomes should be considered invalid.

In the comparative antibiotic trial, the frequencies of scores at intake were about equal for both groups. The frequencies of scores at 24 hours after the intake were:

	Score			
	1	2	3	4
Antibiotic A (code = 0)	16	41	6	0
Antibiotic B (code = 1)	8	40	14	0

Score 4 was not present any more at 24 hours post treatment. Selected output of ordinal logistic regression in SAS is in the table below.

Analysis of Maximum Likelihood Estimates

Variable	DF	Parameter Estimate	Standard Error	Wald Chi-Square	Pr > Chi-square	Odds Ratio
Intercp1	1	-2.1802	0.3441	40.1494	0.0001	.
Intercp2	1	1.0503	0.2723	14.8799	0.0001	.
Treat	1	0.9160	0.3847	5.6689	0.0173	2.499

Score Test for the Proportional Odds Assumption
Chi-Square = 0.0858 with 1 DF (p=0.7696)

Thus, the estimated probability for antibiotic B (coded as 1) to show the higher scores is 2.5 (= OR) times increased as compared to antibiotic A. A seems to be more effective in reducing the score within 24 hours. We also can calculate 2 OR's simply by hand:

	B	A
3	14	6
1 or 2	48	57

--> OR = (14/48) / (6/57) = 2.8

	B	A
2 or 3	54	47
1	8	16

--> OR = (54/8) / (47/16) = 2.3

The ordinal logistic regression procedure calculates a uniform OR of 2.5, which is in between the two manually calculated OR's. Also the proportional odds assumption is insignificant, which could be expected as both OR's were not differing that much. An analysis of variance would reveal that the mean score for group A is 1.84 and for group B is 2.10, the difference being significant with $P < 0.02$. If coding of the categories change, these means would be affected and the significance as well. However, whatever the coding, ordinal logistic regression always produces the same results. This might be undesirable when some categories have a very large impact, e.g., animals that die might get a demeanour score of say, 10. This is then reflecting economic loss and this loss is underestimated when ordinal logistic regression is used.

How can these results be explained in terms of a threshold model? In Fig. 6.4 the logistic probability distributions on the logistic scale are shown (note that the figure has been rotated and that the x-axis actually represents the y-axis). Vertical lines indicate the threshold values, which are identical to the intercepts of the logistic model except for the sign. Below the threshold value of -1.05 the score 1 is assigned while above the value 2.18 the score 3 is reported. Based on the formula for cumulative probabilities, the probability of getting a score of 3 when treated with antibiotic A is estimated as $1/(1+e^{2.1802}) = 0.102$; when treated with antibiotic B this probability is $1/(1+e^{2.1802-0.9160} = 0.220$. The probability of getting a score of 2 or 3 when treated with antibiotic A is: $1/(1+e^{-1.0503}) = 0.741$, thus the probability to get a score of 1 equals 1 - 0.741 = 0.259. Similarly, the probability of getting a score of 1 when treated with antibiotic B is $1 - 1/(1+e^{-1.053-0.9160}) = 0.123$. The probabilities derived directly from the data are resp. 6/63 = 0.095; 14/62 = 0.226; 16/63 = 0.254 and 8/62 = 0.129.

Multivariate analysis of ordinal outcome variables can be applied in the same way as multivariate analysis of binary outcomes.

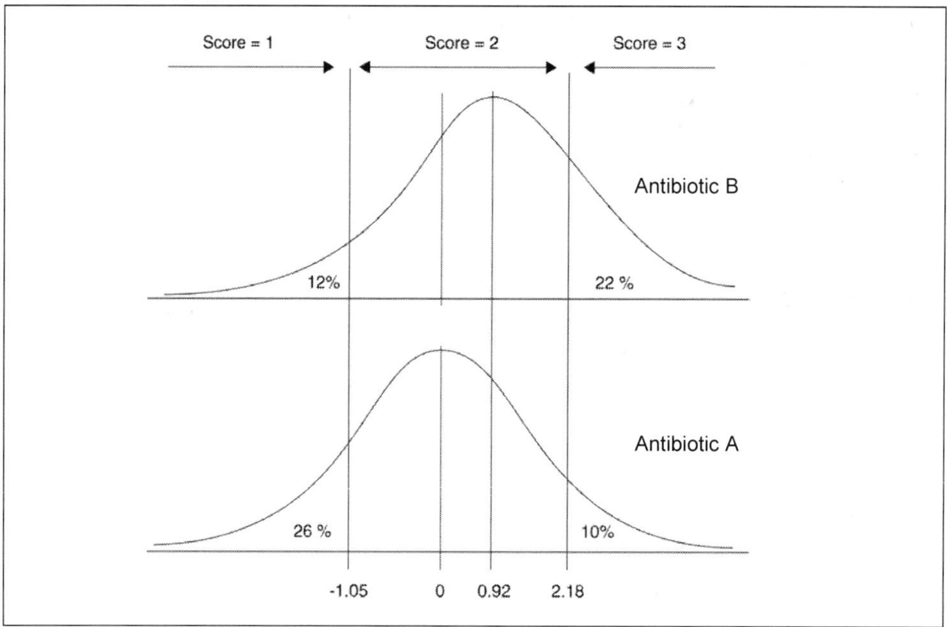

Figure 6.4. Diagram showing the thresholds for an ordinal response variable based on the logistic model.

11. Concluding Remarks

As stated in the beginning, it was needed to treat the logistic regression analysis robustly. The ultimate goal of this part was to show why a multivariate approach is necessary and to get you acquainted with the principles of one of the most frequently used multivariate methods in epidemiology. After (re-)reading this chapter, you should be able to interpret the basic output of logistic regression and to understand and interpret papers in which this methodology is applied. It is unlikely that, by studying only this chapter, you can perform complete logistic regression analyses yourself. Knowledge should be further increased by reading (parts of) the recommended books (see References) or by consulting statisticians that are skilled in this field.

References

Curtis, C.R.; Mauritsen, R.H.; Salman, M.D.; Erb, H.N. (1988). The enigma of herd: a comparison of different models to account for group effects in multiple logistic regression analysis. Acta Veterinaria Scandinavia, 84, 462-465.
Dohoo, I.R.; Ducrot, C.; Fourichon, C.; Donald, A.; Hurnik, D. (1997). An overview of techniques for dealing with large numbers of independent variables in epidemiologic studies. Preventive Veterinary Medicine, 29, 221-239.
Frankena, K.; Keulen, K.A.S. van; Noordhuizen, J.P.; Noordhuizen-Stassen, E.N.; Gundelach, J.; Jong, D.J. de; Saedt I. (1992). A cross-sectional study into prevalence and risk indicators of digital haemorraghes in female dairy calves. Preventive Veterinary Medicine, 14, 1-12.
Hosmer, D.W.; Lemeshow, S. (1989). Applied Logistic Regression. Wiley and Sons, New York.
McCullagh, P.; Nelder, J.A. (1989). Generalized Linear Models. Chapman and Hall, London.

Further Reading

Agresti, A. (1990). Categorical Data Analysis. Wiley and Sons, New York.
Kleinbaum, D.G.; Kupper, L.L.; Muller, K.E. (1988). Applied Regression and Other Multivariable Methods. PWS-KENT Publishing Company, Boston.
Snedecor, G.W.; Cochran, W.G. (1980). Statistical Methods. Iowa State University Press, Ames, Iowa.

Appendix 1. Manual Calculation of Logistic Regression Coefficients

Suppose we have a case-control study with 400 animals: 150 cases and 250 controls. Out of the 150 cases, 100 were exposed to F. Out of the 250 controls, also 100 were exposed.

		F		
		+	-	Total
D	+	100	50	150
	-	100	150	250
	Total	200	200	400

The OR is then: (100/100) / (50/150) = 3.0

The calculation of the β's is as follows:

If F=1 then $P(Y=1 \mid F=1) = \pi(1)$ is equal to 100/200 = 0.5
If F=0 then $P(Y=1 \mid F=0) = \pi(0)$ ie equal to 50/200 = 0.25

$$\text{The logit of } \pi(1) = \ln\left(\frac{\pi(1)}{1-\pi(1)}\right) = \ln(0.5/0.5) = \ln(1)$$

$$\text{The logit of } \pi(0) = \ln\left(\frac{\pi(0)}{1-\pi(0)}\right) = \ln(0.25/0.75) = \ln(1/3)$$

We also know that the logit of $\pi(x) = \beta_0 + \beta_1 x$

Thus:

$\beta_0 + \beta_1 * 1 = ln[1] = 0$; which results in $\beta_1 = -\beta_0$

$\beta_0 + \beta_1 * 0 = \beta_0 = ln[1/3] = -1.0986$

Thus $\beta_1 = -\beta_0 = -(-1.0986) = 1.0986$

And indeed: $e^{\beta} = e^{1.0986} = 3.0$, as we did calculate from the 2x2 table.

Appendix 2. Illustration of an Analysis Using Several Types of Predictor Variables

1185 female dairy calves in the age of 75 to 365 days were diagnosed with regard to red discolorations (RD) in sole horn. RD was diagnosed as being present or absent (Frankena *et al.*, 1992).

2a. AGE as dichotomous variable

LOGISTIC REGRESSION

The LOGISTIC Procedure
Data Set: WORK.EEN
Response Variable: RED
Response Levels: 2
Number of Observations: 1185
Link Function: Logit

Response Profile

Ordered Value	RED	Count
1	0	441
2	1	744

Simple Statistics for Explanatory Variables

Variable	Mean	Standard Deviation	Minimum	Maximum
AGEGROUP	0.526582	0.499504	0	1.00000

Criteria for Assessing Model Fit

Criterion	Intercept only	Intercept and covariates	Chi-Square for Covariates
AIC	1566.416	1483.450	.
SC	1571.493	1493.605	.
-2 LOG L	1564.416	1479.450	84.966 with 1 DF (p=0.0001)
Score	.	.	83.190 with 1 DF (p=0.0001)

Analysis of Maximum Likelihood Estimates

Variable	Parameter Estimate	Standard Error	Wald Chi-Square	Pr > Chi-Square	Standardized Estimate
INTERCPT	-1.1688	0.0993	138.6097	0.0001	.
AGEGROUP	1.1431	0.1275	80.3335	0.0001	0.314808

2b. AGE as polytomous variable

The LOGISTIC Procedure

Data Set: WORK.EEN
Response Variable: RED
Response Levels: 2
Number of Observations: 1185
Link Function: Logit

Response Profile

Ordered value	RED	Count
1	0	441
2	1	744

Criteria for Assessing Model Fit

Criterion	Intercept only	Intercept and covariates	Chi-Square for Covariates
-2 LOG L	1564.416	1432.587	131.829 with 9 DF (p=0.0001)

Analysis of Maximum Likelihood Estimates

Variable	Parameter Estimate	Standard Error	Wald Chi-Square	Pr > Chi-Square	Standardized Estimate
INTERCPT	-2.3979	0.4264	31.6250	0.0001	.
D2	0.4949	0.4994	0.9821	0.3217	0.085597
D3	1.3980	0.4657	9.0113	0.0027	0.252691
D4	1.5755	0.4811	10.7251	0.0011	0.235982
D5	1.7346	0.4758	13.2912	0.0003	0.265944
D6	1.8911	0.4625	16.7218	0.0001	0.329245
D7	2.7473	0.4613	35.4646	0.0001	0.478312
D8	2.2519	0.4566	24.3287	0.0001	0.414173
D9	2.4661	0.4523	29.7292	0.0001	0.483714
D10	2.6027	0.5141	25.6293	0.0001	0.285815

2c. AGE as continuous variable

The LOGISTIC Procedure
Data Set: WORK.EEN
Response Variable: RED
Response Levels: 2
Number of Observations: 1185
Link Function: Logit

Response Profile

Ordered value	RED	Count
1	0	441
2	1	744

Simple Statistics for Explanatory Variables

Variable	Mean	Standard deviation	Minimum	Maximum
AGE	223.468354	80.387391	76.0000	365.000

Criteria for Assessing Model Fit

Criterion	Intercept only	Intercept and covariates	Chi-Square for Covariates
AIC	1566.416	1459.153	.
SC	1571.493	1469.308	.
-2 LOG L	1564.416	1455.153	109.263 with 1 DF (p=0.0001)
Score	.	.	105.225 with 1 DF (p=0.0001)

Analysis of Maximum Likelihood Estimates

Variable	Parameter Estimate	Standard Error	Wald Chi-Square	Pr > Chi-Square	Standardized Estimate
INTERCPT	-2.4251	0.2070	137.2082	0.0001	.
AGE	0.00825	0.00083	98.7662	0.0001	0.365797

12. Exercises

12.1. Trichinosis in pigs

This exercise is based on the paper: "Management factors affecting trichinosis seropositivity among 91 North Carolina swine farms". P. Cowen, R.A. Pacer, P.N. Van Peteghem and J.F.Fetrow. (Preventive Veterinary Medicine 9 (1990): 165-172).

Questions

1. What is the type of study described in this paper?
2. What is your explanation for the fact that the positive tested herds are also the larger herds?
3. Calculate the univariate OR with the 95% confidence interval for variables 2, 6 and 14 from Table 1 (in the paper) for ELISA ≥ 6.
4. What is the OR of herd 1 where are no cats, which do not buy pigs from a commercial company, where tail biting and wildlife is observed compared to herd 2 where cats are walking around, pigs are obtained from a commercial company and where tail biting and wildlife is not observed (Use model ELISA ≥ 6)?

12.2. Epidemiologic observations with respect to *Dermatitis digitalis* (Italian footrot) in dairy cattle

Background information

At the end of the pasture period of 1989, hind claws from all cows on 59 commercial dairy farms with loose housing were trimmed by professional claw trimmers. Disorders in each claw has been recorded by trained observers. In the pasture study (P-study) a total of 2494 cows were trimmed. A similar study was carried out at the end of the housing period of 1990 (H-study). The H-study concerned 2795 animals from 58 dairy farms with loose housing. The objectives of these large-scale studies were: (1) to determine the extent of the presence of claw disorders and (2) to identify possible risk factors and to quantify their effect.

To fulfil these objectives, animals were diagnosed and also characteristics of animals (breed, stage of lactation and parity) and the farm were registered. For the latter one, information was obtained by means of a questionnaire. This questionnaire contained various 'topics' in which information was asked about the farmer, buildings, pasture, hygiene, feed supply, feeding strategy and 'general' (farm size, other diseases etc.). This exercise is restricted to *Dermatitis digitalis* (DD, synonym: Italian footrot, Mortellaro disease) only.

Prevalence of Italian footrot

Table 6.1 shows that DD is more frequent and more severe during the housing period.

Table 6.1. Prevalence of Italian Footrot in two observational studies P and H.

	% of claws affected[b]	
Diagnosis[a]	P	H
DD grade 1	7.7	10.2
grade 2	0.4	3.6
total	8.1	13.8

[a] DD = dermatitis digitalis = Italian footrot
[b] regardless of the number of affected feet

Analysis of potential risk factors

The aetiology of Mortellaro disease still has to be elucidated. Most researchers assume that it is caused by micro-organisms, but this has not been proven by Koch's postulates. Besides that, also environmental factors might be important and therefore a multifactorial causal pathway should be considered.

By means of statistical analysis (multivariate logistic regression, accounting for dependency of animals within a herd) odds ratios of animal and herd factors were calculated. Table 6.2 shows, besides risk factors on the animal level, the importance of various herd and pasture factors. Obviously, animals related to the MRY or 'other' breed (mainly beef type breeds) were less frequently diagnosed as DD positive. Also stage of lactation is important: animals at the top of production had a 1.7 times higher probability to have DD than animals that had past the period of top production. Animals in the dry period showed the lowest prevalence of DD. Farms with an intermediate herd size and production form a group with an increased risk. Free access to pasture is negatively associated to DD. However, a walking distance of >200 meters is, besides a metalled walking path, a risk factor. Also pasture level is significantly related to Mortellaro disease. These are statistical associations, they don't need to be causal. However, for some factors the biological mechanism seems obvious: for example, a metalled walking path will be extra aggravating; when animals have a limited access to pasture they are housed during a relatively long time on a metalled floor surface (slatted floors); in general, high level pasture is more dry, so the claws might be of a better quality. Low level pastures often are well drained and thus might be more dry than pastures with a medium level.

Table 6.2. Estimates of the odds ratio of some factors related to the animal, herd and pasture (P-study).

Parameter	Category	Odds ratio
Parity	1	1.32
	2	1.05
	3	1.00 (ref)
Breed	> 50% HF	1.20
	> 50% FH	1.02
	> 50% MRY	0.12*
	Other	0.34*
	HF/FH 50%	1.00 (ref)
Stage of lactation	Dry	0.34*
	Pre top	0.81
	Top (day 50-70)	1.70*
	Past top	1.00 (ref)
Herd size	< 50 cows	0.61⁰
	≥ 65	0.74
	50 to 65	1.00 (ref)
Production level	< 7000	0.47*
	≥ 8000	0.39*
	7000 - 8000	1.00 (ref)
Access to pasture	limited	1.51*
	free	1.00 (ref)
Walking distance	> 200 meter	5.37*
	< 200 meter	1.00 (ref)
Walking path condition	metalled	2.56*
	non-metalled	1.00 (ref)
Pasture level	low	0.53*
	high	0.59*
	medium	1.00 (ref)

*: $P < 0.05$; ⁰: $P < 0.10$

Note: Causality of factor and presence of disease is hardly to prove with this type of study. For that intervention or experimental studies are needed. However, strong suggestions are obtained regarding the relative importance of some factors. In practice, results of this type of epidemiological study can be used for prevention and control of diseases. However, the more complex a disease or the larger the economic importance of control strategies, the more one should rely on studies revealing causal mechanisms.

Questions

1. A farmer, with huge problems of Italian footrot in his herd, decides to strew sand on his metalled walking path. What is the risk decrease of having Italian footrot for the cows after this measure?

2. A farmer decides to strew sand on the walking path and to give his cows free access to pasture. What is the risk after these measures?
3a. It is summer time and cow Clara 13 is grazing a pasture on farm X. Clara 13 has the following characteristics: parity 1, breed 50%FH/50%HF, in top stage of lactation. Farm X has the following characteristics: herd size 39, herd production level 7500 litres, free access to pasture, walking distance 210 meters, a grass walking path and a medium pasture level. On the neighbour farm Y (herd size 61, herd production level 8150 litres, limited access to pasture, walking distance 190 meters, metalled walking path and a medium pasture level) there is cow Maria 20 (parity 3, >50 %MRY, dry). Calculate the relative risk of Clara 13 *vs.* Maria 20 to have Italian footrot.
3b. The walking distance is an important factor (OR=5.37). The difference in walking distance between Clara 13 and Maria 20 is only 20 metres, however the difference in risk 5.37. Is it justified to put these cows in different categories. If not, how would you account for this problem?

12.3. Salmonellosis in poultry

Re-read exercise 4.2 in Chapter V. Note that the study was not designed with an epidemiological perspective. Thus, information about several, may be important, variables was not present in the data set. Furthermore, the use of the "special" population (great grand parent stock) interferes with the extrapolation to all farms. Also, a large proportion of the flocks was diagnosed as case, which has consequences for interpretation of the OR's as being good estimators for the true relative risks. Moreover, both diagnostic tests were not equal and most likely sensitivity and specificity were different. Thus, the classification into cases and non-cases might not be uniform.

The same analysis as in 4.2 is easier by fitting 3 logistic regression models. All variables were 1,0 coded, the first category mentioned in the table in exercise 4.2 being coded as 1 and the second as 0. In model 1 the variable REGION is included. In model 2, the variable FEEDMILL is added and in model 3 also the interaction term of these 2 variables is added. The estimated logistic regression coefficients and the -2 log likelihood of the variable REGION is presented in Table 6.3 for either model 1, model 2 and model 3.

Table 6.3. Estimated logistic regression coefficients for variable REGION in model 1, 2 and 3 and the -2 log likelihood of the model.

Model	Region	-2 log likelihood
1	1.246	111.87
2	0.517	104.23
3	-0.545	103.80

1a. Is the estimate for REGION confounded by the variable FEEDMILL (given that both have a significant relation with Salmonellosis)?
1b. Is the interaction between REGION and FEEDMILL significant?

Results of several multivariate models are given in Table 6.4.

2a. Calculate the Wald statistics and their significancy for the variables of model C in Table 6.4.
2b. How is the Chi-square of a model calculated?
2c. What is the best model (A, B, C or D), according to you, and why?
2d. Calculate the OR between farm 1 and 2 according to model D in Table 6.3. On farm 1 there is no disinfection tub present, use of hygiene barriers is poor and feed is obtained from a small feed mill. Farm 2 obtains feed from a large feed mill, uses the hygiene barriers good and a disinfection tub is present.
2e. Assume a farm in which a disinfection tub is present and where the hygiene barriers are used very good. Do you think that the risk on salmonellosis is very small then? Explain.
2f. What is notable after completion of the univariate and the multivariate analysis with respect to the risk factors? Give a possible explanation.

Table 6.4. Results of a multivariate analysis.

A. Model containing intercept only: -2 log likelihood = 106.37

B. Model with significant (P < 0.25) variables from the univariate analysis

Variable	β	S.E.
Intercept	0.708	1.100
disinfection tub	1.095	0.806
hygiene barriers	0.838	0.695
region	-0.837	0.777
flock size	-0.292	0.867
farm type	0.277	0.842
feed mill	1.585	0.776
# buildings	-0.728	0.807

-2log likelihood = 81.67; model χ^2 (A-B) = 24.70 with 7 *df.* *P* = 0.0009

C. Model with variables that remain from table B after the process of deleting (P > 0.25), refitting and verifying

Variable	β	S.E.
Intercept	-0.643	0.643
disinfection tub	0.934	0.633
hygiene barriers	1.256	0.610
feed mill	1.992	0.685

-2log likelihood = 84.56; model χ^2 (A-C) = 21.81 with 3 *df.* *P* = 0.0001

D. Model including interaction

Variable	β	S.E.
Intercept	0.477	0.879
disinfection tub (a)	-0.350	0.925
hygiene barriers (b)	-0.485	1.054
interaction (a) ∗ (b)	3.030	1.515
feed mill	1.992	0.686

-2log likelihood = 79.86; model χ^2 (A-D) = 26.51 with 4 *df.* *P* = 0.0001

13. Answers

13.1. Trichinosis in pigs

1. In a prevalence survey the prevalence is estimated. For this survey, 29947 pigs have been screened with an ELISA test. Based on the results of these tests, herds were classified as either seropositive or seronegative. With these data the investigators carried out a case-control study. So, this study is a combined study.

2. There were 29947 samples from individual pigs originating from 343 lots. If at least one pig per lot was seropositive then the whole lot was classified as seropositive. The 343 lots originated from 153 herds. When at least one lot of a herd was tested seropositive, then the herd was classified as positive. If there has been no proportional sampling to lot and herd size, then larger herds are much more likely being classified as seropositive (have a look at paragraph 3.4 of Chapter IV, concerning herd sensitivity). This might be one explanation for the fact that larger herds are more often seropositive. Unfortunately, from the paper it is not clear if proportional sampling was applied.

3. With ELISA≥6, 56% of the herds is positive (0.56∗91=51).

Cats have access to swine house

		yes	no	
status	+	6	45	51
	-	15	25	40
		21	70	91

OR=0.22
[0.08; 0.64]

trichinosis testing important to the producer

		yes	no	
status	+	29	22	51
	-	29	11	40
		58	33	91

OR=0.50
[0.21; 1.22]

swine observed eating rats/mice

		yes	no	
status	+	6	45	51
	-	1	39	40
		7	84	91

OR=5.20
[0.60; 45.09]

4. Note that the β's and OR's do not match! Most likely the OR's are correct, based on univariate outcomes. Then, the first decimal 0 of the factors 'cats' and 'gilts' should be deleted from the regression coefficients. If you present the same information twice, be aware of these typing errors!

   One can not simply enumerate the odds ratios! One can enumerate the regression coefficients and next exponentiate the sum. May be this question is most easily solved by comparing both herds to a herd with all factors at the reference category and dividing both outcomes. The risk for herd 1 is increased with $e^{0+0+0.56+0.50} = 2.89$ and for herd 2 with $e^{-0.78-0.75+0+0} = 0.22$ and their ratio is 2.89/0.22 = 13.1, which is identical to 1.75∗1.66/(0.46∗0.47) = 13.4 (difference due to rounding).

13.2. Epidemiologic observations with respect to *Dermatitis digitalis* (Italian footrot) in dairy cattle

1. The OR for a metalled path is 2.56. Thus, now the cows are walking on a 'soft' path, the probability to have foot rot is 2.56 times less.

2. First, take the ln-value of both OR's, sum these and exponentiate the sum. So, the difference in risk is equal to $e^{\ln 1.51+\ln 2.56} = 3.87$. This is identical to ***multiplying*** the separate OR's (1.51∗2.56 = 3.87).

3a. In principle, the calculation is similar to that in the previous question. With regard to a cow with the reference category for all parameters Clara 13 has an increased risk equal to $e^{\ln 1.32+\ln 1.0+\ln 1.70+\ln 0.61+\ln 1.0+\ln 1.0+\ln 5.37+\ln 1.0+\ln 1.0} = 7.35$ (or 1.32∗1.0∗1.70∗0.61∗1.0∗1.0∗5.37∗1.0∗1.0 = 1.32∗1.70∗0.61∗5.37 = 7.35). Maria 20: $e^{\ln 1.0+\ln 0.12+\ln 0.34+\ln 1.0+\ln 0.39+\ln 1.51+\ln 1.0+\ln 2.56+\ln 1.0} = 0.06$.
    Thus, the probability of Clara 13 with respect to Maria 20 to show Italian footrot is 7.35/0.06 = 122.5 times increased.

3b. This phenomenon is always present when a continuous variable is divided into categories. It is better (if allowed, based on linearity of logits - see goodness-of-fit in paragraph 8 of this chapter) to include such variables in the statistical model as continuous.

13.3. Salmonellosis in poultry

1a. The crude OR can be calculated from model 1 as $e^{1.246} = 3.48$, while the feed mill adjusted OR equals $e^{0.517} = 1.68$. If you think that this is a large adjustment than confounding is present (remember: it is a subjective decision).

1b. Interaction can best be derived from the likelihood ratio test of model 2 versus model 3. The value of this statistic is equal to G = -2log likelihood(without interaction) - 2log likelihood(with interaction) = 104.23 - 103.80 = 0.43. This has a X^2-distribution with 1 degree of freedom. It follows that $P = 0.51$ and thus it is decided that the interaction between FEEDMILL and REGION is not statistically significant.

It follows that use of logistic regression is a quick and efficient way to obtain an adjusted OR and also an easy way to check the homogeneity assumption.

2a. With the Wald Statistic one can determine whether or not a (dummy-)variable in the model is significant or not. It is calculated as $[\beta/SE(\beta)]^2$ and has a X^2-distribution with 1 degree of freedom for all variables in model C. The respective Wald statistics and their significancies (extracted from a Chi-square table) are:

Risk factor	Wald	*P*-value
disinfection tub	2.18	0.14
hygiene barriers	4.24	0.04
feed mill	8.46	0.004

2b. Model Chi-square: (-2 log likelihood model with intercept only) minus (-2 log likelihood of model with intercept and variables)

2c. The complete model explains most (which is intuitively correct); the difference between model B and model C is 84.56 - 81.67 = 2.89 with 4 degrees of freedom. Thus model B and C do not differ significantly and one can stick to model C. The difference between the model with and without interaction (model C and D) is 84.56 - 79.86 = 4.7 with 1 degree of freedom ($P < 0.05$). This is defined as being significant, which means that the model with interaction explains more than the model without. So, model D is the best model.

2d. OR (farm 1 *vs*. farm 2)= $e^{(-0.350*1 + -0.485*1 + 3.030*1 + 1.992*1)}$ = 65.8

2e. No, when a farm obtains feed from a small feed mill it still has an OR of $e^{1.992}$ = 7.3. This is a considerable increase in risk.

2f. In the univariate analysis, absence of disinfection tubs and poor use of hygiene barriers were positively associated with *salmonella* status. However, in the multivariate analysis the OR's were respectively $e^{-0.350}$ = 0.70 and $e^{-0.485}$ = 0.62 and insignificant, but a significant interaction did exist. Thus, the risk of being salmonella positive is increased (due to the strong positive coefficient for the interaction) when both measures are applied together:

OR for disinfection tub present when hygiene barriers are absent is: 0.70
OR for disinfection tub present when hygiene barriers are present is: 14.6
OR for hygiene barriers present when disinfection tubs are absent is: 0.62
OR for hygiene barriers present when disinfection tubs are present is: 12.7

It might be that especially farmers who know that *salmonella* is present, have taken both measures, while others rely on only one method. This is a consequence of the study type in which we cannot say anything about whether the measures have been taken before or after the salmonellosis was diagnosed.

Chapter VII

Analysis of Time at Risk (Survival) Data

K. Frankena
Wageningen University & Research Centre
Department of Animal Sciences
Quantitative Veterinary Epidemiology Group
The Netherlands

E.A.M. Graat
Wageningen University & Research Centre
Department of Animal Sciences
Quantitative Veterinary Epidemiology Group
The Netherlands

1. Introduction

This chapter deals with the analysis of follow-up data when 'time until the event occurs' is important, e.g., in dynamic populations where animals disappear from or enter the study population during the study period. Secondly, this type of analysis is applicable when the total time at risk (see Chapter V) is very different between groups. The analytical method, called survival analysis, is suitable for cohort or experimental studies (e.g., clinical trials) when the time having been at risk is known for each individual. Also, results of survival analysis can be seen as a refinement of results of logistic regression, where the occurrence (yes or no) of the event was analyzed. In this chapter it is assumed that Chapter VI has been studied as many features of logistic regression and survival analysis are comparable. The statistical package used throughout this chapter is STATA (StataCorp, 1997).

2. Event and Time

Survival analysis can be used when the dependent variable not only addresses question, whether or not the event does occur, but also the 'time until the event occurs'. Time can be expressed in days, weeks, months, years, but also in e.g., number of lactations. The event can be every dichotomous outcome. Some examples are:

- becoming sick,
- becoming healthy,
- dying,
- becoming pregnant,
- getting a car accident,
- graduation,
- etc.

At the start of the study all individuals of interest have the same status regarding the event: they are all healthy or all sick or all alive, etc., and are **at risk** to get the event during the study period. Time is normally referred to as **survival time** and the occurrence of the event is called **failure** (though the event can be seen as a success, like graduation or recovery after a therapy). This originates from the fact that the method was initially applied in human medicine to express the success of a therapy.

3. Censored Observations

In a follow-up study, the exact survival time is only known for those individuals that show the event. About the other individuals one can only say that they did not show the event during the study period. These observations are 'censored'. Censoring can occur for two reasons:

1. the event did not happen before the study ended;

2. the event did not happen before the individual was withdrawn from the study, for another reason than the event (e.g., the farmer did not want to cooperate any more or the animal was sold).

This is shown in the following figure, depicting an experiment lasting for 8 weeks.

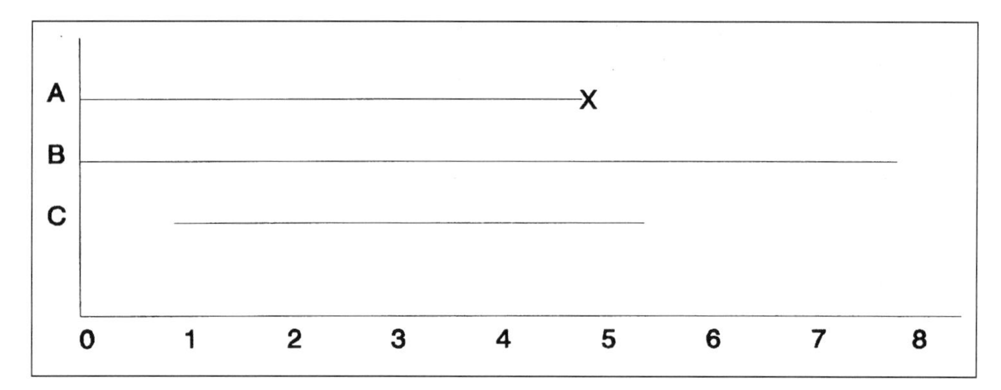

Animal A shows the event (X) after 5 weeks, so it is not censored. The survival time is 5 weeks. Animal B does not show the event and is censored, but its survival time is at least 8 weeks. The survival time of animal C is not known exactly, but it is at least 4.5 weeks. These individuals can be tabulated as:

Individual	Survival time	Event (1 = failed, 0 = censored)
A	5	1
B	8	0
C	4.5	0

Censoring usually occurs at the right side of the follow-up period. The starting point of the time at risk period is known (left side), while the point where the time at risk period ends, due to the occurrence of X, is unknown (e.g., animal B and C). Censoring at the left side is also possible but is not commonly used. An example could be that one is interested in the time between infection and occurrence of clinical disease, while it is only known when the animal tested positive for a pathogen, but it is unknown when it was infected with that pathogen (see figure below).

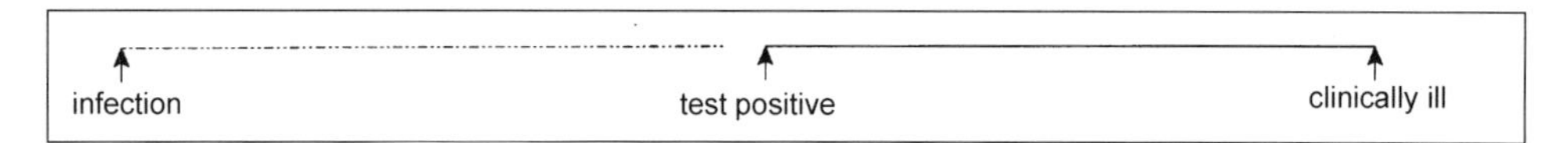

4. The Survival and Hazard Functions

Survival time is usually called T, while t is a specific value for T. One could ask the question: what is the probability that an individual survives at least longer than 5 time units (or what is the probability that an individual will **not** show the event during the first 4 time units): P(T > t=4). The **survivor function S(t)** is defined as:

$$S(t) = P(T > t) \tag{7.1}$$

In words: S(t) gives the probability that an individual will not show the event before time t. The course of S(t) gives the probabilities of the event ***not*** occurring in time. S(0) is equal to P(T>0) which is equal to 1 because it is assumed that at t=0, no individual has shown the event. In theory, the survivor function cannot increase and will, most likely, show a smooth decreasing curve (Figure 7.1.a). In practice however, one usually will have a step-wise function (Figure 7.1.b). Also, t is almost never infinite (∞), so S(t) does not necessarily go to 0. S(t) plotted against time is generally referred to as a Kaplan-Meier graph.

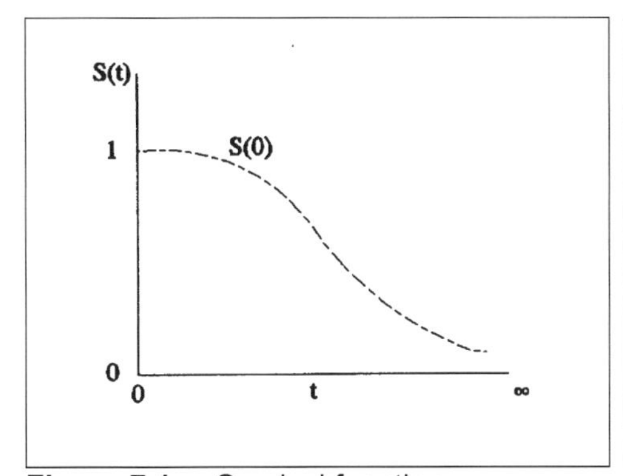

Figure 7.1.a. Survival function (theoretical).

Figure 7.1.b. Survival function (practical example)

The **hazard function h(t)** gives the probability that the event will occur in the ***next*** period of time, given that the individual has not yet shown the event. The hazard function is shown in equation 7.2.

$$h(t) = \lim_{\Delta t \to 0} \frac{P(t \leq T < t + \Delta t \mid T \geq t)}{\Delta t} \tag{7.2}$$

In fact, **h(t)** is not a probability but a **rate:** a **conditional probability per time unit** (see denominator). The hazard function is also known as the instantaneous (or potential) failure rate (or force of morbidity / mortality). Compare it with the speed of a car: if you drive 80 km per hour now, your potential radius for the next hour is 80 km. It is not said you will make that 80 km, you might speed up, slow down or run into a traffic jam: your potential radius for the next hour will change immediately.
The graph of h(t) against time can have several shapes. Figure 7.2 shows a few very well known courses of h(t).

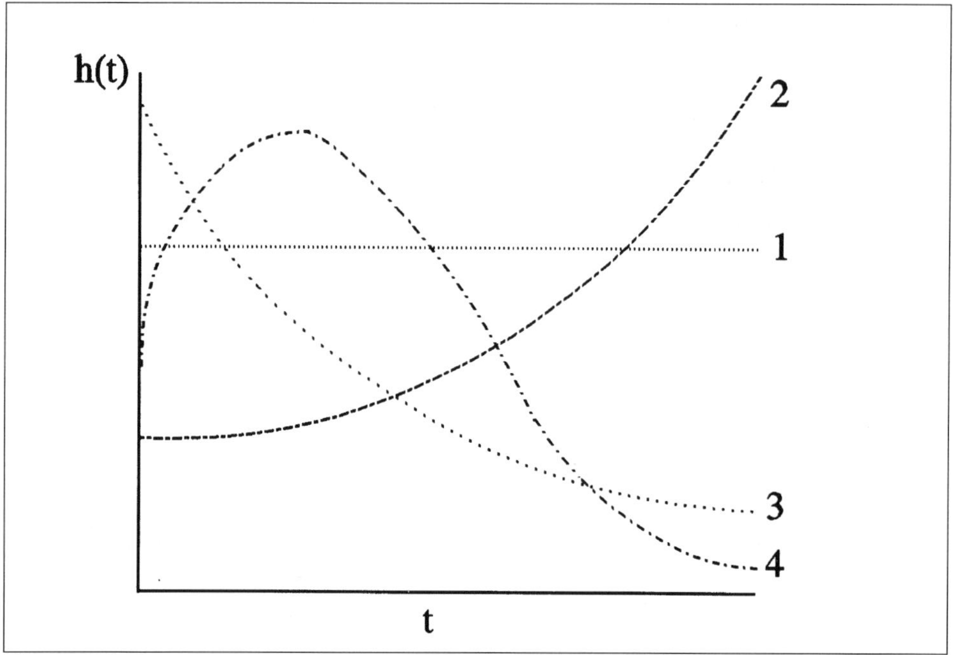

Figure 7.2. Some well known shapes of the hazard function.

1: **Exponential** - h(t) is constant; this means that an individual has a constant potential of showing the event (e.g., lameness due to trauma)

2: **Increasing Weibull** - as survival time increases, the potential of showing the event increases (e.g., being culled for dairy cows)

3: **Decreasing Weibull** - the potential of showing the event decreases as the survival time increases (e.g., dying after an operation: as a patient survives longer after the operation, the probability of dying due to the operation becomes less)

4: **Lognormal** - this type of graph can be expected in some diseases, when the potential of dying after infection first increases, but after some time decreases again (e.g., because of building up immunity)

As the probability of the occurrence of the event is at minimum zero, h(t) ranges from 0 to infinity. Suppose the numerator of h(t) is 0.4 and Δt = 0.5 days: then h(t) is 0.4/0.5 = 0.8 per day. If the time unit is in weeks, then 0.5 days equals 0.07 weeks (1/14) and h(t) is 0.4/0.07 = 5.6 per week (or: 7x0.8). Thus, the value of h(t) depends on the time unit, h(t) is never negative (lower limit is 0) and it has no upper limit.

The survivor function S(t) is focused on the event **not** occurring, while the hazard function h(t) is focused on the event occurring, given that it has not happened until time t. S(t) seems more logical for survival data, because it describes the data directly. h(t) can also be interesting, because:

- it tells something about the conditional failure rate;
- it can be used for mathematical modelling of survival data;
- it can be used to fit a statistical model that suits the data best.

In principle, it does not matter which function, S(t) or h(t), is used, because both are directly related by an ordinary differential equation:

$$h(t) = -\frac{1}{S(t)} * \frac{dS(t)}{dt} \qquad \textbf{(7.3)}$$

Suppose S(t) is described by the exponential function e^{-ct}, in which e is the base of the natural log, c is a positive constant (then S(t) is decreasing) and t denotes the time. Then, h(t) can be calculated as: $(-1/e^{-ct})$ multiplied by the first derivative of e^{-ct} being $-c*e^{-ct}$; thus h(t) = c. This also explains the term 'exponential hazard function' when h(t) is constant. Computer software easily calculates h(t) from S(t) and *vice versa*.

5. Purposes of Survival Analysis

Survival analysis is performed for mainly 3 reasons:

1. to compare survivor and/or hazard functions between groups;
2. to estimate survivor and/or hazard functions and to interpret them;
3. to calculate the relation between predictor variables and survival time.

Purpose 1 and 2 are descriptive, the third one analytical. In veterinary epidemiology, the third application is most common, especially in evaluating clinical trials.

The following example is derived from a vaccination trial in livestock production (see the Appendix for the data). There are two groups of about 115 animals each; one group was vaccinated (group V), while the other received a placebo (group P). The event was the diagnosis of clinical respiratory tract problems (CRTP). The trial lasted for 60 days. In the vaccinated group, 16 (13.9%) animals were diagnosed as positive, while it were 29 (25.0%) in the placebo treated group. During the study, 6 calves were censored because they showed no CRTP but died due to other reasons. The survival times (in days) are summarized in Table 7.1.

Table 7.1. Frequency distribution of survival times (NDAYS) per treatment group (P=Placebo, V=Vaccine), the symbol "+" indicates that one of the observations was censored.

NDAYS	Treat		Total
	P	V	
12	1+	0	1
14	1	0	1
18	1+	1	2
21	1	0	1
23	1+	0	1
25	1	2+	3
27	1	0	1
30	0	3+	3
32	1	0	1
35	1	0	1
37	0	1	1
38	0	1	1
39	1	0	1
40	1	0	1
41	0	4+	4
42	2	0	2
43	1	0	1
44	1	1	2
45	5	2	7
46	2	1	3
47	3	0	3
48	1	1	2
49	0	1	1
50	3	0	3
52	2	0	2
55	1	0	1
59	0	1	1
60	84	96	180
Total	116	115	231

From such a table, the mean and median survival times can be calculated, as is shown below.

Treat = P Category		per subject			
	Total	mean	min	median	max
no. of subjects	116				
(final) exit time		54.41379	12	60	60
time at risk	6312	54.41379	12	60	60
failures	29	.25	0	0	1

Treat = V Category		per subject			
	Total	mean	min	median	max
no. of subjects	115				
(final) exit time		56.46087	18	60	60
time at risk	6493	56.46097	18	60	60
failures	16	.1391304	0	0	1

The median survival time is equal to the study length, indicating that in both groups less than 50% of the animals have shown the event. The mean survival time is 2 days longer for group V. However, the proportion of failures is almost twice as high in the placebo group (0.25) compared to the vaccinated group (0.139).

In Table 7.2 on the next page, the results are structured further. Such a table is called a ***life table***. The number of observations showing the event in a specific interval is in the column headed as 'Deaths' while censored observations are in the column headed as 'Lost'.

Table 7.2. Life table vaccination trial data for vaccinated and placebo group.

Interval		Begin Total	Deaths	Lost	Survival	Std. Error	[95% Conf. Int.]	
TREAT P								
12	13	116	0	1	1.0000	0.0000	.	.
14	15	115	1	0	0.9913	0.0087	0.9399	0.9988
18	19	114	0	1	0.9913	0.0087	0.9399	0.9988
21	22	113	1	0	0.9825	0.0122	0.9320	0.9956
23	24	112	0	1	0.9825	0.0122	0.9320	0.9956
25	26	111	1	0	0.9737	0.0150	0.9206	0.9914
27	28	110	1	0	0.9648	0.0173	0.9090	0.9867
32	33	109	1	0	0.9560	0.0193	0.8975	0.9814
35	26	108	1	0	0.9471	0.0210	0.8861	0.9759
39	40	107	1	0	0.9383	0.0226	0.8749	0.9701
40	41	106	1	0	0.9294	0.0241	0.8638	0.9641
42	43	105	2	0	0.9117	0.0267	0.8421	0.9515
43	44	103	1	0	0.9029	0.0279	0.8315	0.9450
44	45	102	1	0	0.8940	0.0289	0.8209	0.9384
45	46	101	5	0	0.8498	0.0336	0.7695	0.9038
46	47	96	2	0	0.8321	0.0351	0.7494	0.8894
47	48	94	3	0	0.8055	0.0372	0.7198	0.8674
48	49	91	1	0	0.7966	0.0379	0.7100	0.8599
50	51	90	3	0	0.7701	0.0396	0.6810	0.8372
52	53	87	2	0	0.7514	0.0406	0.6619	0.8219
55	56	85	1	0	0.7435	0.0411	0.6525	0.8141
60	61	84	0	84	0.7435	0.0411	0.6525	0.8141
TREAT V								
18	19	115	1	0	0.9913	0.0087	0.9399	0.9988
25	26	114	1	1	0.9826	0.0122	0.9321	0.9956
30	31	112	2	1	0.9649	0.0172	0.9093	0.9867
37	38	109	1	0	0.9561	0.0192	0.8977	0.9815
38	39	108	1	0	0.9472	0.0210	0.8863	0.9759
41	42	107	3	1	0.9206	0.0254	0.8539	0.9579
44	45	103	1	0	0.9116	0.0267	0.8419	0.9514
45	46	102	2	0	0.8937	0.0290	0.8205	0.9382
46	47	100	1	0	0.8848	0.0301	0.8099	0.9314
48	49	99	1	0	0.8759	0.0311	0.7994	0.9245
49	50	98	1	0	0.8669	0.0320	0.7890	0.9176
59	60	97	1	0	0.8580	0.0329	0.7787	0.9105
60	61	96	0	96	0.8580	0.0329	0.7787	0.9105

Plotting the survival probabilities (in the column headed as 'Survival') against time gives the survival graph for both groups (synonym: Kaplan-Meier plot), which is very illustrative (Figure 7.3.a). Alternatively, the failure curve can be plotted, the failure probability being 1 minus the survival probability (Figure 7.3.b).

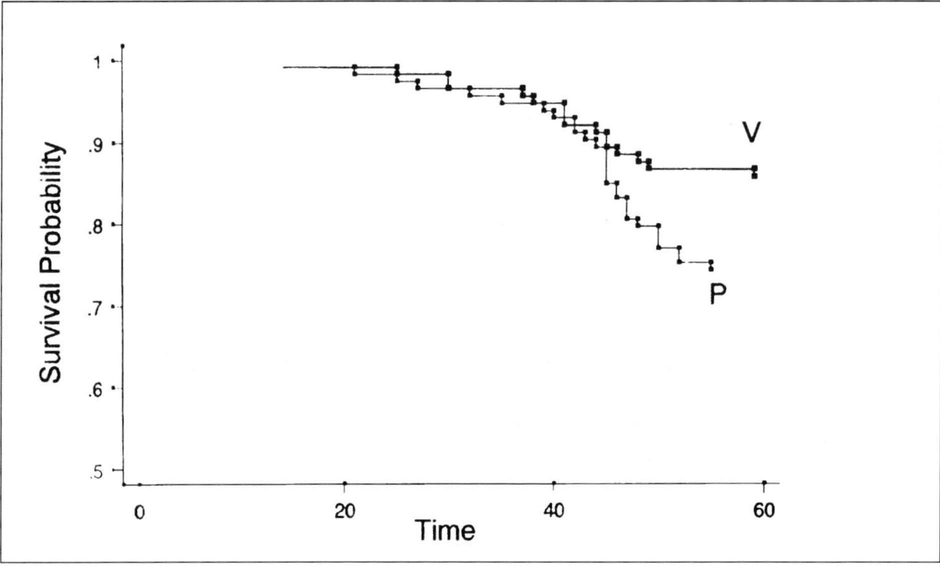

Figure 7.3.a. Kaplan-Meier survival curve of both treatment groups.

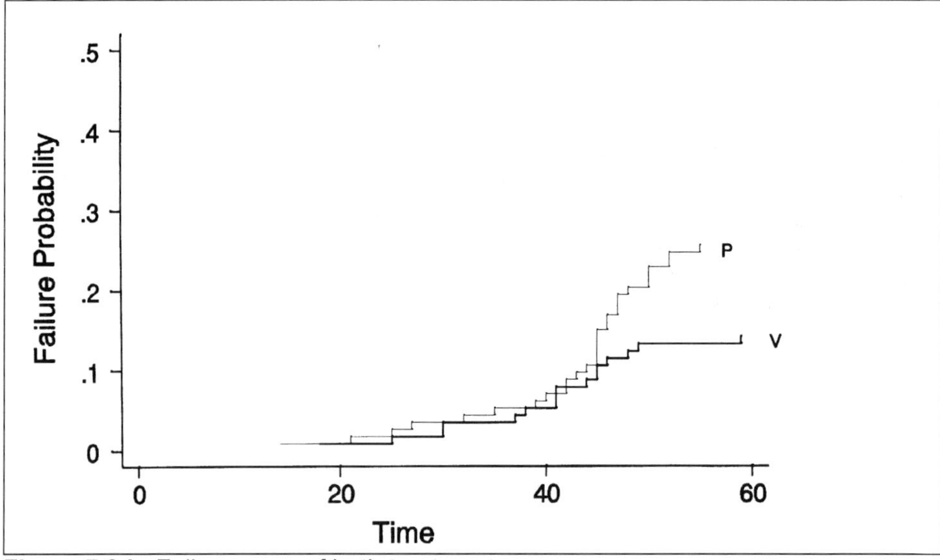

Figure 7.3.b. Failure curve of both treatment groups.

CRTP occurred especially in the period between 40 to 50 days of age. The curves are descriptive in nature (purpose 1) and several standard rank tests are available to say whether or not these curves are statistically equal (Table 7.3).

Table 7.3. Statistical evaluation of equality of survivor functions using the log-rank and the Wilcoxon test.

Log-rank test:			Wilcoxon (Breslow) test:			
Treat	Events observed	expected	Treat	Events observed	expected	Sum of ranks
P	29	22.11	P	29	22.11	1350
V	16	22.89	V	16	22.89	-1350
Total	45	45.00	Total	45	45.00	0
	chi2(1) =	4.25		chi2(1) =	3.89	
	Pr>chi2 =	0.0391		Pr>chi2 =	0.0487	

The tests indicate that both survival functions differ significantly ($P < 0.05$).

Subsequently we may look if the survival times follow a specific distribution (purpose 2), e.g., a Weibull or exponential distribution. The Weibull survival and hazard functions are given by formula 7.4 and 7.5 (Weibull, 1951), respectively.

$$S(t) = e^{-(a\,t)^p} \quad \textbf{(7.4)}$$

$$h(t) = a\,p\,(a\,t)^{p-1} \quad \textbf{(7.5)}$$

The 'p' is called the shape parameter and 'a' is the scale parameter. Both parameters need to be estimated from the data. Exponential regression is a special form of Weibull regression, namely when p equals 1. In Figure 7.4, both the Kaplan-Meier survival estimates and the Weibull survival curves are shown for each group separately. For the placebo group 'a' was estimated as 0.0109 and 'p' as 2.7946 while these estimates were 0.0076 and 2.3647 for group 2. In Figure 7.5 both hazard functions are shown.

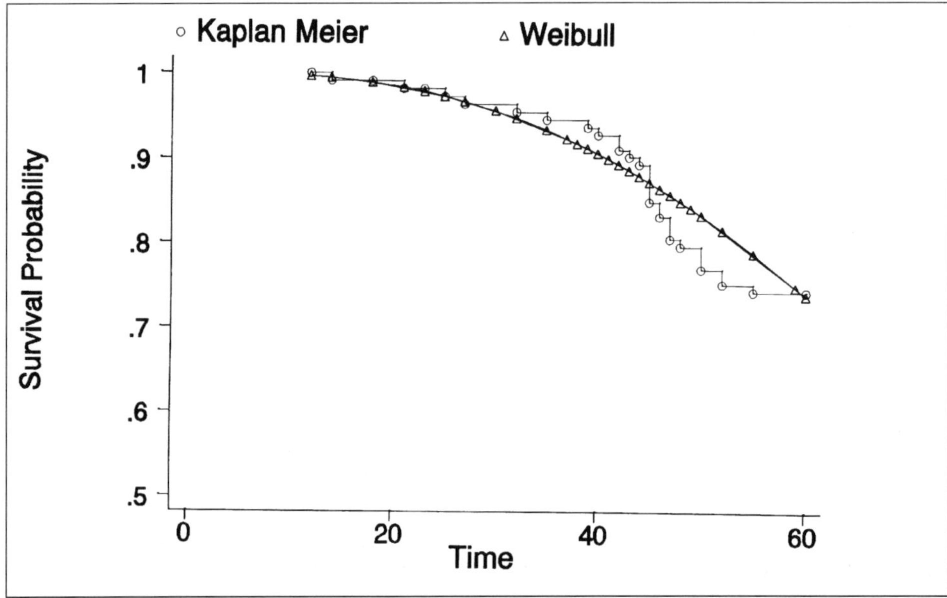

Figure 7.4.a. Kaplan-Meier and Weibull survival curve for placebo group.

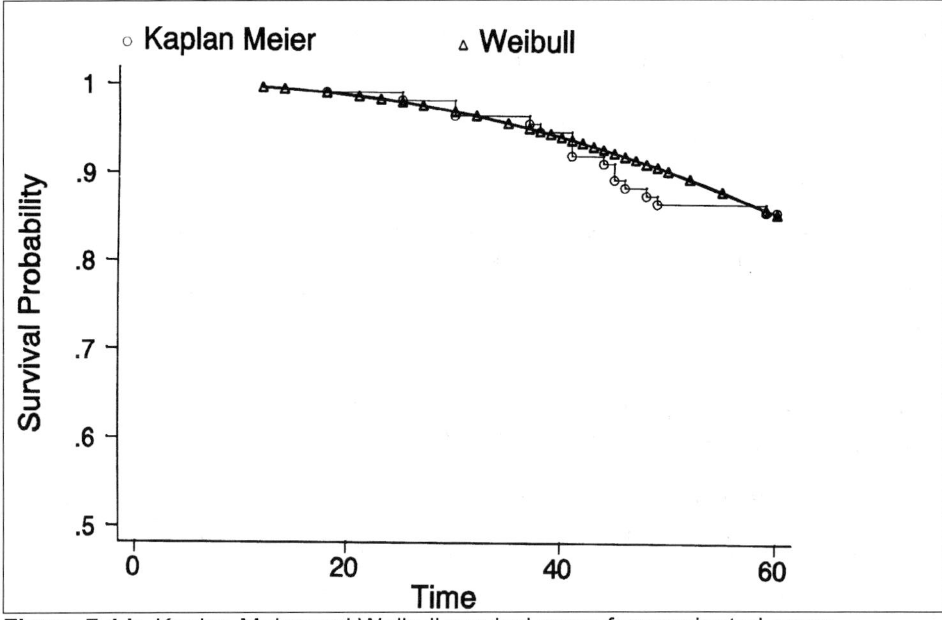

Figure 7.4.b. Kaplan-Meier and Weibull survival curve for vaccinated group.

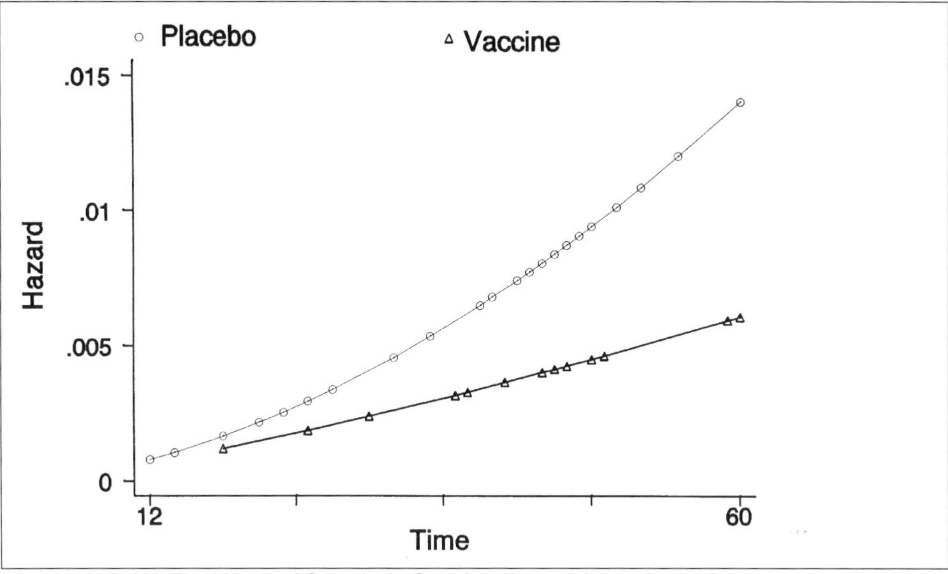

Figure 7.5. Weibull hazard functions for placebo and vaccinated group.

However, the main goal of a vaccination trial is not to describe the survivor functions in each group or to compare them in a qualitative way (purpose 1 and 2), but to obtain a quantitative measure (with its confidence interval) of the association between vaccination and CRTP (purpose 3). A simple measure would be the '**average hazard rate**' which can be calculated as:

$$h_i = \frac{\#\text{ failures}}{\sum t_i}$$

For group P, h_p equals 29/6312=0.00459, h_v equals 16/6493=0.00246 (see output on page 180). The relation between both, the **hazard ratio**, is 0.00246/0.00459 = 0.54. This is identical to the incidence rate ratio (IRR, Chapter V). The hazard ratio (HR) can be interpreted in the same way as the IRR:

HR = 1: the factor has no effect;
HR > 1: the factor is positively associated to the occurrence of the disease;
HR < 1: the factor is negatively associated to the occurrence of the disease.

One should take care about the length of the study period in relation to the moment when the last case occurred in that period. If during the last part of the study period no cases occurred, the IRR (and HR) will be underestimated. Suppose you have a small 10 day experiment with 2 treatment groups of 10 animals each. In both groups 5 cases occur, in group A on day 1, 2, 3, 4 and 5 and in group B on day 6, 7, 8, 9 and 10. Then, the time at risk in group A is 1 + 2 + 3 + 4 + 5 + 5∗10 = 65 and in group B the time at risk equals 6 + 7 + 8 + 9 + 10 + 5∗10 = 90. Thus, the IRR equals (5/65) / (5/(90) = 1.4. Extending the study with another 10 days, without any extra cases occurring, will give times at risk of 115 and 140, the IRR being 1.2. Extending the period further will force the IRR more to 1.0. Therefore, the length of the study period should be based on what is known about the epidemiology of the disease.

To calculate the HR, regression methods might be used in which the survival time is the outcome variable, taking censoring into account. In general, it is assumed that the hazard functions of individuals with different covariate patterns are proportional in time. This means that the hazard ratios do not change with time. Then, the hazard function might be described as: $h(t|x) = h_0(t) * g(x)$, where $g(x)$ is a function of the covariates and $h_0(t)$ is the baseline hazard, which is obtained when $g(x)$ equals 1. An exponential function is frequently used for $g(x)$ and then the hazard is given by:

$$h(t,x) = h_0(t) * e^{\beta_1 x_1 + \dots + \beta_k x_k} \qquad \textbf{(7.6)}$$

The hazard is described by the product of the baseline hazard $h_0(t)$ and an exponential function of k predictor variables. The baseline hazard is the hazard where all the predictor variables have the value 0 (recall: $e^0 = 1$). Now, the methods to calculate the HR, differ in how this baseline hazard is approached. In the following paragraphs, 3 approaches will be shown:

1. Cox proportional hazard regression (Cox, 1972): $h_0(t)$ is not specified;
2. Exponential regression: $h_0(t)$ equals 1;
3. Weibull regression: $h_0(t) = ap(at)^{p-1}$; a and p are estimated from the data.

6. Cox Proportional Hazard Model

$h(t,x)/h_0(t)$ (see formula 7.6) is a relative risk and thus $\beta_1 x_1 + \dots + \beta_k x_k$ is the natural log of that relative risk. Quite often one is not interested in the hazard of factor X compared to the theoretical baseline, but rather in the ratio of the hazards in the situation where factor X is present versus the situation where X is absent. In this case, that relative risk, called hazard ratio, is given by:

$$\frac{\dfrac{h(t,x=1)}{h_0(t)}}{\dfrac{h(t,x=0)}{h_0(t)}} = \frac{h(t,x=1)}{h(t,x=0)} = e^{\beta_1 x_1}$$

We see that the baseline hazard is cancelled out and it is not needed to specify it; it can have any shape. That is why the Cox model is called 'non-parametric' (and the reason why it is so popular). When a known baseline hazard is used (e.g., Weibull), the model is called parametric. The β's can be estimated with an iterative Maximum Likelihood method, just as in logistic regression. Exponentiation of the β's gives the HR. Predictor variables might be dichotomous, polytomous or continuous. The analysis strategy is in principle the same as in logistic regression (see Chapter VI).

One condition that needs to be satisfied in order to make a valid use of the Cox proportional hazard model is that the hazards of group x=0 and of group x=1 should be proportional in time (or: the HR should be constant in time). The proportionality can be assessed by plotting the survival curves on a log-log scale with ln[-ln(S(t)] on the Y-axis and ln(t) on the X-axis. The two resulting curves for group x=0 and x=1 should be more or less parallel.

Using the data of the vaccination trial data again, the output of Cox regression is:

```
Iteration 0:  Log Likelihood =        -239.35531
Iteration 1:  Log Likelihood =        -237.22132
Iteration 2:  Log Likelihood =        -237.21987

No. of subjects =    231                          Log likelihood =   -237.21987
No. of failures =     45                          chi2(1) =               4.27
Time at risk    =  12805                          Prob > chi2 =         0.0388
```

	Haz. Ratio	Std. Err.	z	P>|z|	[95% Conf. Interval]	
TREATN	.5329778	.1660088	-2.020	0.043	.2894556	.9813781

(TREATN is coded as 0 for the placebo group and as 1 for the vaccinated group).

In iteration 0, the log likelihood of a model without any parameters (L_0) is calculated. The last iteration (in this case iteration 2) is the final solution giving the log likelihood (L1) of the model with parameter TREATN. Now, recall the -2log likelihood ratio (or deviance difference) in logistic regression (Chapter VI). This can be calculated from this output as:

$$-2L_0 - -2L_1 = 478.71 - 474.44 = 4.27$$

This value is directly in the output as chi2(1), with its probability. The hazard ratio equals 0.54, indicating that the HR in the vaccinated group is almost half of that in the placebo group. The HR is significantly smaller than 1.0 as this value is excluded from the 95% confidence interval. An output with regression coefficients, standard errors, a Z value (being the square root of the Wald statistic), a *P*-value (based on the Chi-square distribution and using Z^2) and a 95% confidence interval for the regression coefficient can be obtained as well, as is shown below.

```
No. of subjects =       231                       Log likelihood =   -237.21987
No. of failures =        45                       chi2(1) =               4.27
Time at risk =        12805                       Prob > chi2 =         0.0388
```

	Coef.	Std. Err	z	P > |z|	[95% Conf. Interval]	
TREATN	- .6292755	.3114741	-2.020	0.043	-1.239753	- .0187975

This output is quite similar to the output of logistic regression, the difference being that exponentiation of the coefficient will give an hazard ratio instead of an odds ratio.

Now, we introduce the covariate IgG (immunoglobulin G, derived from colostrum) as a potential confounder. It might well be that IgG level has a significant relation with

CRTP and that the distribution of the IgG level is not equal for both groups. Then, the outcome for the variable TREATN might be biased. IgG has been categorized into 4 classes (IgG1: ≤ 5, IgG2: 5-10, IgG3: 10-15 and IgG4: > 15 mmol/l). Categorization was necessary because the logits where not linear (see paragraph 4 of Chapter VI). The class of 5-10 mmol/l was chosen as reference category.

No. of subjects =	231			Log likelihood =	-231.83572	
No. of failures =	45			chi2(4) =	15.04	
Time at risk =	12805			Prob > chi2 =	0.0046	
	Haz. Ratio	Std. Err.	z	P > |z|	[95% Conf. Interval]	
TREATN	.5443988	.1699791	-1.958	0.051	.2952189	1.003899
IgG1	2.621342	1.178825	2.143	0.032	1.085765	6.328654
IgG3	1.548873	.7544785	0.898	0.369	.5961881	4.023912
IgG4	3.619782	1.585998	2.936	0.003	1.533665	8.543468

From this output we learn that the HR for TREATN is almost identical to the model without the IgG dummy variables, indicating that IgG is no confounder. IgG is significantly related to CRTP as the deviance difference is 15.04 - 4.27 = 10.77 with 3 *df* (*P* = 0.013). There seems to be an optimal IgG level as at both very low and very high levels there is an increased risk of CRTP. This was also the reason why using IgG as a linear variable was not valid.

It is needed to check whether or not the use of the Cox model was justified, as the hazards should be proportional in time. For that purpose the log-log plot is needed, in which ln(-ln(S(t)) is plotted against the ln(time). Figure 7.6 shows that the 2 lines are reasonably parallel and that the proportional hazard assumption is not violated.

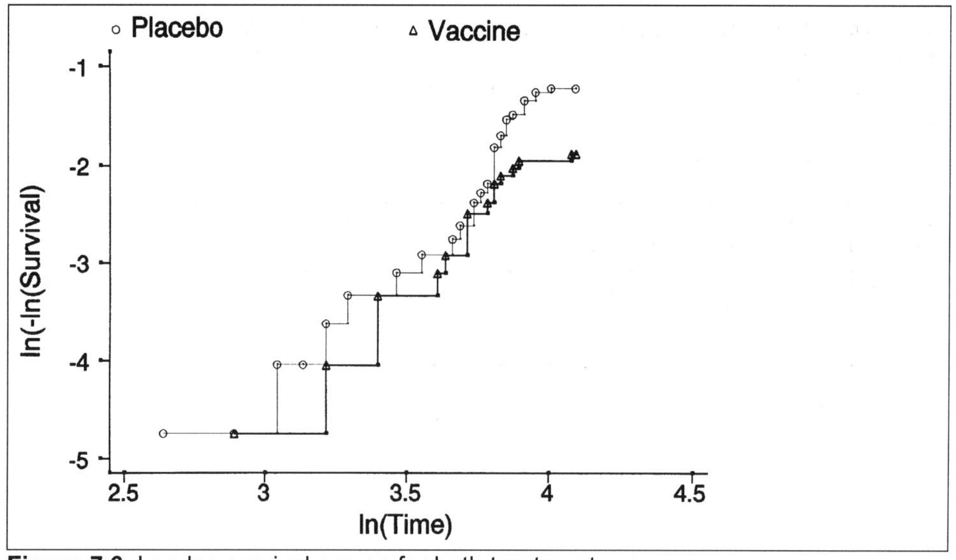

Figure 7.6. Log-log survival curves for both treatment groups.

7. Weibull and Exponential Regression

Using the nonparametric Cox survival model, it was not necessary to make inferences about $h_0(t)$. In the exponential regression model it is assumed that $h_0(t) = 1$ and in Weibull regression $h_0(t) = a*p*(a*t)^{p-1}$ (if p = 1, this reduces to the exponential model). If the survival distributions follow a known pattern, parametric tests are more powerful than non-parametric ones. However, their computation is more difficult. After Cox regression (or Kaplan-Meier calculations) it is possible to make inferences about whether or not to use a parametric model. If the line of the ln(-ln(Survival)) against ln(Time) is about linear, a Weibull distribution might be the best solution. If this straight line has a slope of about 1, it reduces to the exponential distribution.

If the data of the vaccine trial is fitted in a Weibull regression, the output is as shown below.

Weibull regression

No. of subjects =	231	Log likelihood =	-114.88976
No. of failures =	45	chi2(1) =	4.64
Time at risk =	12805	Prob > chi2 =	0.0312

	Haz. Ratio	Std. Err.	z	P > |z|	[95% Conf.	Interval]
TREATN	.5190938	.1616874	-2.105	0.035	.2819119	.9558246
ln p	.9662456	.1434726	6.735	0.000	.6850444	1.247447
p	2.628059				1.98386	3.481443
1/p	.3805089				.2872372	.5040678

We see that vaccination reduces the hazard of CRTP with about 0.5. 'p' equals 2.63, indicating that the hazard increases with time (see also Figure 7.5). We can make the treatment effect more visible in a hazard plot; for that purpose the output with the coefficients is needed:

	Coef.	Std. Err.	z	P > |z|	[95% Conf.	Interval]
TREATN	-.6556707	.3114801	-2.105	0.035	- 1.266161	- .0451809
cons	-11.96438	1.541081	-7.764	0.000	-14.98484	-8.943917
ln p	.9662456	.1434726	6.735	0.000	.6850444	1.247447
p	2.628059				1.98386	3.481443
1/p	.3805089				.2872372	.5040678

From this output the scale parameter 'a' is calculated as $e^{(cons/p)} = 0.0105$. Then, the hazard function for the placebo group is given by:

$$0.0105*2.6281*(0.0105*NDAYS)^{2.6281-1}*e^{-0.6557*0} = h_0(t)$$

and for the vaccine group by:

$0.0105*2.6281*(0.0105*NDAYS)^{2.6281-1}*e^{-0.6557*1} = h_0(t)*e^{\beta_1}$

If the hazards of both groups are plotted against time (Figure 7.7), about the same graph as Figure 7.5 is obtained. It can be seen that the hazard in the vaccinated group is about half of the hazard in the placebo group at each point in time.

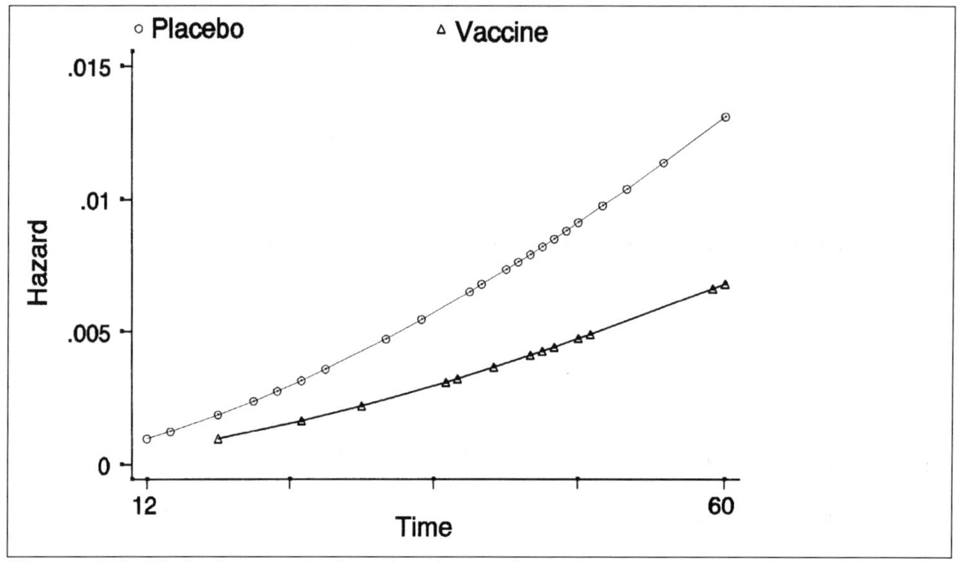

Figure 7.7. Weibull hazards for placebo and vaccine group as estimated from the Weibull regression model.

Though p is 2.63, the exponential regression (using p = 1) can be fitted as well:

Exponental regression

No. of subjects =	231	Log likelihood =	-131.48046
No. of failures =	45	chi2(1) =	4.19
Time at risk =	12805	Prob > chi2 =	0.0408

	Haz. Ratio	Std. Err.	z	P > |z|	[95% Conf.	Interval]
TREATN	.5363442	.1670286	-2.000	0.045	.2913144	.987473

The exponential HR is identical to the IRR (see Chapter V). The IRR equals (16/6493) / (29/6312) = 0.5363. For the calculation of the confidence interval for this IRR, the following steps were needed:

1. take the natural logarithm of the IRR (which is equal to the exponential regression coefficient), ln(0.5363) = -0.6231;
2. calculate the standard deviation of this transformed IRR, $\sqrt{(1/29 + 1/16)} = 0.3114$;

3. calculate the confidence interval of the transformed value: $-0.6231 \pm 1.96*0.3114 = [-1.2334; -0.0128]$;
4. calculate the confidence interval of the IRR by exponentiating the outcome of step 3: $[e^{-1.2334}; e^{-0.0128}] = [0.2913; 0.9873]$.

Comparing the output of Cox, Weibull and exponential regression:

	Hazard ratio 95%	Confidence interval	Deviance difference
Cox	0.53	[0.29; 0.98]	4.27
Weibull	0.52	[0.28; 0.96]	4.64
Exponential	0.54	[0.29; 0.99]	4.19

It shows that the hazard ratios and the confidence intervals are about equal. From the deviance difference it can be concluded that Weibull has a slightly better relative goodness of fit.

8. Concluding Remarks

In veterinary epidemiology, survival analysis is most frequently used for analytical purposes (estimation of hazard ratios) and far less in a descriptive setting (estimating the course of a survival curve for prognostic purposes). Also in studies regarding animal reproduction, the technique of survival analysis is applied (e.g., factors affecting the time interval between parturition and insemination). See the list of further readings for some references in this field.

The proportional hazard model of Cox is most frequently used and will give satisfactory results if the proportional odds assumption holds. The use of parametric models (Weibull, exponential) is less common, though the (univariate) exponential model yields the incidence rate ratio (IRR), which is one of the basic measures of association.

The development of survival analysis techniques is still going on, resulting in further refinements. For example, one can take into account a covariate which value changes over time (a *time-varying* covariate). An example might be, that an animal is preventively treated (e.g., routine claw trimming) during the study which affects the occurrence of the disease of interest (e.g., sole ulcer). Then, this animal will be present with 2 records in the data set: one record ending (exit) at the moment the claw trimming is carried out and the second record starts (entry) at the moment the first one ends. If the animal was trimmed at day 24 and showed a sole ulcer at day 63, then the records would be as presented below.

Rec. no.	Animal id.	Entry	Exit	Trim	Sole ulcer
1	9	0	24	0	0
2	9	24	63	1	1

A last remark is that still much work needs to be done on regression diagnostics (e.g., goodness-of-fit) in relation to survival analysis models.

References

Studies. John Wiley and Sons, New York.
Thomson, B.L.; Jorsal, S.E.; Andersen, S.; Willeberg, P. (1992). The Cox regression model applied to risk factor analysis of Cox, D.R. (1972). Regression models and life tables. Journal of the Royal Statistical Society B, 34, 187-195.
StataCorp. (1997). Stata Statistical Software: Release 5.0. College Station, TX: Stata Corporation.
Weibull, W. (1951). A statistical distribution of wide applicability. Journal of Applied Mechanics, 18, 293-297.

Further Reading

Suggested further reading (examples of survival analysis in veterinary epidemiology and/or reproduction):

Barkema, H.W.; Schukken, Y.H.; Guard, C.L.; Brand, A; Weyden, G.C. van der (1992). Fertility, production and culling following cesarean section in dairy cattle. Theriogenology, 38, 589-599.
Beaudeau, F.; Ducrocq, V; Fourichon, C.; Seegers, H. (1995). Effect of disease on length of productive life of French Holstein dairy cows assessed by survival analysis. Journal of Dairy Science, 78, 103-117.
Ducrocq, V.; Quaas, R.L.; Pollack, E.J.; Casella, G. (1988). Length of productive life of dairy cows. 1. Justification of a Weibull model. Journal of Dairy Science, 71, 3061-3070.
Kleinbaum, D.G. (1996). Survival Analysis: a Self-learning Text. Springer, New York.
Lee, E.T. (1992). Statistical Methods for Survival Data Analysis. John Wiley and Sons, New York.
Lee, L.A.; Ferguson, J.D.; Galligan, D.T. (1989). Effect of disease on days open assessed by survival analysis. Journal of Dairy Science, 72, 1020-1026.
Marubini, E; Valsecchi, M.G. (1995). Analysing Survival Data from Clinical Trials and Observational infections in the breeding and multiplying herds in the Danish SPF system. Preventive Veterinary Medicine, 12, 287-297.
Thysen, I. (1988). Application of event time analysis to replacement, health and reproduction data in dairy cattle research. Preventive Veterinary Medicine, 5, 239-250.

Appendix: Vaccination Trial Data

Vaccination trial data group P.

group	ndays[1]	CRTP[2]	IgG[3]	group	ndays	CRTP	IgG	group	ndays	CRTP	IgG
P	12	0	8	P	60	0	6	P	60	0	10
P	14	1	28	P	60	0	14	P	60	0	5
P	18	0	12	P	60	0	22	P	60	0	14
P	21	1	5	P	60	0	2	P	60	0	14
P	23	0	4	P	60	0	12	P	60	0	7
P	25	1	16	P	60	0	12	P	60	0	24
P	27	1	6	P	60	0	12	P	60	0	10
P	32	1	3	P	60	0	12	P	60	0	6
P	35	1	3	P	60	0	16	P	60	0	12
P	39	1	22	P	60	0	10	P	60	0	6
P	40	1	12	P	60	0	4	P	60	0	5
P	42	1	4	P	60	0	28	P	60	0	14
P	42	1	9	P	60	0	12	P	60	0	3
P	43	1	6	P	60	0	5	P	60	0	8
P	44	1	8	P	60	0	8	P	60	0	12
P	45	1	7	P	60	0	14	P	60	0	4
P	45	1	18	P	60	0	21	P	60	0	7
P	45	1	20	P	60	0	9	P	60	0	8
P	45	1	5	P	60	0	2	P	60	0	6
P	45	1	5	P	60	0	12	P	60	0	3
P	46	1	10	P	60	0	12	P	60	0	24
P	46	1	8	P	60	0	14	P	60	0	8
P	47	1	18	P	60	0	5	P	60	0	10
P	47	1	4	P	60	0	9	P	60	0	15
P	47	1	12	P	60	0	5	P	60	0	22
P	48	1	18	P	60	0	8	P	60	0	8
P	50	1	14	P	60	0	8	P	60	0	7
P	50	1	11	P	60	0	12	P	60	0	12
P	50	1	14	P	60	0	4	P	60	0	8
P	52	1	26	P	60	0	4	P	60	0	22
P	52	1	20	P	60	0	18	P	60	0	10
P	55	1	2	P	60	0	12	P	60	0	12
P	60	0	26	P	60	0	8	P	60	0	12
P	60	0	3	P	60	0	8	P	60	0	7
P	60	0	14	P	60	0	10				
P	60	0	4	P	60	0	4				
P	60	0	6	P	60	0	16				
P	60	0	15	P	60	0	9				
P	60	0	4	P	60	0	16				
P	60	0	9	P	60	0	14				
P	60	0	26	P	60	0	3				

[1] ndays = time at-risk,
[2] CRTP = clinical respiratory tract problems,
[3] IgG = Immunoglobulin G level (in mmol/l)

Vaccination trial data group V.

group	ndays[1]	CRTP[2]	IgG[3]	group	ndays	CRTP	IgG	group	ndays	CRTP	IgG
V	18	1	11	V	60	0	9	V	60	0	4
V	25	1	26	V	60	0	10	V	60	0	14
V	25	0	4	V	60	0	16	V	60	0	7
V	30	1	3	V	60	0	12	V	60	0	10
V	30	0	8	V	60	0	5	V	60	0	8
V	30	1	12	V	60	0	10	V	60	0	8
V	37	1	1	V	60	0	10	V	60	0	12
V	38	1	3	V	60	0	12	V	60	0	8
V	41	1	25	V	60	0	12	V	60	0	6
V	41	1	2	V	60	0	6	V	60	0	7
V	41	0	6	V	60	0	18	V	60	0	6
V	41	1	8	V	60	0	8	V	60	0	12
V	44	1	16	V	60	0	16	V	60	0	10
V	45	1	20	V	60	0	6	V	60	0	2
V	45	1	20	V	60	0	8	V	60	0	4
V	46	1	16	V	60	0	2	V	60	0	8
V	48	1	12	V	60	0	12	V	60	0	20
V	49	1	15	V	60	0	6	V	60	0	15
V	59	1	2	V	60	0	17	V	60	0	6
V	60	0	3	V	60	0	11	V	60	0	14
V	60	0	12	V	60	0	8	V	60	0	16
V	60	0	17	V	60	0	14	V	60	0	7
V	60	0	18	V	60	0	8	V	60	0	9
V	60	0	11	V	60	0	12	V	60	0	4
V	60	0	9	V	60	0	18	V	60	0	8
V	60	0	10	V	60	0	1				
V	60	0	18	V	60	0	8				
V	60	0	5	V	60	0	20				
V	60	0	2	V	60	0	21				
V	60	0	8	V	60	0	4				
V	60	0	28	V	60	0	5				
V	60	0	12	V	60	0	8				
V	60	0	4	V	60	0	1				
V	60	0	14	V	60	0	5				
V	60	0	20	V	60	0	12				
V	60	0	6	V	60	0	15				
V	60	0	18	V	60	0	7				
V	60	0	7	V	60	0	12				
V	60	0	8	V	60	0	7				
V	60	0	7	V	60	0	3				
V	60	0	11	V	60	0	24				
V	60	0	5	V	60	0	10				
V	60	0	2	V	60	0	8				
V	60	0	4	V	60	0	8				
V	60	0	2	V	60	0	9				

[1] ndays = time at-risk,
[2] CRTP = clinical respiratory tract problems,
[3] IgG = Immunoglobulin G level (in mmol/l)

9. Exercise: Probiotic Trial

(Data were extracted with permission from report 90.015: 'A study into the effect of a probiotic on the course of an induced infection with enteropathogenic *Escherichia coli* in piglets', Animal Health Service, Boxtel, The Netherlands, 33 pages, in Dutch).

9.1. Introduction

In a pilot study it was shown that the addition of probiotics to feed of piglets exerts a preventive effect on infection with entero-pathogenic *E. coli* bacteria. These agents are frequently involved in diarrhoea around weaning. A general description of a 'probiotic' is: organisms or substances that, in an effective dose, contribute to the microbiological equilibrium in the gastro-intestinal tract by reducing the colonization of pathogenic organisms. The administration of this specific probiotic seems, at least partly, to prevent the symptoms of the weaning diarrhoea complex under laboratory conditions. In the study below, the efficacy of this probiotic is tested under field conditions. The aim was to determine whether or not the probiotic, administered via the feed, could reduce the severity of an induced *E. coli* infection in weaned piglets under field conditions. Piglets were obtained from herds with and without a relatively high incidence of weaning diarrhoea (problem and non-problem herds).

9.2. Material

In total 180 piglets were available, 90 came from 2 problem herds and 90 from 2 non-problem herds. Four days before weaning (at an average age of 3 weeks), 4 groups were created: a probiotic treated group and a control group (without probiotic) one of each within problem herds and non-problem herds. From this moment on, piglets in the treatment groups received the probiotic. At an average age of 25 days, the piglets were weaned by removing the sow. Piglets stayed for another 3 days in the farrowing pen and were then moved to another barn with 2 units. Piglets of non-problem herds were allocated to unit 1, piglets of problem herds to unit 2. The number of piglets per group and per pen were not exactly equal because the number of piglets per sow and the number of places available per pen and per unit did not fit exactly.

From weaning until 16 days after arrival in the barn, piglets received the same feed as at the farm of origin (with or without the probiotic of course). Then, all piglets were fed the same feed (but still with or without the probiotic). Ten days after arrival, a dose of entero-pathogenic *E. coli* was administered orally to all piglets. The trial succeeded for another 23 days.

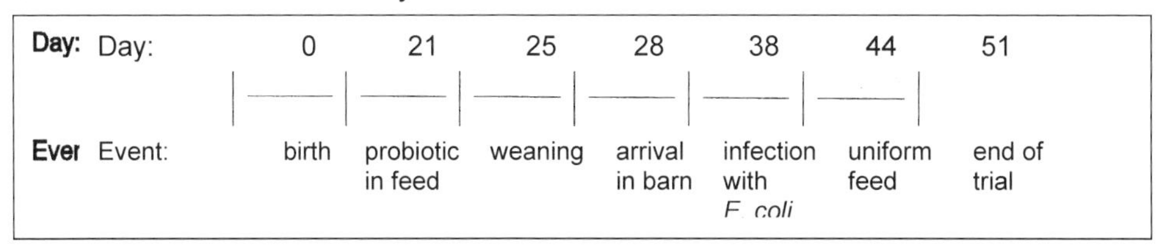

9.3. Results

Table 7.4 shows some descriptive figures of the trial. The exact day of death of animals in each group is shown in Table 7.5.

Table 7.4. Description of design (columns 1 to 5) and results (column 6).

Unit 1 non-problem herds						Unit 2 problem herds					
pen	group	herd	feed	n	dead	pen	group	herd	feed	n	dead
11	prob.	3	3	13	6	21	prob.	1	1	13	8
12	prob.	3	3	13	5	22	prob.	1	1	13	7
13	prob.	4	4	13	1	23	prob.	2	2	13	1
14	prob.	4	4	7	0	24	prob.	1+2	2	12	4
15	contr.	3	3	14	0	25	contr.	1	1	13	4
16	contr.	4	4	14	0	26	contr.	2	2	13	0
17	contr.	3+4	3	16	0	27	contr	1+2	2	13	3

Table 7.5. Number of animals that died per day in each group.

	Probiotic group herd of origin		Control group herd of origin	
Day	non-problem	problem	non-problem	problem
1				
2				
3				
4				
5				1
6				
7				
8				
9		1		
10				
11				
12				
13	1			
14	1			
15	2	1		
16	3	3		
17	3	3		1
18	1	5		1
19		5		3
20				
21				
22	1	1		1
23		1		
Total	12	20	0	7

Notes:* No separate effects of unit and herd of origin can be calculated. Furthermore, feed is nested with herd of origin. It would have been better to provide the animals the same feed from the start of the experiment (maybe even from moment of weaning).

* There should be a correction for pen effects. It is obvious (see Table 7.4) that in some pens the mortality was higher than in other pens. Nevertheless, in this exercise it is assumed that all observations were independent.

9.4. Questions

Relative risk calculation based on cumulative incidences

1a. Calculate the cumulative incidence ratio (CIR) for the use of probiotic from the cumulative incidence with its 95% confidence interval.
1b. As 1a, but now per stratum (non-problem herds, problem herds).
1c. Calculate the herd-of-origin adjusted CIR for the use of probiotic from the cumulative incidence with its 95% confidence interval using some multivariate technique.
1d. Draw your conclusion.

Relative risk calculation based on incidence rates

2a. Calculate the incidence rate ratio (IRR) for the use of probiotic from the incidence rates with its 95% confidence interval. First, calculate the number of days at risk per group.
2b. As 2a, but now per stratum (non-problem herds, problem herds).
2c. What does it mean that the CIR (in 1a) and IRR (in 2a) are not equal?
2d. Which measure of association is best to use, the CIR or the IRR? Account for your answer.

3a. Produce the life table and Kaplan-Meier survival curves for the control and the probiotic group.
3b. Calculate the crude and the herd-of-origin adjusted hazard ratio for the use of probiotic with its 95% confidence interval using Cox, Weibull and exponential regression.
3c. Draw your conclusion.

10. Answers

This exercise cannot be solved easily by manual calculations, a statistical software package is recommended.

1a. The CIR is in the row denoted as Risk ratio and is calculated as (32/97)/(7/83) = 3.91. The confidence interval indicates that the Exposure (= feeding probiotics) significantly increases the risk of dying because 1.0 is excluded from the 95% confidence interval.

	Exposed	Unexposed	Total
Cases	32	7	39
Noncases	65	76	141
Total	97	83	180

Risk	.3298969	.0843373	.2166667	
	Pt. Est.		[95% Conf. Interval]	
Risk difference	.2455596		.1345239	.356592
Risk ratio	**3.911635**		**1.822939**	**8.393525**
Attr. frac. ex.	.7443524		.4514354	.8808605
Attr. frac. pop	.6107507			
	chi2(1) =15.78		Pr > chi2 =0.0001	

1b. 'Origin' was coded as 0 for non-problem herds and as 1 for problem herds. As no control animals originating from non-problem herds died (see Table 7.5 in exercise description), the CIR of treatment cannot be calculated within this group.

origin	CIR	[95% Conf. Interval]		M-H Weight
0	.	.	.	0
1	**2.184874**	1.028955	4.639343	3.966667
Crude	3.911635	1.822939	8.393525	
M-H combined	.	.	.	
Test for heterogeneity (M-H)		chi2 (1) = 0.000	Pr>chi2 = 1.0000	

1c. We could either use a Mantel-Haenszel formula or logistic regression. The Mantel-Haenszel estimator is already given in 1b but is not calculated due to a zero cell frequency. Logistic regression gives:

Logit Estimates — Number of obs = 180; chi(2) = 24.09; Prob > chi2 = 0.0000; Log Likelihood = - 82.032879; Pseudo R2 = 0.1280

died	Odds Ratio	Std. Err.	z	P>|z|	[95% Conf. Intervall]	
treat	5.37137	2.455077	3.678	0.000	2.192951	13.15653
origin	2.805742	1.130249	2.561	0.010	1.273956	6.179322

The OR equals 5.4, but is a biased estimator of the CIR. If we have the regression coefficients, we can calculate the CIR directly (but not its confidence interval), from the coefficients:

Iteration 0: Log Likelihood = -94.078184
Iteration 2: Log Likelihood = -82.045318
Iteration 3: Log Likelihood = -82.032885
Iteration 4: Log Likelihood = -82.032879

Logit Estimates — Number of obs = 180; chi(2) = 24.09; Prob > chi2 = 0.0000; Log Likelihood = - 82.032879; Pseudo R2 = 0.1280

died	Coef.	Std. Err.	z	P>|z|	[95% Conf. Intervall]	
treat	1.681083	.4570671	3.678	0.000	.7853479	2.576918
origin	1.031668	.4028343	2.561	0.010	.2421272	1.821209
cons	-2.978653	.4832768	-6.163	0.000	-3.925858	-2.031448

The probability of disease (see Chapter VI) equals:

$$P(Y=1 \mid X) = \frac{e^{\beta_0 + \beta_1 x}}{1 + e^{\beta_0 + \beta_1 x}}$$

For the probiotic group, x was coded as 1, for the control group as 0 (and only β_0 remains in the formula). Then the probabilities for each group can be calculated:

P(died | probiotic) = 0.215
P(died | no probiotic) = 0.048

and the CIR is the ratio of these 2 probabilities:

CIR = 0.215 / 0.048 = 4.48

1d. Feeding of this probiotic increases (!) the risk to die about 4 fold. The next (and most important) step is to explain this outcome in terms of causality. The most likely explanation was an interaction with another additive in the feed, making both less effective.

2a. The time at risk is shown in the row denoted as 'Person-time' and the IRR equals (32/2044)/(7/1867) = 4.18, which is in the row 'Inc. rate ratio'. The IRR is significantly larger than 1.0 as this value is excluded from the 95% confidence interval. This confidence interval was calculated using an exact method instead of a large sample size approximation.

	Exposed	Unexposed	Total	
Cases	32	7	39	
Person-time	2044	1867	3911	
Incidence Rate	.0156556	.0037493	.0099719	
	Pt. Est.		[95% Conf. Interval]	
Inc. rate diff.	.0119062		.0058122	.0180003
Inc. rate ratio	**4.175566**		**1.810441**	**11.20545(exact)**
Attr. frac. ex.	.7605115		.4476484	.9107577(exact)
Attr. frac. pop	.6240094			

2b. Again the IRR for the non-problem herds is not calculated due to the zero cell frequency. Also the Mantel-Haenszel estimator is not calculated:

origin	IRR	[95% Conf. Interval]		M-H Weight	
0	.	2.875195	.	0	(exact)
1	**2.291611**	.9320197	6.414161	3.884435	(exact)
Crude	4.175566	1.810441	11.20545		(exact)
M-H combined	.	.	.		
Test for heterogeneity (M-H)		chi2 (1) = 0.00		Pr > chi2 = 1.0000	

2c. The difference between CIR and IRR indicates that mortality in both groups has not an equal distribution over time. Since the IRR (4.2) is larger than the CIR (3.9), mortality starts somewhat ***earlier*** in the exposed group (probiotic group), which can be seen directly from Table 7.5 in the exercise description.

2d. It is better to use the risk estimator based incidence rates, since animals that died are not at risk any more. However, in this specific trial the difference between CIR and IRR is relatively small.

3a. In a life table the data are summarized and the survival probabilities are calculated.

Interval		Begin Total	Deaths	Lost	Survival	Std. Error	[95% Conf. Int.]	
Control								
5	6	83	1	0	0.9880	0.0120	0.9175	0.9983
17	18	82	1	0	0.9759	0.0168	0.9071	0.9939
18	19	81	1	0	0.9639	0.0205	0.7821	0.9882
19	20	80	3	0	0.9277	0.0284	0.8462	0.9669
22	23	77	1	0	0.9157	0.0305	0.8312	0.9589
23	24	76	0	76	0.9157	0.0305	0.8312	0.9589
Probiotic								
9	10	97	1	0	0.9897	0.0103	0.9291	0.9985
13	14	96	1	0	0.9794	0.0144	0.9201	0.9948
14	15	95	1	0	0.9691	0.0176	0.9072	0.9899
15	16	94	3	0	0.9381	0.0245	0.8675	0.9717
16	17	91	6	0	0.8763	0.0334	0.7924	0.9278
17	18	85	6	0	0.8144	0.0395	0.7218	0.8788
18	19	79	6	0	0.7526	0.0438	0.6540	0.8267
19	20	73	5	0	0.7010	0.0465	0.5992	0.7816
22	23	68	2	0	0.6804	0.0473	0.5777	0.7632
23	24	66	1	65	0.6601	0.0501	0.5520	0.7480

The final Survival probabilities (0.9157 for the control group and 0.6601 for the probiotic group) are equal to 1 minus the CIR for each group (see table in answer 1a).

The Kaplan-Meier survival curves are shown in Figure 7.8, they represent the survival probabilities from the life table in a graphical form. The probability to survive is much higher in the control group.

3b. Before using Cox regression, the proportional hazard assumption needs to be verified by plotting the log-log curves for each treatment group. These curves need to be parallel (see Figure 7.9).

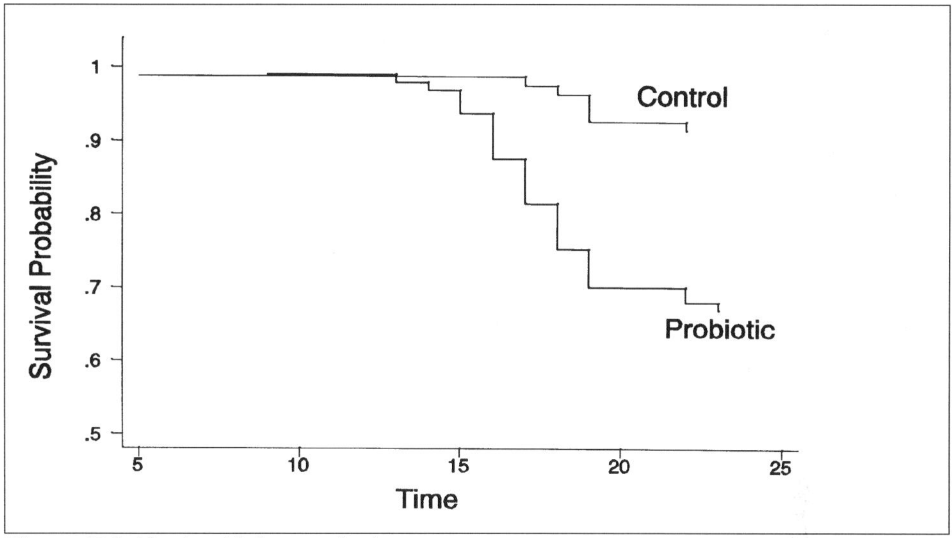

Figure 7.8. Kaplan-Meier survival curves.

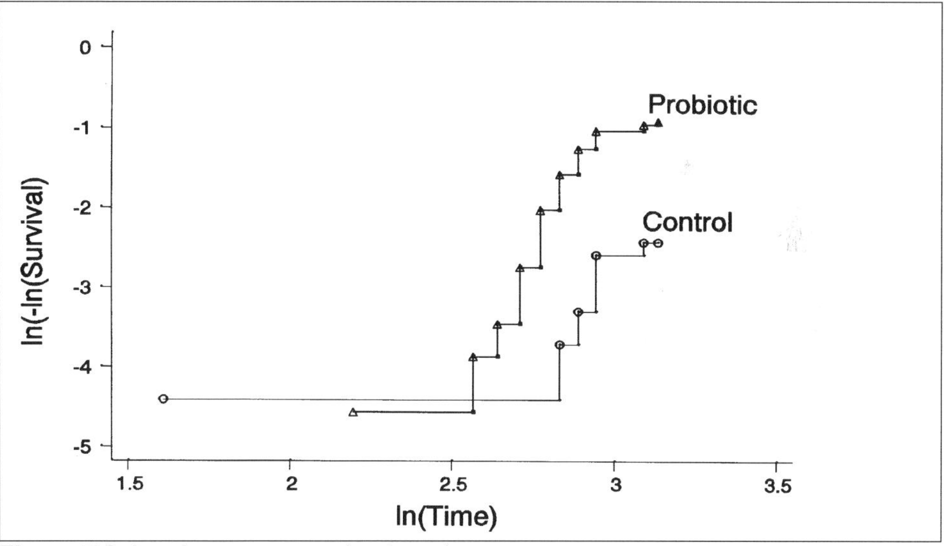

Figure 7.9. Log-log curves per treatment group.

Both lines are reasonably parallel and thus the proportional hazards assumption is not heavily violated. The output of the Cox proportional hazard analyses are shown on the next page:

Crude (univariate) Cox:

No. of subjects = 180				Log likelihood = -190.11119		
No. of failures = 39				chi2(1) = 17.08		
Time at risk = 3911				Prob > chi2 = 0.0000		
	Haz. Ratio	Std. Err.	z	P > |z|	[95% Conf. Interval]	
treat	4.527363	1.890374	3.617	0.000	1.997244	10.26265

Origin-adjusted (multivariate) Cox:

No. of subjects = 180				Log likelihood = -187.59571		
No. of failures = 39				chi2(1) = 22.11		
Time at risk = 3911				Prob > chi2 = 0.0000		
	Haz. Ratio	Std. Err.	z	P > |z|	[95% Conf. Interval]	
treat	4.29499	1.795923	3.486	0.000	1.892508	9.747353
origin	2.11848	.7364014	2.160	0.031	1.071864	4.18706

The origin-adjusted HR (4.3) for treatment with antibiotic is about equal to the crude estimate (4.5), indicating that Origin is not a serious confounder. Survival analysis using the Weibull survival function:

Crude (univariate) Weibull:

No. of subjects = 180				Log likelihood =-79.166672		
No. of failures = 39				chi2(1) = 17.80		
Time at risk = 3911				Prob > chi2 = 0.0000		
	Haz. Ratio	Std. Err.	z	P > |z|	[95% Conf. Interval]	
treat	4.655111	1.943297	3.684	0.000	2.05396	10.55038
ln p	1.245951	.1522937	8.181	0.000	.9474608	1.544441
p	3.476239				2.579152	4.685353
1/p	.2876672				.2134311	.3877243

Origin-adjusted (multivariate) Weibull:

No. of subjects = 180				Log likelihood = -79.178231		
No. of failures = 39				chi2(1) = 23.77		
Time at risk = 3911				Prob > chi2 = 0.0000		
	Haz. Ratio	Std. Err.	z	P > |z|	[95% Conf. Interval]	
treat	4.421359	1.847952	3.556	0.000	1.94889	10.55038
origin	2.260474	7853688	2.347	0.019	1.144095	4.466189
ln p	1.255598	.1520147	8.260	0.000	.9576541	1.553541
p	3.509935				2.605577	4.728183
1/p	.2849056				.2114978	.3837922

Again the HR is not much affected by adding Origin to the model. Note that the value of p is rather large (3.5), indicating that the hazard of dying exponentially increases with time.

Survival analysis using the exponential function:

Crude (univariate) exponential:

No. of subjects =	180	Log likelihood =	-101.32536
No. of failures =	39	chi2(1) =	15.17
Time at risk =	3911	Prob > chi2 =	0.0001

	Haz. Ratio	Std. Err.	z	P > |z|	[95% Conf.	Interval]
treat	4.175566	1.742303	3.425	0.001	1.84307	9.459953

Origin-adjusted (multivariate) exponential:

No. of subjects =	180	Log likelihood =	-98.65428
No. of failures =	39	chi2(1) =	20.52
Time at risk =	3911	Prob > chi2 =	0.0000

	Haz. Ratio	Std. Err.	z	P > |z|	[95% Conf.	Interval]
treat	3.983233	1.663843	3.309	0.001	1.756624	9.032181
origin	2.16464	.7518203	2.223	0.026	1.095841	4.275866

Note that the crude exponential HR is identical to the IRR as calculated in **2a**.

3c. In summary:

Hazard ratios and 95% confidence intervals:

	Crude (univariate)		Origin-adjusted (multivariate)	
IRR	4.18	[1.8; 11.2]	---	(Mantel-Haenszel)
Cox	4.53	[2.0; 10.3]	4.29	[1.9; 9.7]
Weibull	4.66	[2.0; 10.6]	4.42	[1.9; 10.1]
Exponential	4.18	[1.8; 9.4]	3.98	[1.8; 9.0]
deviance differences:	Univariate		Multivariate	
Cox	17.08		22.11	
Weibull	17.80		23.77	
Exponential	15.17		20.52	

From the deviance differences it can be concluded that Cox and Weibull fit the data better than the exponential. The exponential and Weibull regression would yield similar deviances if the shape parameter 'p', given in the Weibull output, equals 1. As the value of 'p' is 3.5, it is clear that the Weibull fits better, though the final outcome and conclusion do not differ in this particular trial.

Chapter VIII

Veterinary Clinical Trials

Part I

Introduction[19]

Michael Thrusfield
University of Edinburgh
Department of Veterinary Clinical Studies
United Kingdom

[19] Reproduced, in part, from Thrusfield (1997), with the permission of the publishers.

1. The Need for Clinical Trials

There is now an awareness of the need for clinical trials in both human and veterinary medicine, and new chemotherapeutic preparations usually require mandatory formal testing before they are licensed[20]. Although the effects of some treatments are so marked that they are obvious (e.g., the intravenous administration of calcium to cases of acute bovine hypocalcaemia), this is not true for many prophylactic and therapeutic procedures, where, for example, the advantages of a new drug over an established one may be small. Moreover, the observations of individual veterinarians provide insufficient evidence for determining efficacy[21]. In the past, treatment was often based on beliefs that had never been scientifically assessed; and anecdotal or unattested cures entered the veterinary and medical literature. Indeed, it has been estimated that only about 20% of human medical procedures have been evaluated properly (Konner, 1993), and many veterinary procedures have also been poorly evaluated (Smith, 1988). Conclusive evidence of efficacy is provided by a **clinical trial**.

1.1. Definition of a clinical trial

A clinical trial is a systematic study in the species, or in particular categories of the species, for which a procedure is intended (the target species) in order to establish the procedure's **prophylactic** or **therapeutic** effects. In veterinary medicine, effects may include improvements in production as well as amelioration of clinical disease. The procedure may be a surgical technique, modification of management (e.g., diet), or prophylactic or therapeutic administration of a drug. If the latter is being assessed, a clinical trial would also include studies of its pattern of absorption, metabolism, distribution within the body and excretion of active substances. With these aims in mind, the assessment of drugs can be classified chronologically into four categories, according to the purpose of the assessment (Friedman *et al.*, 1996):

1. **pharmacological and toxicity trials,** usually conducted on either the target species or laboratory animals to study the safety of a drug;
2. **initial trials of therapeutic effect and safety**, usually conducted on the target species on a small scale in a controlled environment (e.g., on research establishments), and often with the object of selecting the potentially most attractive drugs from those that are available;
3. **clinical evaluation of efficacy**, undertaken on a larger scale in the field, that is, under **operational conditions**, where management and environment can affect the result of the trial;
4. **post-authorization surveillance** of a drug after it has been licensed, to monitor adverse drug reactions.

[20] Some paradoxes, however, remain. For example, although chemotherapeutic agents are subject to mandatory assessment, homeopathic remedies commonly are not.

[21] A distinction is sometimes made between *effectiveness* and *efficacy*. The former is the extent to which a procedure does what it is intended to do when applied in the day-to-day routine of medical or veterinary practice. The latter is the extent to which a procedure produces beneficial results under ideal conditions. A procedure may be efficacious but relatively ineffective if it is not taken up widely (e.g., if owners' compliance with the advice of the veterinarian is low).

This chapter focuses on the third type of trial: clinical evaluation of **efficacy**.

1.2. Field trials

The term **field trial** is commonly used in veterinary medicine. Two characteristics of field trials have been identified:

A. the trial is undertaken on subjects 'in the field', that is, under husbandry and management practices typical of those under which the procedure is intended to be used (operational conditions);

B. the trial is frequently prophylactic and therefore relies on natural challenge to the treatment that is being assessed (e.g., assessment of the efficacy of a bacterial pneumonia vaccine would rely on vaccinated animals being naturally exposed to infection with the relevant bacterium during the period of the trial).

However, these characteristics only represent related circumstances under which clinical trials may be conducted (B is a logical consequence of A), and so a distinction between clinical and field trials is not maintained here; the latter are essentially instances of trial type 3, above.

1.3. Community trials

A **community trial** is a trial in which the 'experimental unit' (*see* part 2: 'Design and conduct of clinical trials') is an entire community. Community trials have been undertaken in human medicine, for example, the fluoridation of the public water supply to prevent dental caries.

2. Basic Terms

2.1. Controlled trials

The clinical condition of sick animals can be compared before and after treatment. However, interpretation of such an **uncontrolled** trial may be difficult because any observed changes could result either from the treatment or from natural progression of the disease. An essential feature of a well designed clinical trial therefore is a comparison of a group receiving the treatment with a **control** group not receiving it.

The control group may be selected at the same time as the group receiving the treatment (a **concurrent** control group) or generated using historical data (a **historical** control group). Early clinical trials, such as Lister's assessment of antiseptic surgery (see Chapter I), utilized historical controls, but this approach is open to criticism because of the various factors, unrelated to treatment, that can produce observed differences over a period of time (e.g., improvements in husbandry, changes in diagnostic criteria, disease classification and selection of animals, alterations in virulence of infectious agents, and reduction in the severity of disease). The net result of these problems is that studies with historical controls tend to exaggerate the value of a new treatment. Concurrent control groups are therefore usually advocated.

The control group may receive another (standard) treatment with which the first treatment under trial is being compared (a 'positive' control group), no treatment (sometimes called a 'negative' control group), or a **placebo** (an inert substance that is visually similar to the treatment under trial, and therefore cannot be distinguished from the treatment by those administering and those receiving the treatment and placebo). Groups can also serve as their own controls.

2.2. Randomization

Bias (*systematic*, as opposed to *random* variation) can occur in a trial if there is preferential assignment of subjects to treatment or control groups, differential management of the groups, or differential assessment of the groups. For example, a veterinarian may allocate animals only with a good prognosis to the treatment group. A central tenet of a controlled clinical trial is that subjects are assigned to treatment and control groups **randomly** so that the likelihood of bias due to preferential allocation is reduced. This process of **randomization** should also balance the distribution of other variables that may be outcome-related (e.g., age), and guarantees the validity of the statistical tests used in the analysis of the trial.

2.3. Blinding

Bias may also occur if owners of animals (patients in human trials) are aware of their group allocation. For instance, if an owner knows that his or her animal has been allocated to the treatment group, then he/she may be tempted to think that improvement has occurred when, in fact, it has not. This bias can be avoided by keeping owners ignorant of the allocation schedule (to treatment or control group). This procedure is **blinding**.

A good clinical trial is therefore: **controlled**, **randomized**, and **blind**.

References

Friedman, L.M.; Furburg, C.D.; Demets, D.L. (1996). Fundamentals of Clinical Trials, 3rd edn. Mosby, St. Louis.

Konner, M. (1993). The Trouble with Medicine. BBC Books, London.

Smith, R.D. (1988). Veterinary clinical research: a survey of study designs and clinical issues appearing in a practice journal. Journal of Veterinary Medical Education, 15, 2-7.

Thrusfield, M. (1997). Veterinary Epidemiology. Revised 2nd edn. Blackwell Science Limited, Oxford.

Part II

The Design and Conduct of Clinical Trials[22]

Michael Thrusfield
University of Edinburgh
Department of Veterinary Clinical Studies
United Kingdom

[22] Reproduced, in part, from Thrusfield (1997), with the permission of the publishers.

1. Trial Protocols

The goals and design of a clinical trial should be documented in a **trial protocol**. This is required by regulatory organizations who assess the value and validity of the proposed trial, and also provides background information to veterinarians and owners who are asked to participate in the trial. The main components of a protocol are listed in Table 8.1.

2. The Primary Hypothesis

The first step in writing a protocol for a clinical trial is determination of its **major objective**, so that a **primary hypothesis** can be formulated. Thus, a primary hypothesis could be 'evening primrose oil has a beneficial effect against canine atopy' (Scarff and Lloyd, 1992). Several principal criteria of response might be assessed, but it is helpful if one particular response variable can be identified as the main criterion for testing the primary hypothesis; this is the **primary end point**. The following topics must be addressed in determining this end point:

1. which end points are the most **clinically** and **economically** important?
2. which of these can be measured in a reasonable manner?
3. what practical constraints (e.g., budgetary limits) exist?

Thus, the primary end point in the evening primrose oil trial might be the level of pruritus. Other end points could include the levels of oedema and erythema; these constitute **secondary end points**.

The response variables that are used to measure the end points should adequately represent the effect that is being studied in the trial, and therefore address the primary hypothesis (**construct validity**). Thus, there is a relationship between plasma essential fatty-acid levels and the inflammatory response (Horrobin, 1990), and so changes in plasma phospholipid levels could be monitored, but these are less clinically relevant than the actual clinical signs which may, therefore, be more appropriate response variables for ensuring construct validity. However, clinical signs are often measured subjectively on an ordinal or visual analogue scale, whereas fatty-acid levels can be measured on the ratio scale. Therefore, a compromise between strength of measurement and relevance (construct validity) may be necessary. However, subjective scales of measurement may be unreliable. For example, if a post-mortem pulmonary-lesion scoring system (i.e., an ordinal variable) were being used to assess the efficacy of an antibiotic against bacterial pneumonia, differences between pulmonary scores in treated and untreated animals might arise from an inability of the pathologist to score lesions consistently, rather than a true treatment effect. The reliability of such measures therefore should be assessed before adopting them.

A suitable procedure is to quantify the **agreement** between repeated observations (undertaken blindly) of the same individuals. Appropriate statistical methods are calculation of *kappa,* for discrete variables (*see* Chapter IV); weighted *kappa* for ordinal variables (Ciccetti and Allison, 1971); and the intraclass correlation coefficient (Bartko, 1994) and limits of agreement (Altman, 1991) for Normally-distributed continuous variables.

Table 8.1. Components of a protocol for a clinical trial (modified and reduced from Noordhuizen et al., 1993).

General information	Title of trial Names and addresses of investigators and sponsors Identity of trial site(s)
Justification and objectives	Reason for execution of the trial Primary hypothesis to be tested

Design	Response variables:
	    Nature of response variables (level of measurement) (*see* Chapter IV)
	    Definition of efficacy (magnitude of the difference to be detected between treatment and control groups)
	Duration:
	    Date of beginning and end
	    Duration of disease under study
	    Period for recruitment of cases
	    Duration of treatment
	    Drug withdrawal period (for food-producing animals)
	    Decision rules for terminating a trial
	Experimental population:
	    The experimental unit (*see* also Chapter V and VI)
	    Inclusion/exclusion criteria
	    Post-admission withdrawal criteria
	    Definition of cases/diagnostic criteria
	    Selection of controls
	    Sample size determination (see also Chapter III)
	Therapeutic or prophylactic procedure:
	    Dosage
	    Product formulation and identification
	    Placebo/standard treatment formulation and identification
	    Method of administration
	    Definition of stage at which administration stops
	    Blinding technique
	    Compliance monitoring
	Type of trial:
	    Randomization
	    Stratification variables
	    Implementation of allocation process
	Data collection:
	    Data to be collected
	    Method for recording adverse drug reactions
	    Identification of experimental units
	    Confidentiality
	Data analysis:
	    Description of statistical methods
	    Interpretation of significance levels/confidence intervals (see Chapter V, VI and VII)
	    Approach to withdrawals and animals 'lost to follow up'

3. Defining Efficacy

The primary end point defines the **outcome** that is assessed, and therefore the nature of the trial's response variables (Table 8.2), and efficacy can be determined either by hypothesis-testing or estimation procedures. In either case, measures of efficacy may be based either on *absolute differences* or *relative measures* (e.g., the relative risk - *see* also Chapter IV). Examples of measures are morbidity (prevalence; incidence; cumulative incidence), mortality (case fatality), survival (see Chapter VII) and relative risk.

Table 8.2. Response variables assessed in clinical trials.

Response variable		Efficacy	
Level of measurement	Examples	Definition	Description of method and sample size determination
Nominal	Mortality	Difference between proportions	Pocock (1983)
	Incidence Prevalence	Relative risk	Gardner and Altman (1989)
		Attributable proportion (exposed)	Elwood (1988) Elwood (1988)
Ordinal	Scores of clinical severity Condition scores	Difference between medians	Siegel and Castellan (1988) Gardner and Altman (1989) Khmaladze (1975)
Interval and ratio, and the visual analogue scale	Liveweight gain Milk cell counts Visual analogue assessment of clinical severity	Difference between means (if variables are Normally distributed)	Pocock (1983) Gardner and Altman (1989)

3.1. Vaccinal efficacy

A common measure of vaccinal efficacy is the **attributable proportion (exposed)**, λ_{exp}, - also called the aetiological fraction (exposed). This measure - like the relative risk - is sometimes computed in observational studies (see Chapter V). Using the notation in Table 8.3, it is defined as:

$$\frac{\frac{a}{a+b} - \frac{c}{c+d}}{\frac{a}{a+b}}$$

Table 8.3. The 2x2 contingency table constructed in observational studies.

	Diseased animals	Non-diseased animals	Total
Hypothesized risk factor present	a	b	a + b
Hypothesized risk factor absent	c	d	c + d
Total	a + c	b + d	a + b + c + d = n

In the context of vaccine trials, unvaccinated animals are defined as 'exposed' to the risk factor. Table 8.4 shows the results of a clinical trial of the efficacy of a *Bacteroides nodosus* vaccine against foot rot in sheep, where:

$$\lambda_{exp} = \frac{\text{prevalence}_{exposed} - \text{prevalence}_{unexposed}}{\text{prevalence}_{exposed}}$$

$$= \frac{\frac{94}{422} - \frac{21}{317}}{\frac{94}{422}} = \frac{0.157}{0.223} = 0.704$$

Table 8.4. Efficacy of a Bacteroides nodosus vaccine against foot rot (84 days after vaccination). (Raw data derived from Hindmarsh et al., 1989).

	Foot rot present	Foot rot absent	Totals
Non-vaccinated sheep	94	328	422
Vaccinated sheep	21	296	317

Therefore, 70.4% of foot rot in unvaccinated sheep is attributable to not being vaccinated; this is alternatively the percentage of disease prevented by the vaccine in vaccinated animals.

Confidence intervals for the attributable proportion (exposed) can, and should, be calculated, to indicate the precision of the estimate of vaccinal efficacy achieved by the trial. The 95% confidence interval for λ_{exp} for the foot rot vaccine (using the formula of Kahn and Sempos, 1989), is 53.4%, 81.0%, indicating that one is 95% confident that the vaccine's efficacy lies within this range. (If a more precise estimate were needed, a larger trial would be required.)

3.2. Efficacy of ectoparasitic preparations

Efficacy of ectoparasitic products can be calculated thus (CVMP, 1993):

$$\%efficacy = \frac{C - T}{C} * 100$$

where:

C = mean (the mean may be the arithmetic mean, or an appropriate transformation (e.g., logarithmic transformation)) number of ectoparasites/animal in the control group;

T = mean number of ectoparasites/animal in the treated group.

3.3. Standards for efficacy

There is not always a fixed standard for acceptable therapeutic effect or efficacy. In the European Union, for example, the therapeutic effect of a veterinary medicinal product is generally understood by the relevant regulatory body to be the effect 'promised by the manufacturer' (Beechinor, 1993). European regulatory guidelines for the efficacy of ectoparasitic preparations (CVMP, 1993), using the formula above, are 'approximately 100%' for flea and louse infestations; '80-100% (preferably more than 90%)' for infestations with Diptera; and 'more than 90%' for tick infestations. Note, however, that the value of a therapeutic effect lies ultimately in its clinical and economic impact.

4. The Experimental Unit

The **experimental unit** is the smallest **independent** unit to which the treatment is randomly allocated. It may be elementary units (usually individual animals) or aggregates such as pens or herds. Most companion animal and human clinical trials involve allocation to individuals. Some trials in livestock, however, may involve allocation of treatments to groups. In contrast, the experimental unit may be the udder quarter when locally administered intramammary preparations are being assessed; the elementary unit is then the *quarter,* not the *animal.*

The experimental unit may be a group because events at the individual level cannot be measured, even though they are of interest. For instance, in trials of in-feed compounds likely to affect weight gain in poultry and pigs, either the amount eaten by, or the weight increase of, individuals within a house or pen is not recorded. This often arises because it is not practical to identify individual animals at weighing. Consequently, liveweight gain *per house* or *pen* is the response variable. Moreover, when animals are penned together, external factors (e.g., farm hygiene) may affect the group, and such 'group effects' cannot be separated from individual treatment effects; therefore the group must be identified as the experimental unit (Donner, 1993).

Thus, the efficacy of in-feed antibiotic medication in reducing the incidence of streptococcal meningitis in pigs could be assessed by dividing a herd into pens containing a specified number of animals. The treatment is then randomly allocated to the pens, and medicated and 'placebo' diets supplied to pigs in the respective treatment and control pens. In this circumstance, each pen only contributes the value 1 in sample size determination for the trial because variability can only be legitimately assessed between pens, rather than between individuals.

A particular problem arises with trials involving some infectious diseases. If the treatment could reduce excretion of infectious agents (e.g., vaccination in poultry houses or anthelmintic trials on farms) then treated and control animals should not be kept together because any reduction in infection 'pressure' will benefit treated **and** control animals; similarly, control animals constitute a source of infection to treated animals. This can lead to similar results in both categories (Thurber *et al.*, 1977), therefore reducing the likelihood of detecting beneficial therapeutic effects. The practice of mixing animals in each group is therefore unacceptable when herd immunity or group immunity is being assessed. In these circumstances, an appropriate independent unit must be identified. Thus, separate houses could be used on an intensive poultry enterprise, or separate tanks on a fish farm. Dairy farms, in contrast, usually have a continuous production policy with mixing of animals, and so the herd may become the experimental unit.

5. The Experimental Population

The population in which a trial is conducted is the **experimental population**. This should be representative of the **target population**. Differences between experimental and target populations may result in the trial not being generalizable (**externally valid**); that is, unbiased inferences regarding the target population cannot be made. For example, findings from a trial of an anaesthetic drug conducted only on thoroughbred horses may not be relevant to the general horse population because of differences in level of fitness between thoroughbreds and other types of horse. External validity (which is facilitated by conducting trials 'in the field') contrasts with **internal validity**, which indicates that observed differences between treatment and control groups in the **experimental population** can be legitimately attributed to the treatment. Internal validity is obtained by good trial design (e.g., randomization). The evaluation of external validity usually requires much more information than assessment of internal validity.

Prophylactic trials require selection of an experimental population that is at high risk of developing disease so that natural challenge can be anticipated during the period of the trial. Previous knowledge of disease on potential trial sites may be sufficient to identify candidate populations. However, the period of natural challenge may vary, reflecting complex patterns of infection. Many infections are seasonal; others may be poorly predictable.

6. Admission and Exclusion Criteria

Criteria for inclusion of animals in a trial (**admission criteria**, **eligibility criteria**) must be defined. These should be listed in the protocol, and include:

1. a precise **definition of the condition** on which the treatment is being assessed;
2. the **criteria for diagnosis** of the condition.

For example, in the trial of the efficacy of evening primrose oil in the treatment of canine atopy, chronically pruritic dogs were included only if they conformed to a documented set of diagnostic criteria (Willemse, 1986) and reacted positively to the relevant intradermal skin tests. Similarly, specific types of mastitis may need to be defined in bovine mastitis trials; other admission criteria could include parity and stage of lactation.

Exclusion criteria are the corollaries of admission criteria. Thus, dogs with positive reactions to flea allergens were excluded from the trial of evening primrose oil. Cows might be excluded from a mastitis trial if they had been previously treated for mastitis during the relevant lactation, if they had multiple mammary infections, or if they also had other diseases which could affect treatment. Trials of non-steroidal anti-inflammatory drugs would require exclusion from the treatment group of animals to which corticosteroids were being administered. However, too many exclusion criteria should be avoided; otherwise external validity may be compromised. It may be prudent to accommodate factors either in the trial design by stratification (see below), or during the analysis.

7. Informed Consent

The objectives and general outline of a trial should be explained to owners of animals that are included in the trial, and then their willingness to participate documented. This is **informed consent**.

8. Blinding

Blinding (**masking**) is a means of reducing bias. In this technique, those responsible for measurements or clinical assessment are kept unaware of the treatment assigned to each group. The classification of blinding into **single** or **double** is based on whether the owner or attendant (patient in human medicine) or investigator is 'blinded' (Table 8.5). 'The investigator can be more than one category of person; for example, participating veterinary practitioners and the principal investigators that analyze the results (the term 'treble-blinding' has been advocated in this situation).

Table 8.5. Summary of the types of blinding to assignment of treatment.

Type of blinding	Knowledge of assignment of treatment	
	Owner	Investigator
None	Yes	Yes
Single	No	Yes
Double	No	No

Blinding should be employed wherever possible, and is facilitated by the use of a placebo in the control group. However, there may be circumstances in which blinding is not feasible; for example, if two radically different treatments are being compared (e.g., a surgical and chemotherapeutic procedure) or if formulation of visually identical 'trial' and 'standard' drugs is impracticable.

9. Randomization

9.1. Simple randomization

Simple randomization is the most basic type of randomization. When there are only two treatments, tossing a coin is an elementary method. However, it is usually more convenient to randomize in advance using random numbers (these can be obtained from published tables, and can also be generated on most pocket calculators and many statistical software packages), allocating units identified by odd numbers to one group, and evenly numbered units to the other. Randomization should be undertaken **after** eligible units have been identified.

When comparing a new treatment with an established one, and there is evidence that the new treatment is superior, it can be allocated to twice the number of units as the established one (Peto, 1978). This can increase the benefit to participating animals. For example, if a new treatment was expected to reduce mortality by 50%, 2:1 randomization would be expected to produce an equal number of deaths in the two groups. This randomization ratio can be obtained by using twice as many random numbers for allocation of the new treatment as those used to allocate the established one. There is no advantage in increasing the ratio further, because of the resultant loss of statistical *power* which can only be counteracted by increasing the total sample size.

9.2. Block randomization

Simple randomization can produce grossly uneven totals in each group if a small trial is undertaken. This problem can be overcome using **block** (**restricted**) randomization. This limits randomization to blocks of units, and ensures that within a block equal numbers are allocated to each treatment. For example, if randomization is restricted to units of 4 animals, receiving either treatment A or treatment B, the numbers 1 - 6 are attached to the six possible treatment allocations in a block: ABAB, AABB, BBAA, BAAB, ABBA, and BABA. One of these numbers is then selected from a random number table for the next block of 4 individuals entering the trial, and gives its treatment allocation.

9.3. Stratification

Some factors (e.g., age, parity or severity of disease) may be known to affect the outcome of a trial and may bias results if they are unevenly distributed between the treatment and control groups. This can be taken into account during initial randomization by **stratifying** (i.e., matching) both groups according to these confounding factors. The experimental units are then allocated to treatment and control groups within the strata, using simple or block randomization. The most extreme case is individual matching, with subjects in the matched pairs being randomly allocated to the treatment and control groups.

Stratification leads to related samples and therefore decreases the number of units that are required to detect a specified difference between treatment and control groups (*see* also in Chapter III).

9.4. Alternatives to randomization

Some alternatives to randomization include allocation according to date of entry (e.g., treatment on odd days, placebo on even days), clinic record number, wishes of the owner, and preceding results. An example of the last method is the 'play-the-winner' approach (Zelen, 1969): if a treatment is followed by success, the next unit receives the same treatment; if it is followed by failure, the next unit receives the alternative treatment. This limits the number of animals receiving an inferior treatment. All of these techniques have disadvantages and should never be considered as acceptable alternatives to randomization (Bulpitt, 1983).

10. Trial Designs

There are three main trial designs:

1. standard;
2. cross-over;
3. sequential.

10.1. Standard trials

In the basic **standard trial**, experimental units are randomized to a single treatment group using either simple or block randomization, and each group receives a single treatment. A specified number of units enter the trial and are followed for a predetermined period of time, after which the treatment is stopped. The basic design can be refined by stratification.

The analytical techniques employed in a standard trial involving two unstratified groups are listed in Table 8.2. Estimation of parameters with associated confidence intervals is preferred to hypothesis testing. Confidence intervals should also be quoted for negative, as well as positive, results.

10.2. Cross-over trials

In a **cross-over trial**, subjects are exposed to more than one treatment consecutively, each treatment regimen being selected. Experimental units therefore serve as their own controls and treatment and control groups are therefore *matched*. Groups that are compared may be **related** or **independent**. Samples are related **paired**) when:

1. they are **matched** for other variables;
2. comparisons are made between **repeated** measurements on the same individuals.

Matching is the process of evenly distributing factors that might affect outcome (e.g., age) between the groups that are being compared, and different analytical procedures are required for these two circumstances. Paired samples require *smaller* sample sizes than unpaired samples to detect a specified difference.This design is useful when treatments are intended to alleviate a condition, rather than effect a cure, so that after the first treatment is withdrawn the subject is in a position to receive a second. Examples are comparisons of anti-inflammatory drugs in arthritis, and hypoglycaemics in diabetes. Moreover, a comparison on the same individuals is likely to be more precise than a comparison between subjects because the responses are *paired*. The cross-over trial is therefore valuable if the number of experimental units is limited. However, analysis of results is complex if a treatment effect carries over into the next treatment period. If there is any doubt, conclusions should be based only on the first period, using analyses of unpaired samples. Alternatively, more complex methods that identify interactions between treatment effect and period of treatment can be applied (Hills and Armitage, 1979).

10.3. Sequential trials

A **sequential trial** is one whose conduct at any stage depends on the results so far obtained. Two treatments are usually compared, and experimental units (usually individuals) enter the trial in pairs; one individual being given one treatment, and one the other. Results are then analyzed sequentially according to the outcome in the pairs, and boundaries are drawn to define levels at which specified differences are obtained at the desired level of statistical significance. The trial may be terminated when these levels are reached. If the desired level is not reached, the investigator may decide to increase the sample size indefinitely until the former is reached; this is an **open** trial. Alternatively, the trial may be terminated if a specified difference is not reached by a certain stage; this is a **closed** trial.

Sequential trials facilitate early detection of beneficial treatment effects and can require fewer experimental units. However, they may be difficult to plan because their duration is initially unknown. They are also unsuited to trials in which treatment response times are long because responses need to be analyzed quickly so that a decision can be taken to enlist more subjects, if necessary.

A key feature of sequential trials therefore is that significance tests are conducted repeatedly on accumulating data. This tends to **increase** the overall significance level (Armitage *et al.*, 1969). For example, if 5 interim analyses are conducted, the chance of at least one analysis showing a treatment difference at the 5% level (α = 0.05) increases to 0.23 (i.e., $1 - [1 - \alpha]^5$); if 20 interim analyses are undertaken, it increases to 0.64 ($1 - [1 - \alpha]^{20}$). The overall Type 1 error therefore increases if α = 0.05, for any single interim analysis, is used as the trial's stopping criterion. If data are analyzed frequently enough, a value of $P < 0.05$ is likely, regardless of whether there is a treatment difference.

This problem can be overcome by choosing a more stringent *nominal* significance level for each repeated test, so that the overall significance level is kept at a reasonable value such as 0.05 or 0.01. Table 8.6 can be used for this purpose under two-tailed conditions. A one-tailed test assumes that a difference can only be in *one direction*, for example, that a treatment can only produce a decrease in disease frequency, and not an increase, relative to the control protocol. Two-tailed tests, in contrast, accept that differences may be in *either* direction. One-tailed comparisons require *fewer* animals than two-tailed comparisons, to detect a specified difference. This discrimination therefore should be maintained in trial design and analysis. Unless there is strong evidence that a one-tailed test is justifiable, it is prudent to estimate sample sizes for two-tailed conditions.

Table 8.6. Nominal significance level required for repeated two-tailed significance testing with an overall significance level α = 0.05 or 0.01 and various values of N, the maximum number of tests (from Pocock, 1977).

N	α = 0.05	α = 0.01
2	0.0294	0.0056
3	0.0221	0.0041
4	0.0182	0.0033
5	0.0158	0.0028
6	0.0142	0.0025
7	0.0130	0.0023
8	0.0120	0.0021
9	0.0112	0.0019
10	0.0106	0.0018
15	0.0086	0.0015
20	0.0075	0.0013

Appropriate parametric statistical tests, under various conditions and assumptions, are described by Armitage and Berry (1994). Non-parametric tests are detailed by Siegel and Castellan (1988). For example, if the overall significance level is set at α = 0.05, and if a maximum of three analyses is anticipated, $P < 0.022$ is used as the stopping rule for a treatment difference at each analysis; similarly, if a maximum of 5 analyses is anticipated, $P < 0.016$ is used. Suitable values for one-sided tests are given by Demets and Ware (1980).

Clinical trials, which are usually conducted prospectively, closely resemble cohort studies, in which the risk factor is replaced by treatment status.

11. What Sample Size should be Selected

The number of experimental units in treatment and control groups should be determined *before* a trial is undertaken. The measure of efficacy determines the method for calculating sample size, and the probability of committing a Type I and Type II error must be considered (see Table 8.5[23]). The following parameters must be specified (see Chapter III for more details):

1. the acceptable level of **Type I error**, α, (the probability of erroneously inferring a difference between treatment and control group);
2. test **power**, $1 - \beta$, - the probability of correctly inferring a difference between treatment and control group - where β = the probability of Type II error (the probability of erroneously missing a true difference between treatment and control group);
3. the **magnitude** of the treatment effect (i.e., the difference between proportions, medians or means);
4. the choice of **alternative hypothesis**: 'one-tailed' or 'two-tailed'; additionally, for ordinal, interval and ratio response variables:
5. the **variability** (e.g., the standard deviation) of the response variable between treatment and control groups.

Type I error is traditionally set at 0.05, but a value as low as 0.01 can be justified if a trial is unique and its findings are unlikely to be repeated in the future. Power can vary considerably (values between 0.50 and 0.95 have been quoted in human clinical trials; 0.80 is common when $\alpha = 0.05$, and 0.96 when $\alpha = 0.01$ conventionally, β is set at four times α). The magnitude of the treatment effect depends on its clinical and economic relevance.

If a placebo or no treatment has been administered to the control group, and there is therefore intuitive evidence that the treatment can cause only an improvement in comparison with the control group, a one-tailed test is justifiable, and the sample size can be determined accordingly. However, the use of placebos or 'negative' control groups is now ethically debatable; consequently many contemporary clinical trials use a 'positive' control group and it is therefore prudent to assume two-tailed conditions (i.e., the treatment under test may be either better, or worse, than the

[23] In clinical trials in which treatment and control groups are **matched** the formulae for sample size in the references in Table 8.2 will tend to overestimate the number of units required.

standard treatment). Additionally, the magnitude of the difference between treatment and 'positive' control groups may be small; thus large sample sizes may be specified. See also paragraph 14 (exercises) and Chapter III.

Sometimes investigators may wish to determine sample size to demonstrate that there is *no* difference between the efficacy of treatments (e.g., when comparing a new drug with an acceptable, but more expensive, established one). An appropriate formula for comparing proportions cured in this circumstance is given by Donner (1984).

11.1. Power calculation

The number of animals required may not be recruited (e.g., for financial reasons). Moreover, animals may be 'lost' during the trial (*see* below). Additionally, the actual difference between treatment and control groups is most likely to be different than that hypothesised when calculating sample size, and a statistically significant difference may not be identified. In such circumstances, the **power** of the trial should be calculated, so that the ability of a trial to detect a treatment effect can be reported. Surprisingly, this is frequently not done. Appropriate formulae for power calculation are given by Cohen (1988), Elwood (1988) and Lipsey (1990).

12. Losses to 'Follow-Up'

The outcome of a trial may not be recorded in some experimental units because they are lost to 'follow-up'. For example, owners may move house or refuse to continue with the trial. The exent of this loss to follow-up needs to be assessed, and is frequently based on the experience of the investigator. The sample size then needs to be increased by multiplying the sample size by $1/(1 - d)$, where d is the anticipated proportion of experimental units lost. For example, if $d = 10/100$, the sample size would need to be multiplied by 1.11 (1/0.9) to compensate. Losses to follow-up cannot be included in subsequent analyses.

13. Compliance

The success of a trial depends on participants acting in accordance with the instructions of the trial's designers; that is, **complying** with treatment. For example, they may decide to switch from the treatment under trial to an alternative treatment. Poor compliance will decrease the statistical power of the trial because the observed difference in outcome between treatment and control groups will be reduced, but it will not produce spurious differences between groups. Reasons for poor compliance include: unclear instructions; forgetfulness; inconvenience of participation; cost of participation; preference for alternative procedures; disappointment with results; side effects.

Participants cannot be forced to comply, and so **regular contact** should be maintained with them, so that they can be encouraged to comply, and the degree of compliance **regularly assessed**. For example, if a treatment is formulated as a tablet, the number of tablets remaining can be counted regularly by the veterinarian. Assessment may be difficult (e.g., with in-feed medication) but should, nevertheless, be attempted. Other methods of improving compliance include: enroling motivated participants; assessing the willingness of participants to comply; providing incentives (e.g., free treatment); supplying simple, unambiguous instructions; limiting duration of the trial.

If non-compliance is substantial, the required sample size should again be modified in the same way as adjustment for loss to follow-up. If both losses to follow-up and non-compliance are anticipated, a composite value for *d* is required.

14. Terminating a Trial

The number of experimental units entering a trial and the duration of treatment are specified during the design of a trial; therefore a trial will usually last as long as it takes to enlist the units and for the last unit to complete the trial. However, it may be necessary to terminate a trial (particularly a long-term one) prematurely if there are serious adverse side effects in the treatment group, and such a **decision rule** should be written into the trial's protocol. In sequential trials another decision rule may be that a trial will be terminated when the specified difference is detected to the predetermined level of significance (see above).

15. Meta-analysis

Meta-analysis is the statistical analysis of data pooled from several studies to integrate findings. The technique originated in educational research, has been widely applied in social sciences, and has become popular in medicine and, more recently, veterinary medicine. Applications include the evaluation of diagnostic tests (e.g., Greiner *et al.*, 1997) and observational studies, but, notably, the assessment of clinical trials. Pooling of results can improve the precision of estimates of therapeutic effect, and increase statistical power and external validity. Commonly, the different studies are treated as separate strata for the purpose of analysis. Thus, for example, when categorical data analysed, the strata can be analysed using Mantel-Haenszel stratified analysis (*see* Chapter V). However, the technique is not without its disadvantages, such as the tendency to mix different trials unwittingly and ignore differences. (*See* Thrusfield 1997, pages 413-416, for more details.)

References

Altman, D.G. (1991) Practical Statistics for Medical Research. Chapman and Hall, London
Armitage, P.; Berry G. (1994). Statistical Methods in Medical Research. 3rd edn. Blackwell Science, Oxford.

Armitage, P.; McPherson, C.K.; Rowe, B.C. (1969). Repeated significance tests on accumulating data. Journal of the Royal Statistical Society, Series A, 132, 235-244.
Bartko, J.J. (1994) Measures of agreement: a single procedure. Statistics in Medicine, 13, 737-745.
Beechinor, G. (1993). Regulatory and administrative implications of clinical trials. In: Field Trial and Error. Proceedings of the International Seminar with Workshops on the Design, Conduct and Interpretation of Field Trials, Berg en Dal, Netherlands, 27-28th April 1993. Noordhuizen, J.P.T.M.; Frankena, K.; Ploeger, H.; Nell, T. (Eds.). pp. 29-35. Epidecon, Wageningen, The Netherlands.
Bulpitt, C.J. (1983). Randomised Controlled Clinical Trials. Martinus Nijhoff Publishers, The Hague.
Ciccetti, D.V. and Allison, T. (1971) A new procedure for assessing reliability of scoring EEH sleep recordings. American Journal of EEG Technology, 11, 101-109
Cohen, J. (1988). Statistical Power Analysis for the Behavioral Sciences. 2nd edn. Lawrence Erlbaum, Hillside.
CVMP (1993). Demonstration of efficacy of ectoparasiticides. CVMP Working Party on the Efficacy of Veterinary Medicines. Notes for Guidance. Document No. III/3682/92-EN. Commission of the European Communities, Brussels.
Demets, D.L.; Ware, J.H. (1980). Group sequential methods in clinical trials with a one-sided hypothesis. Biometrika, 67, 651-660.
Donner, A. (1984). Approaches to sample size estimation in the design of clinical trials - a review. Statistics in Medicine, 3, 199-214.
Donner, A. (1993). The comparison of proportions in the presence of litter effects. Preventive Veterinary Medicine, 18, 17-26.
Elwood, J.M. (1988). Causal Relationships in Medicine. A Practical System for Critical Appraisal. Oxford University Press, Oxford.
Gardner, M.J., Altman, D.G. (1989). Statistics with Confidence. British Medical Journal, London.
Greiner, M., Böhning, D. and Dahms, S. (1997) Meta-analytic review of ELISA tests for the diagnosis of human and porcine trichinellosis: which factors are involved in diagnostic accuracy? In: Proceedings of the Society for Veterinary Epidemiology and Preventive Medicine, Chester, 7th-11th April 1997. Eds. and Goodall. E.A. and Thrusfield, M.V. Pp 12-21
Hills, M.; Armitage, P. (1979). The two-period cross-over clinical trial. British Journal of Clinical Pharmacology, 8, 7-20.
Hindmarsh, F.; Fraser, J.; Scott, K. (1989). Efficacy of a multivalent Bacteroides nodosus vaccine against foot rot in sheep in Britain. Veterinary Record, 125, 128-130.
Horrobin, D.F. (Ed.) (1990). Omega-6 Essential Fatty Acids: Pathophysiology and Roles in Clinical Medicine. Alan R. Liss, New York.
Kahn, H.A.; Sempos, C.T. (1989) Statistical Methods in Epidemiology. Oxford University Press, New York.
Khmaladze, E.V. (1975). Estimation of the necessary number of observations for discriminating simple close hypotheses. Theory of Probability and its Applications, 20, 116-126.
Lipsey, M.W. (1990). Design Sensitivity. Statistical Power for Experimental Design. Sage Publications, Newbury Park.
Noordhuizen, J.P.T.M.; Frankena, K.; Ploeger, H.; Nell, T. (Eds.) (1993). Field Trial and Error. Proceedings of the International Seminar with Workshops on the Design, Conduct and Interpretation of Field Trials, Berg en Dal, The Netherlands, 27-28th April 1993. Epidecon, Wageningen, The Netherlands.
Peto, R. (1978). Clinical trial methodology. Biomedicine Special, 24-26.
Pocock, S.J. (1977). Group sequential methods in the design and analysis of clinical trials. Biometrika, 64, 191-199.
Pocock, S. (1983). Clinical Trials: A Practical Approach. John Wiley and Sons, Chichester.
Scarff, D.H.; Lloyd, D.H. (1992). Double blind, placebo-controlled, crossover study of evening primrose oil in the treatment of canine atopy. Veterinary Record, 131, 97-99.
Siegel, S.; Castellan, N.J. (1988). Nonparametric Statistics for the Behavioral Sciences. 2nd edn. McGraw-Hill, New York.
Thrusfield, M. (1997). Veterinary Epidemiology. Revised 2nd edn. Blackwell Science, Oxford.
Thurber, E.T.; Bass, E.P.; Beckenhauer, W.H. (1977). Field trial evaluation of a reo-coronavirus calf diarrhoea vaccine. Canadian Journal of Comparative Medicine, 41, 131-146.
Willemse, T. (1986). Atopic skin disease: a review and a reconsideration of diagnostic criteria. Journal of Small Animal Practice, 27, 771-778.
Zelen, M. (1969). Play the winner rule and the controlled clinical trial. Journal of the American Statistical Association, 264, 97.

16. Exercises

For the following exercises you can use most statistical software packages, such as STATISTIX, STATA or WINEPISCOPE. The latter is a public domain software package under Windows for epidemiology which is particularly suited to self-teaching. WINEPISCOPE can be downloaded from the Website: http://www.zod.wau.nl/qve.

A clinical trial is a systematic study in the species, or in a particular category of the species, for which a procedure is intended in order to establish the procedure's prophylactic or therapeutic effect. There are several study designs but, in veterinary medicine (particularly when assessing a drug before it is licensed) a simple trial design is used, in which a group of treated individuals is compared with a group of either:

1. untreated individuals;
2. individuals to which a placebo has been administered, or;
3. individuals to which an alternative, well-established treatment has been given.

16.1. General

1. Why is a control group necessary?
2. What is a placebo?
3. Are there reasons why administration of either no treatment or a placebo might be considered unacceptable?

16.2. Continuous response variable

The two columns of (hypothetical) data from the table below represent a trial in which the safety of a vaccine is evaluated - that is, does the vaccine have an adverse effect on milk production? (see e.g., Bosch *et al.*, 1997). The data concern the total milk production of dairy cows over a 4-day period after treatment with either a placebo (group P) or the vaccine (group V). Enter the data into your statistical software package.

V	P	V	P	V	P	V	P
85	86	95	96	99	101	105	105
86	89	96	96	99	101	106	107
86	89	96	97	99	103	107	107
88	90	96	98	100	103	113	108
89	91	97	99	101	103	114	109
91	91	97	99	102	104		110
93	93	98	99	102	104		110
94	94	98	100	103	104		112
94	95	98	100	103	105		115
95	95	99	101	104	105		119

1. Display the frequency distribution of the milkproduction for each group. Is there any indication that the data are not Normally distributed?

2. Compute the mean and median values for each group. Is the mean an appropriate measure of central tendency? Why?

3. Is there evidence that the vaccine has an effect on milk production?

4. A rigorous inference about effect on milk production can only be made by conducting a statistical significance test. Why?

5. This question assumes basic statistical knowledge about the analysis of continuous data and significance tests (see, for example, Thrusfield 1997, pages 201-205).

5a. The appropriate significance test for these data is a Student's *t*-test. Why?
5b. What hypothesis is being tested?
5c. Is this test one-tailed or two-tailed? Why?
5d. Is this test for independent or related samples?

Now conduct a *t*-test.

5e. The output from the test produces a *P*-value. To what does this value refer and what is your interpretation of the result?

16.3. Discrete response variable

The table below presents the results of a clinical trial of a bovine pneumonia virus vaccine. The trial was conducted on a farm with a regular history of outbreaks of respiratory disease in the winter (this approach is necessary to ensure that animals are naturally challenged with virus during the period of the trial). A control group of animals was not vaccinated, and vaccine was administered to each animal in the treatment group.

	Control group	Vaccinated group
Number of cases of pneumonia	12	7
Total number of animals in group	47	40

This question assumes basic statistical knowledge about the analysis of discrete data (see, for example, Thrusfield 1997, pages 211-212).

1a. An appropriate significance test for these data is a Chi-square test. Why?

Using your statistical software package, conduct a Chi-square test.

1b. What is your interpretation of the result (i.e., can you infer that the vaccine is efficacious)?

2. Another method of statistical analysis is to calculate the cumulative incidence ratio (CIR) and its confidence interval (see Chapter 5). Using WINEPISCOPE (Analysis, Cohort (Cum. incidence)), perform this analysis and interpret the results.

3. In principle, the Chi-square analysis and the analysis using the CIR allow a similar inference. However, which one do you prefer, and why?

4. An appropriate measure of vaccinal efficacy is the aetiological fraction (exposed) - also called, the attributable proportion (exposed). Using WINEPISCOPE (Analytical observational studies, cohort studies, cumulative incidence), calculate the aetiological fraction (exposed) - in WINEPISCOPE it is called the attributable proportion (exposed).

5. Interpret the attributable proportion (exposed).

6. Vaccinated and control animals were kept in separate pens in this trial. Why would it not be correct to mix animals from the two groups in the same pen?

17. Answers

17.1. General

1. A control group is necessary to ensure that any change in condition in the treated group is attributable only to treatment. If a control group was not included, one could not be certain that any improvement in condition in the treated group was not due to other factors such as natural progression of the disease.

2. A placebo is a procedure with no known therapeutic or prophylactic effect, which is administered to the control (untreated) group. It is used to balance, between treatment and control groups, the possibility that the power of suggestion (simply knowing that something is being given) will, in itself, produce a cure (or, in veterinary medicine, give animals' owners the impression that an improvement has occurred).

3. Administration of either no treatment or a placebo might be considered ethically unacceptable when an alternative treatment, which is already known to be efficacious (even to the point of reducing mortality), is already available.

17.2. Continous response variable

1. The mean is an appropriate measure of central tendency because (1) the data are continuous measurements, and (2) the histograms indicate that the frequency distribution of milk production levels in both groups are approximately Normally distributed. If this were not the case, an appropriate transformation (e.g. logarithmic) might be attempted to produce Normality.

2. The mean and median milk production levels (kg) are:

	V	P
Mean	97.9	101.8
Median	98.0	102.0

As the mean and median are almost identical, the mean is an appropriate measure of central tendency.

3. There is some evidence that the vaccination has an adverse effect on milk production because the mean milk production level in the group treated with the vaccine is about 4 kg lower than the mean level in the placebo group.

4. A rigorous inference about efficacy can only be made by conducting a statistical significance test because a simple comparison only of the mean milk production levels in the two samples that were studied does not account for sampling variation: the difference between the sample means may have arisen by chance because of such sampling variation. Significance tests, however, allow us to quantify the probability (*P*-value) that the differences arose by chance, a small probability therefore providing strong evidence in favour of a real difference (i.e., treatment effect). (Conventionally, 0.05 is taken as a critical *P*-value in interpreting the results of significance test, values of *P* below 0.05 being reported as "statistically significant").

5a. Two means of continuous, Normally distributed data are being compared; the appropriate significance test for this comparison is Student's two-sample *t*-test. (If the data were not Normally distributed on their natural scale of measurement, but logarithmic transformation produced Normality, then the *t*-test could be used validly to compare the logarithmic means).

5b. The hypothesis that there is no difference between the mean of the two groups is being tested. Remember that significance tests test an hypothesis of no difference (the null hypothesis).

5c. This test should be one-tailed because one is assessing whether the vaccine has an adverse effect. It is difficult to explain why a vaccine would have a beneficial effect on milk production in such a short time period.

5d. This test is for independent samples because the two groups are neither paired nor matched.

5e. The *P*-value refers to the probability, α, of a Type I error: wrongly inferring that there is a true difference in means in the populations of dogs from which the two samples have implicitly been assumed to have been drawn. The *P*-value is 0.01 (one-sided), this is the probability that the difference between the two means has arisen by chance. Thus, there is substantial evidence that the vaccine has an adverse effect on milk production. Note that significance tests DO NOT indicate if there either IS or IS NOT a difference - they give the probability of there not being a difference (and therefore also, by implication, of there being a difference: 1 - α): they present a balance of probabilities.

17.3. Discrete response variable

1a. The Chi-square test is an appropriate test because two *independent proportions* are being compared.

1b. How to enter the data depends on the possibilities of your software package. A short-hand method is to create three variables:

PNEU pneumonia present (1)
pneumonia absent (0)

TREAT vaccinated (1)
unvaccinated (0)

FREQ frequency of each instance of the classification.

The data should therefore read:

PNEU	TREAT	FREQ
1	0	12
0	0	35
1	1	7
0	1	33

The Chi-square test shows a *P*-value of 0.366, indicating that there is little evidence that the vaccine reduces the rate of pneumonia in vaccinated animals compared with unvaccinated ones: there is a 37% chance that the difference between the rate of pneumonia in the vaccinated group (7/40 = 0.175) and the unvaccinated group (12/47 = 0.255) arose by chance.

2. The 2x2 table in WINEPISCOPE should read:

7	12
33	35

Then, the CIR is (7/40) / (12/47) = 0.69 and its 95% confidence interval limits are [0.30; 1.57]. The 95% confidence interval for the CIR includes the value 1, indicating no difference (at the 5% level of statistical significance) between the rates of pneumonia in the two groups. Thus the trial does not provide evidence that vaccination reduces the occurence of pneumonia.

3. The CIR is preferable to the Chi-square test. The latter only generates a probability (*P*-value) that the observed effect arose by chance (0.37, in this exercise). The CIR, in contrast, indicates the magnitude of the effect (0.69, in the trial sample in this exercise) and the direction of the effect (the CIR is smaller than one, and therefore pneumonia has been observed less frequently in the vaccinated group than in the vaccinated group). Note, that the result of the Chi-square test, and the confidence intervals for the CIR are related. If the 95% interval includes one (as it does in this exercise), the result is not

significant at the 5% level (i.e., the *P*-value is greater than 0.05). Similarly, if the 99% interval includes one, the result is not significant at the 1% level (i.e., the *P*-value is greater than 0.01); and if the 90% interval includes one, the result is not significant at the 10% level (i.e., the *P*-value is greater than 0.10).

4. When calculating the attributable proportion (exposed) as a measure of vaccinal efficacy, the exposed group (the group at risk) is clearly the unvaccinated group. The 2x2 table in WINEPISCOPE should therefore read:

12	7
35	33

The attributable proportion (exposed) is 0.31. The vaccine's efficacy in the sample is therefore 31%. The 95% confidence interval limits are [-0.57; 0.70] (obtained with the software package STATA, StataCorp, 1997), indicating that the attributable proportion (exposed) could be zero in the larger population from which this sample was drawn.

5. The attributable proportion (exposed) means that 31% of all cases in the non-vaccinated group is attributed to non-vaccination. Thus, 31% of all pneumonia cases in this group could have been saved by vaccination (which is 31% of 12 = 4 animals). However. the confidence interval indicates that efficacy cannot be generalized to the target population from which the trial animals were drawn.

6. It would have been incorrect to mix vaccinated and unvaccinated animals in the same pens because, if the vaccine had any effect at all, vaccinated individuals would decrease the infection pressure on the control animals. Similarly, control animals would increase the infection pressure on vaccinated animals. The next effect would be ***to decrease the observed efficacy*** of the vaccine (in practice, a farmer is likely to vaccinate either all, or none, of his animals).

References

Bosch, J.C.; Frankena, K.; Oirschot, J.T. van (1997). The effect of vaccination with a bovine herpesvirus 1 gene-deleted vaccine on milk production. Veterinary Record, 140, 196-199.
Thrusfield, M. (1997). Veterinary Epidemiology. Revised 2nd edn. Blackwell Science, Oxford.

Further reading

Suggested for further reading and self-teaching:

Noordhuizen, J.P.T.M.; Frankena, K.; Ploeger, H.; Nell, T. (Eds.) (1993). Field Trial and Error. Proceedings of an International Seminar with Workshops on the Design, Conduct and Interpretation of Field Trials, Berg en Dal, The Netherlands, 27-28th April, 1993. Epidecon, Wageningen, The Netherlands.

Examples and exercises in Chapter VII.

Chapter IX

Introduction To Theoretical Epidemiology

E.A.M. Graat
Wageningen University
Department of Animal Sciences
Quantitative Veterinary Epidemiology Group
The Netherlands

K. Frankena
Wageningen University
Department of Animal Sciences
Quantitative Veterinary Epidemiology Group
The Netherlands

1. Introduction

The previous chapters covered, in essence, two different types of research: observational and experimental studies. In observational studies, the status with regard to disease (infection) and exposure are recorded, but no interventions or experimentations are applied. The primary goal of these studies is to investigate the causes and distribution of disease in order to optimize prevention and control strategies. This chapter covers a third type of research which makes use of ***mathematical models*** in order to describe characteristics of disease in populations. It is aimed for showing the essence of modelling and hence this chapter is restricted to relatively simple models. First, some background information about models will be given. In the following paragraphs, we will start out with some well known models (Markov Chains and Reed-Frost) and end up in a more general description of mathematical infectious disease models.

A model is any representation or abstraction of a system or process (Starfield and Bleloch, 1991). As a model is made to be used for a specific goal, e.g., prediction of whether or not an epidemic will occur, only key elements of a system or process are included in the model. Therefore, a model is by definition a simplification of the real system or process. Models are developed in order to:

1. define the problem more accurately;
2. organise our knowledge;
3. better understand the data that are available;
4. test knowledge;
5. predict;
6. support decision-making.

From this list it is clear that 'data' and 'knowledge' are central in modelling, and a 2x2 table can be used for further classification of models (modified from Holling, 1978).

		quantity/quality of data	
		poor	good
knowledge	poor	4	3
	good	2	1

Category 1 is the most desirable one with high quality data and with a good knowledge of the process. Such models might be used routinely e.g., in physics (for example, flight simulators, models to plot tracks of missiles or satellites). If good data are available, but understanding is (still) poor (category 3), mathematical and or statistical techniques are very well suited to detect patterns, to test hypotheses and by that increasing knowledge. Compared to physics, many of the problems concerning causes and effects of diseases are in category 4. Then, one may follow 2 ways: first collect sufficient data and then start modelling or to start modelling and see which data are likely to be of major importance. The first approach might easily lead to **not** collecting information that, afterwards, shows to be important (remember that *a priori* the knowledge level was poor). In the se-cond approach one starts with a, most likely weak, model based on poor understanding of the problem. Next, the model is improved in time by adding relevant data that are collected because the initial weak model indicated that such data were important. This second approach is called mechanistic (synonyms are: theoretical, explanatory, biological, heuristic). Mechanistic research aims to understand the behaviour of a system and based on that to model the system. *Vice versa*, the development of a model can be useful to help to understand the system.

Epidemiological models might play an important role by generating and testing theories about the spread of disease in a population and by the development of detection, control and prevention programmes. These models respect the basic principles of the population dynamics of a disease (Hethcote, 1989).

2. Model Types and Model Building

2.1. Types of models

An example of a simple model is:

$$M = p * C$$

which can be used to calculate the amount of money (M) a farmer has to pay his practitioner, who has performed a treatment at price p to a number of cows (C). To get M (the output) one needs to specify some input (p and C). M and C are variables, p is a parameter (it relates C to M). The structure of the model above is ***linear*** : for each extra cow treated, the extra cost is p. The model above is an oversimplification of reality as it excludes the costs for driving to and from the farm and disregards the fact that the price per treatment might decrease if many cows on the same farm are treated. Models are always an oversimplification; they never describe reality in an exact way and in fact that is not necessary as long as they fulfil the purpose they were developed for. This means that each model has its own constraints and a model should be used only within its own limits and under defined conditions.

Finally, the model above is ***deterministic*** because p is defined as a constant. If p would vary between a minimum and maximum value, e.g., by chance, then we would have a ***stochastic*** model. In such a model the value of p is determined by a randomly chosen value each time the model is run. This value is chosen from a given distribution (e.g., a Normal distribution) between a specified minimum and maximum value.

Another example of a simple model is:

$$X_{t+1} = X_t + (a * X_t) - (b * X_t)$$

This model is linear as well, but opposite to the first static model, this model is ***dynamic***. In a dynamic model the outcome (X_{t+1}, e.g., population size) depends on X_t (the population size in the previous time period) plus $a*X_t$ (the number of newborns, 'a' being the birth rate) minus $b*X_t$ (the number of deaths, 'b' being the mortality rate).

Besides the classification in linear/non-linear, static/dynamic, deterministic/ stochastic, there is a second classification according to how 'time' is treated in the model. Time can be treated either as ***discrete*** or ***continuous***. The dynamic model above is discrete as one can only have outcomes at specific points in time (t, t+1 etc.) and the model is described by **difference equations**. If time is treated continuously, the model consists of **differential equations**. In the latter integration and differentiation of mathematical formulae are central.

Model solutions can be obtained in 2 ways:

1. analytically, i.e., making calculations using pencil and paper (e.g., taking the second derivative of the formula of a growth curve and calculating the moment of maximal growth by putting the equation to 0);
2. numerically, i.e., calculate the outcomes of a growth curve for a large number of moments and determine the moments t and $t+\delta$ between which the difference in weight is maximal.

Only simple models, i.e., with specified behaviour and with few parameters, are to be solved analytically. Complex models are solved numerically and are called simulation models.

2.2. Model building process

The model building process consists of several steps:

- description of the system
- testing and improving
- experimentation

Description of the system

First of all, one has to define what is going to be modelled and why. This needs an accurate description of the problem and a clear formulation of the goals. Each part of the system to be modelled should be described, as well as the relation between parts and what inputs and outputs are important. In general, one should start with a simple model. If necessary, the model can be made more complex in a later stage. The borders of the system to be modelled and the main parameters and processes should be formulated/determined. Next, the type of model is chosen and model building can start. Often it is not clear which type of model suits best or how to develop a model that is suitable. In literature, only very general criteria are given as guidelines to choose the preferable model type. The next summary of criteria is according to Den Ouden (Personal Communication, 1990):

1. The mechanisms that form the basis of the model should be intuitively acceptable;
2. The model should behave reasonably in both biological and mathematical sense;
3. The model should be sensitive to known important parameters and insensitive to known less important parameters;
4. The model should mimic real-life situations;
5. The model should be simple enough for robust tests, but still have enough complexity to represent the modelled aspect of the system in an adequate way;
6. If the model is going to be used as an additional tool in decision making, the goal and limits of the model should be fully understood by the decision maker.

The diversity of the problems makes it impossible to formulate guidelines in a very strict way.

Testing and improving

If all mathematical equations are described, the model should be validated both internally and externally. A synonym for internal validation is verification.

verification: the assessment of precision and accuracy of the developed model. In other words: is the model doing, what you think it should do?

validation: validation is testing how well the model reflects reality. If suitable data are not available then only parts of the model can be validated. If validation shows that the model reflects reality in an insufficient way, the structure of the model or the parameters need to be improved. Sensitivity analysis might be part of the validation process. Sensitivity analysis means that values of parameters are systematically varied and it is examined how these changes affect the output of the model. Sensitivity analysis can be used to see whether or not the conclusion(s) from the output remain valid if the original parameter estimates are far from the true parameter values in the population.

The process of testing and improvement will continue until the model is found to reflect reality in a sufficient way. Validation might be done using field data.

Experimentation with the model

Only after the acceptance of the model, it can be used for its final purpose; e.g., a model might be used for evaluation and comparison of alternative control strategies of a disease in an epidemiological or economic sense. If a stochastic model is used, the model needs to be runned several times to evaluate an alternative. This will result in an average outcome and a variance which are both necessary for a formal statistical evaluation.

Use of model output

The ultimate goal of building a model is the development and application of specific theories or strategies. This indicates that the results of the model need to be combined with existing knowledge. Possible consequences of alternative parameter values can be evaluated. If a model is very sensitive to a specific parameter and the real value of this parameter is unknown, research to assess this specific value might be given a higher priority. By application of sensitivity analyses, the importance of inaccurate or missing knowledge about diseases or control strategies might be further specified. For example, outcomes of a simulation model might be used as a guide to determine which field data should be collected to increase insight in the transmission of a disease.

An example of a simple model is given by Frankena *et al.* (1997). The purpose of this model was to assess the probability of detection of the introduction of a bovine herpesvirus type 1 (BHV-1) seropositive animal on to a negative herd based on an antibody test in bulk milk. This information is essential if it is decided that a monitoring programme of a BHV-1 negative status is performed on bulk milk. This probability depends on the amount and titre of the positive milk and to what extent this positive milk is diluted by the herd mates. The minimal titre that converts the bulk milk to positive can then be calculated. A deterministic model returns the proportion of positive cows that have a titre larger or equal than this calculated minimal titre. For this, the titre distribution of positive cows needs to be known. A stochastic model randomly selects one cow (one titre) from the titre distribution and determines whether this titre exceeds the minimal titre. If the latter process is repeated several times, one can calculate the proportion of runs that resulted in a positive bulk milk status and this is the probability that a single positive cow will convert the bulk milk status. In the long run, the deterministic outcome and the average of all stochastic outcomes should be equal. However, from stochastic outcomes, variability can be assessed. E.g., if 100 runs were made and the stochastic probability to convert the bulk milk status was 0.25 (25%), then a 95% confidence interval would be $0.25 \pm \sqrt{(0.25*0.75)} / \sqrt{100} = [0.16; 0.34]$.

3. Infectious Disease Models

Mathematical models are also useful in investigations of the spread of infectious diseases in populations. A discrimination is made between models for macroparasitic and microparasitic infections. Microparasites are those agents that multiply within the host, that are relatively small, that have a short generation interval (sum of latent and infectious period) compared to the hosts' lifespan and that provoke an immune response in the host. Viral, bacterial and protozootic organisms can be seen as microparasites. Macroparasites do not directly multiply within the host (like gastro-intestinal nematodes), duration of infection is relatively long when compared to the hosts' lifespan and reinfection is common, because immunity is incomplete and/or is only effective during a short period of time (Anderson and May, 1991).

In models concerning microparasitic infections, the host plays a central role and the presence or effect of the parasite is included in the model in a qualitative way (host is infected or not, host is immune or not). In macroparasitic infections, the number of parasites is far more relevant. The level of infection is more important than the positive infection status. Hence, macroparasitic models are quantitative in nature. It should be mentioned that the division in micro- and macroparasites is not absolute, but the characteristics should be seen as an approximation. For example, a coccidiosis infection is, according to above mentioned characteristics, a microparasitic infection, since it is caused by a protozoan organism. However, the duration of a coccidiosis infection in broilers is relatively long when compared to the length of the hosts' life, and immunity development and production losses are influenced by the level of infection. This could be a reason for classifying coccidiosis as being caused by a macroparasite. Dependent on the modelling goals one should develop a micro- or macroparasitic model. This chapter mainly deals with modelling microparasitic infections. In paragraph 4 some attention is paid to macroparasitic infections.

3.1. Basic models in microparasitic infections

In microparasitic infections, the population of hosts might be split in a number of distinguishable classes. The distribution of the hosts over the classes changes in time. Individuals that are susceptible, but not yet infected are allocated to class S (Susceptible). Hosts that are infectious and are able to pass the infection to other hosts are assigned to class I Infectious). The class denoted as R consists of hosts that are Removed or Recovered (e.g., immune). Individuals in class R do not play a role any more in the interaction between susceptible and infectious individuals, because they are either (completely) immune, isolated or have died. $S_{(t)}$, $I_{(t)}$ and $R_{(t)}$ are expressions of the **proportions** of the total host population (N) in the several classes at time t. Models using these three classes are called SIR models.

3.2. SIR models using a constant probability of infection

At a constant probability of infection, individuals move between classes according to a specified, fixed probability, e.g., p_{si} (the probability that an animal moves from class S to class I). For example, in a SIR model without birth and mortality, the proportion of animals that is still in class S at time t + 1 is given by:

$$S_{(t+1)} = (1-p_{si})*S_{(t)} \text{with } 0 \leq p_{si} \leq 1$$

This system with fixed transition probabilities can be represented by a Markov chain. A Markov chain has two components: states and transitions, which are synonyms for variables and parameters. The probability of the transition from the current state to another state is solely determined by the current state. This means that the number of individuals that is becoming infected only depends on the number of susceptibles multiplied by a fixed probability ($p_{si}*S_{(t)}$). All the transition probabilities can be tabulated in a transition matrix (Table 9.1). The rows indicate the current state ('from') and the columns the next state ('to'). The probability of transition from a state in period i to another state in period j = i + 1, is denoted as p_{ij}. The sum of all probabilities in a row is always equal to one (each individual has to be in some class in the next time period). The unit of time and unit of modelling depend on the goals of the model. The unit of time can be days, weeks, months or even years. The unit of modelling might vary from individual animals to complete herds.

Table 9.1. Example of Markov chain transition matrix with 3 states.

	S[a]	I	R
S[b]	p_{ss}[c]	p_{si}	p_{sr}
I	p_{is}	p_{ii}	p_{ir}
R	p_{rs}	p_{ri}	p_{rr}

[a] Columns denote the state in period t + 1
[b] Rows denote the state in period t
[c] p_{ij}'s are the transition probabilities of a state at time t to another state at time t + 1

A simple numerical example of the Markov chain model is in the next table.

Transition matrix:

		To: Susceptible	Infectious	Recovered
	Susceptible	0.90	0.10	0.00
From:	Infectious	0.00	0.80	0.20
	Recovered	0.00	0.00	1.00

If in the start situation 100 susceptible animals are present and one infectious animal is introduced, then the number of animals in each category can be calculated based on the probabilities in the transition matrix. In the list below this is done for the first three time periods.

Period	Susceptible	Infectious	Recovered
0	200	1	0
1	200∗.9+1∗0+0∗0=180	200∗.1+1∗.8+0∗0=20.8	200∗0+1∗.2+0∗1=0.2
2	180∗.9+20.8∗0+0.2∗0=162	180∗.1+20.8∗.8+0.2∗0=34.6	180∗0+20.8∗.2+0.2∗1=4.36
3	162∗.9+34.6∗0+4.36∗0=73	162∗.1+34.6∗.8+4.36∗0=43.9	162∗0+34.6∗.2+4.36∗1=11.3

Figure 9.1 shows the graph obtained for the first 60 time periods. Figure 9.2 shows results from a more complicated model where a fourth state (Dead) is included with an equal transition probability of 0.1 from all three other states (be aware that all the probabilities in the transition matrix change, because all rows should sum up to one - see Table below). The population size is kept constant by the influx of newborns to the state Susceptible. Figure 9.2 shows that by the introduction of susceptible newborns, the infection sustains in the population (becomes endemic).

		To:			
		Susceptible	Infectious	Recovered	Dead
From:	Susceptible	0.81	0.09	0.00	0.10
	Infectious	0.00	0.72	0.18	0.10
	Recovered	0.00	0.00	0.90	0.10
	Dead	1.00	0.00	0.00	0.00

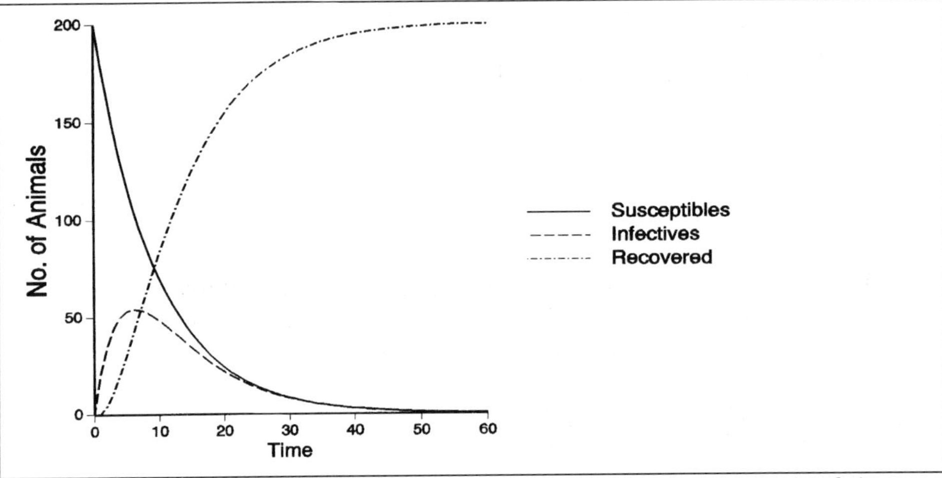

Figure 9.1. The course of number of animals in a population in each of the classes S, I, and R when a model is used with fixed transition probabilities.

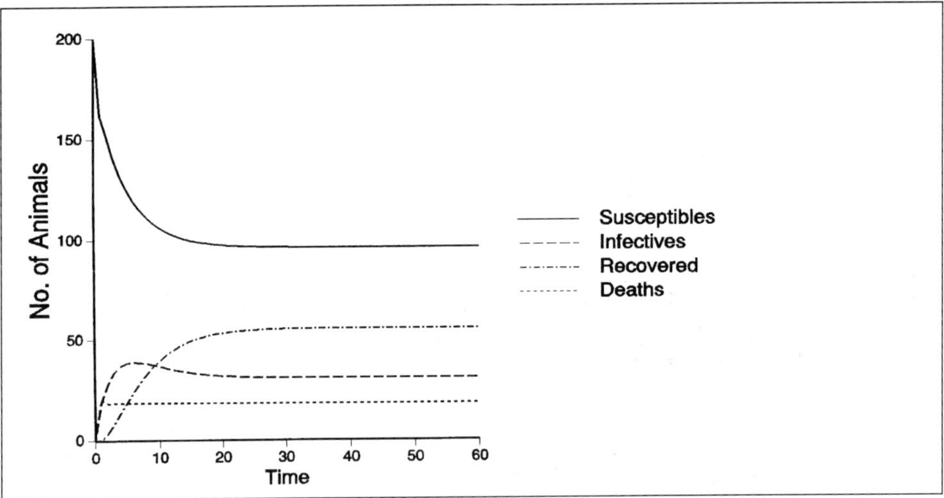

Figure 9.2. The course of number of animals in a population in each of the classes S, I, R, and a fourth state D when a model is used with fixed transition probabilities. Note that the disease becomes endemic.

3.3. SIR models with variable transition probabilities

The transition probabilities between states might vary according to the number of infectious animals in the previous period. This is a more general state transition model as the transition probabilities are not constant in time (as in the Markov chain model). A well known example is the Reed-Frost model in which it is assumed that infection of a susceptible animal occurs by direct contact (a contact with a specified intensity), with an infectious animal. Opposite to the Markov chain model, the number of infectious animals has an effect on the transition probabilities. It is assumed that each infectious animal has contact with a specified number of animals, regardless of their status, (S, I or R). The mathematical equation of such a model is:

$$I_{(t+1)} = S_{(t)} * \left(1 - Q^{I_{(t)}}\right)$$

t	=	time period (usually the time unit is chosen in a way that it reflects the length of the incubation period)
$I_{(t+1)}$	=	number of (new) infectious animals at the start of time period t+1
$I_{(t)}$	=	number of infectious animals at the end of time period t
$S_{(t)}$	=	number of susceptibles at the end of period t
Q	=	1 - p in which:
p	=	the probability of an effective contact (effective means that infection will occur if one of both is infectious and the other is susceptible); Q is therefore the probability of avoiding such a contact.

By assuming that cases become immune (R) after one time unit and immunity is permanent, all proportions can be determined:

$$S_{(t+1)} = S_{(t)} - I_{(t+1)}$$

$$R_{(t+1)} = \sum_{t=0}^{t=t} I_t$$

$$\text{with } S_{(t+1)} + I_{(t+1)} + R_{(t+1)} = 1$$

By multiplying the proportions by the population size, absolute numbers in each class are obtained. The data in Table 9.2 serve as an illustration. In a population of 200 susceptible animals, one infectious animal is introduced. It is assumed that there are six effective contacts per time unit, thus p equals 6/201 = 0.03 and Q = 0.97. In general, when x infectious animals are introduced p equals 6/(200 + x).

Table 9.2. Example of a Reed-Frost model.

t	$S_{(t)}*N$	$I_{(t)}*N$	$R_{(t)}*N$	$p*S_{(t)}*N$
0	200	1	0	5.97
1	194	6	1	5.79
2	162	32	7	4.83
3	61	101	39	1.83
4	3	58	140	0.09
5	1	2	198	0.02
6	1	0	200	0.03
7	1	0	200	0.03

The column $p*S_{(t)}*N$ indicates whether or not an epidemic (increasing number of cases) will occur when one infectious animal is introduced in the population. Note that the number of new cases decreases as soon as $p*S_{(t)}*N$ becomes smaller than one. This result can be used in control strategies, e.g., by making $S_{(t)}$ small (for example by vaccination) or by affecting p (for example other type of housing resulting in fewer effective contacts). The epidemic curve is shown in Figure 9.3.

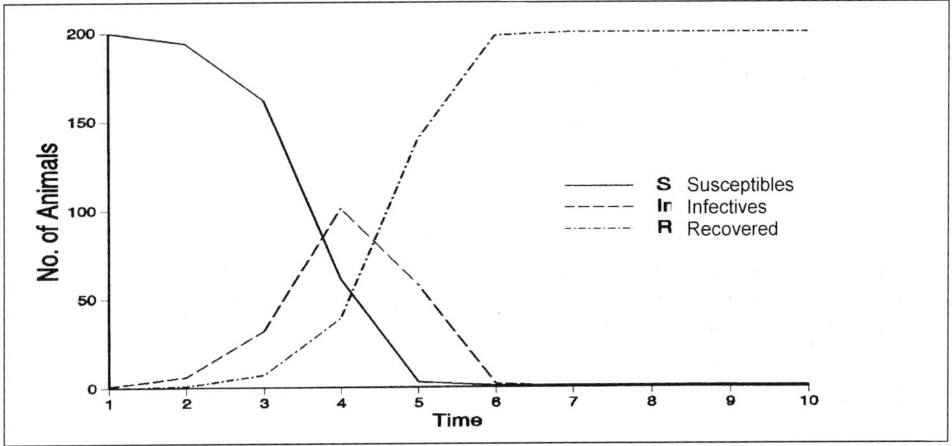

Figure 9.3. The course of number of animals in a population in each of the classes S, I, and R when variable transition probabilities are used (Reed-Frost model).

Exercise: suppose the population in the Reed-Frost example above is a population of sows. The purchase of one sow results in an outbreak of porcine respiratory and reproductive syndrome (PRRS). Of all the animals in the unit in which the purchased sow is placed, 50% was immune as a result of an earlier vaccination. You might use WINEPISCOPE (http://www.zod.wau.nl/qve) to solve this exercise and to obtain the epidemic curve.

Question 1: after how many weeks is the peak of the epidemic?
Question 2: as the vaccine is out of stock, the farmer tries to reduce the number of effective contacts. What is the maximum value of the number of effective contacts guaranteeing that, at average, an outbreak will not occur?

Answers: Question 1. The following table shows the number of animals in each class for the first eight time periods.

Exercise of a Reed-Frost model

t	$S_{(t)}*N$	$I_{(t)}*N$	$R_{(t)}*N$	$p*S_{(t)}*N$
0	100	1	100	2.99
1	97	3	101	2.90
2	89	8	104	2.64
3	70	19	112	2.08
4	39	31	131	1.17
5	15	24	167	0.46
6	7	8	186	0.22
7	5	2	194	0.16
8	5	0	196	0.14

Note that in this partly immune population, the number of cases decreases dramatically and that the peak of the epidemic is somewhat later (at t = 4) compared to Table 9.2 (a fully susceptible population with $S_{(t=0)}$ = 200 and $R_{(t=0)}$ = 0).

Question 2: $p*S_{(t)}*N$ should be equal to one at t = 0. As $S_{(t=0)}$ equals 100, p = 0.01 and the number of effective contacts is then $p*N = 0.01*200 = 2$ (this means that, at average, one effective contact is with a susceptible animal and one with an immune animal).

The Reed-Frost model is particularly suitable for diseases with a short infectious period (compared to the incubation period), direct disease transmission, complete immunity after infection, and when the group of individuals is homogeneous. Markov chain models are especially used to model a system or process in time (dynamic models). Transition probabilities might be estimated from e.g., longitudinal studies. By changing these probabilities it is possible to estimate effects of prevention and control strategies.

The Reed-Frost and Markov chain models can be adapted and/or combined in such a way that it makes the model fit better for the situation to be modelled. Instead of using fixed transition probabilities in Markov chain models, one can use a dynamic transition probability according to the Reed-Frost equation. Carpenter (1988a; 1988b) showed examples of classical Reed-Frost models and of modified Markov chains with a dynamic component according to the Reed-Frost model.

In the models considered until now, each run resulted in the same output (deterministic models), because the probabilities were used as fixed proportions flowing to the next state (e.g., 10% of the susceptibles became infected). However, probabilities might be used as such as well: each susceptible individual has a probability of 0.10 to become infected, but whether or not an animal will become infected is determined in a random way. An example is the "MoloCOF" model, a state transition model for cystic ovarian disease (COD) in dairy cattle (Hogeveen *et al.*, 1994). Five states were discriminated: fresh, cyclic, COD, pregnant and culled. In MoloCOF, the transition of one state to another depends on the previous state(s) of the cow and the transitions between states are determined using a randomizer. Suppose that the transition probability of state 'COD' to state 'pregnant' is 2% (0.02). MoloCOF draws a random number between 0 and 1; if this number is smaller than 0.02, the cow will flow to state 'pregnant'; if not the cow stays in state 'COD'. At average, 2% of the animals will then change from 'COD' to 'pregnant'. Because the transition probabilities are stochastic, each run will have a (slightly) different outcome. Such a model needs to be run several times to get a mean outcome and its variance.

3.4. Elaboration of SIR models

In the previous paragraphs, two specific types of SIR models were shown, the Markov chain model and the Reed-Frost model. SIR models may vary depending on characteristics of the agent (e.g., virulence), immunologic characteristics of the host, environmental characteristics affecting contacts between animals etc. In the following, a general approach is followed for SIR models in which newborns and mortality do not play an essential role and for SIR models with birth and mortality.

Figure 9.4 is a general diagram illustrating a SIR model with birth and mortality. In this diagram, the boxes contain numbers of individuals and the flow of animals, indicated by arrows, also represent numbers of animals.

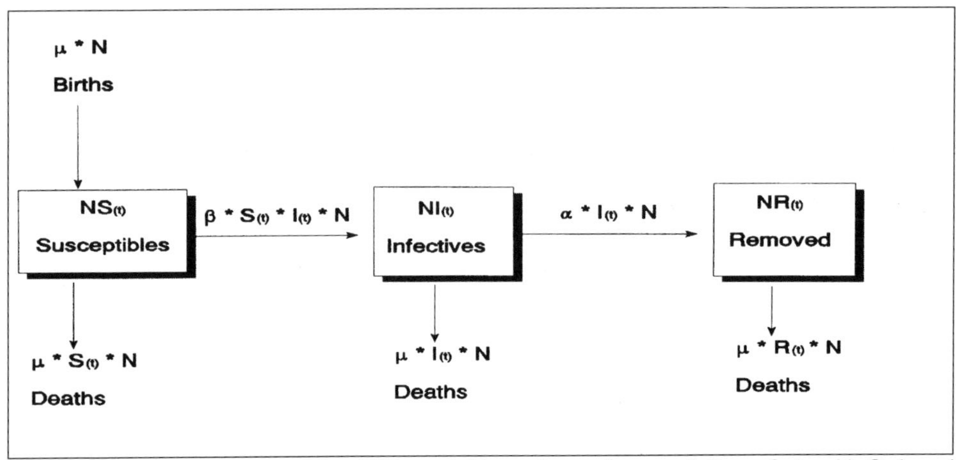

Figure 9.4. The diagram of the SIR model in a dynamic population of size N; S, I and R are proportions; α, β and μ are positive constants

We start with the most simple model: a SIR model with constant population size N and without mortality and birth (or without culling and purchase). Thus μ in Figure 9.4 is set to 0. This is a realistic model for infections that spread so rapidly that birth and mortality have no or very little effect on transmission of the disease (e.g., foot-and-mouth disease, infectious bovine rhinotracheitis (IBR)). In these models the following assumptions are made:

1. a single infection triggers the disease process in the host (just for microparasitic models);
2. an infectious animal is equally infectious during its infectious period;
3. infection results in complete immunity;
4. the environment of the host is constant;
5. the number of contacts of each animal with other animals is assumed to be independent of the population size (note that this logically implies that the chance of encountering one particular animal becomes smaller as the population size increases);
6. all individuals are assumed to be identical with regard to susceptibility and infectivity;
7. the size of the host population can be regarded as infinite.

When $\mu = 0$, the ***number*** of animals that flow per time unit from class S to class I depends on the infection rate β, the proportion of infectious animals ($I_{(t)}$) and the proportion of susceptible animals ($S_{(t)}$). This number equals:

$$\beta * S_{(t)} * I_{(t)} * N \qquad \textbf{(9.1)}$$

Then, the ***proportion*** of susceptibles in time decreases (recall that no new susceptibles enter the population):

$$\frac{dS_{(t)}}{dt} = \frac{-\beta * S_{(t)} * I_{(t)} * N}{N} = -\beta * S_{(t)} * I_{(t)}$$

This is the mass-action formulation in the form originally written by Lotka (1956), based upon the similarity with chemical reaction kinetics. That mass-action can also be applied to animals that mix randomly, has been demonstrated experimentally by Bouma *et al.* (1995).

In this formula, $dS_{(t)}$ denotes the change in the proportion of susceptible animals in a specific time interval of length dt.

Individuals that become infected recover each time period with a rate α, the recovery rate. This implies that the mean length of the infectious period is $1/\alpha$. The change in the proportion of animals in class R is described by:

$$\frac{dR_{(t)}}{dt} = \frac{\alpha * I_{(t)} * N}{N} = \alpha * I_{(t)}$$

Finally, the change in the proportion of infectious animals can be written in terms of the infection rate and the recovery rate:

$$\frac{dI_{(t)}}{dt} = \frac{\beta * S_{(t)} * I_{(t)} * N}{N} - \frac{\alpha * I_{(t)} * N}{N} = \beta * S_{(t)} * I_{(t)} - \alpha * I_{(t)}$$

The change in the proportion of infectious animals ($dI_{(t)}$) between time t and t + dt is determined by the proportion of animals that come from class S and that leave to class R.

From the three differential equations, the number of cases can be calculated at each point in time after an infectious individual is brought into a completely susceptible population. As stated before, the population size was defined as constant and thus $S_{(t)} + I_{(t)} + R_{(t)} = 1$.

In a completely susceptible population in which one infectious animal is introduced, $S_{(t=0)}$ equals 1, $I_{(t=0)} = 1/N$ and $R_{(t=0)} = 0$. Thus, the average ***number of effective contacts*** (σ) of an infectious individual with other individuals (any class) is:

$$\sigma = (\beta * S_{(t)} * I_{(t)} * N) * \frac{1}{\alpha} = \left(\beta * 1 * \frac{1}{N} * N\right) * \frac{1}{\alpha} = \frac{\beta}{\alpha}$$

In this formula $1/\alpha$ is the average length of the infectious period. The parameter σ is called the **basic reproductive rate R_0** (R nought), although it is not a rate but a number. Therefore, it is often called basic reproduction number. It expresses how many new cases arise, at average, from one infectious animal. Also basic reproduction ratio is used for R_0, in which ratio means the total number of newly infected individuals per infectious animal (De Jong and Diekmann, 1992). After introduction of an infectious animal in a (partly) susceptible population a minor or major outbreak may occur. Minor and major indicate the size of the outbreak. If R_0 is larger than 1, the probability to get a major outbreak is higher than the probability of getting a minor outbreak. If R_0 is smaller than 1, the outbreak will be, at average, of limited size and the infection cannot sustain itself in the population. This is only true if $\mu > 0$, since in a closed population with SIR dynamics an infection always disappears. Only in SIS models (no immunity after infection) an infection can become endemic.

The proportion of the population in class I will not change any more if $dI_{(t)}/dt = 0$, thus if $(\beta * S_{(t)} * I_{(t)}) - (\alpha * I_{(t)}) = 0$. This is true if $I_{(t)} = 0$ or if $S_{(t)} = \alpha/\beta$. The latter is equivalent to $S_{(t)} = 1/\sigma$ or $S_{(t)} * \sigma = 1$. Strictly, this is only true in the specific case that one infectious animal is brought into an infinitely large population of susceptible animals. Hence, the addition of the subscript 0 in R_0 and 'basic' in basic reproduction number. If not all members of the population are initially susceptible, the use of R instead of R_0 is recommended. In Anderson and May (1991), the relation between R and R_0 is given as: $R = R_0 * x$, where x is the proportion of initially susceptibles.

How can the value of σ be obtained? First of all, challenge experiments can be carried out, in which infectious animals are put among susceptible ones (De Jong and Kimman, 1994). By daily sampling, it can be determined if and when susceptibles become infected and the length of the infectious period can be determined as well. In this way, R values (after a single and a double vaccination respectively) for Aujeszky's disease were estimated to be 3.4 and 1.5, respectively (Stegeman *et al.*, 1995). Secondly, R_0 can be estimated from longitudinal field data, in which the number of susceptibles at the beginning of the time period ($S_{(t=0)}$) and the number at the end ($S_{(t=\infty)}$) are known (Bosch, 1997). If $S_{(t=0)}$ and $S_{(t=\infty)}$ are not equal and it is assumed that $I_{(t=\infty)}$ is zero (the infection has died out) a relatively simple formula approximates R (Hethcote, 1989).

$$\sigma = \frac{\left(\ln\left(\frac{S_{(t=0)}}{S_{(t=\infty)}}\right)\right)}{S_{(t=0)} - S_{(t=\infty)}}$$

Example: imagine a multiplier farm with 130 sows experiencing an outbreak of disease. Before the outbreak, all animals were negative. After the outbreak, only 10 animals remained negative, while no infectious animals were left. Now: calculate σ (answer: $S_{(t=0)} = 130/130 = 1$ and $S_{(t=\infty)} = 10/130$, then $\sigma = 2.8$).

The value of R_0 is very basic in mathematical epidemiology and can be used for evaluating different strategies for disease control. If the control strategy consists of a vaccination programme, it can be calculated whether or not the infection still spreads in the population. The ultimate result of vaccination (assuming that it is 100% effective) is that individuals flow directly from state S to state R. Then, $S_{(t)}$, and thus $\sigma * S_{(t)}$, will be lower as fewer new infectious cases arise from one infectious individual. This implies that unvaccinated animals are protected from infection if (a considerable) part of the herd mates are immune. Thus, in a vaccination programme it is not needed to vaccinate the entire population to eradicate the disease (although it is most effective if only the time scale of the eradication programme is considered).

Using the value of R_0, it is possible to calculate the proportion of individuals which needs to be immune in order to achieve eradication of the infectious agent. Anderson and May (1991) called this the 'critical proportion' and it is calculated as:

$$\text{Critical Proportion} = 1 - \frac{1}{R_0}$$

Thus, the higher R_0, the higher the proportion of individuals that needs to be immune in order to prevent spread of the disease (see also Figure 9.5). Use of the critical proportion is only valid when contacts between animals are random, implying a homogeneous distribution of immune animals over the population.

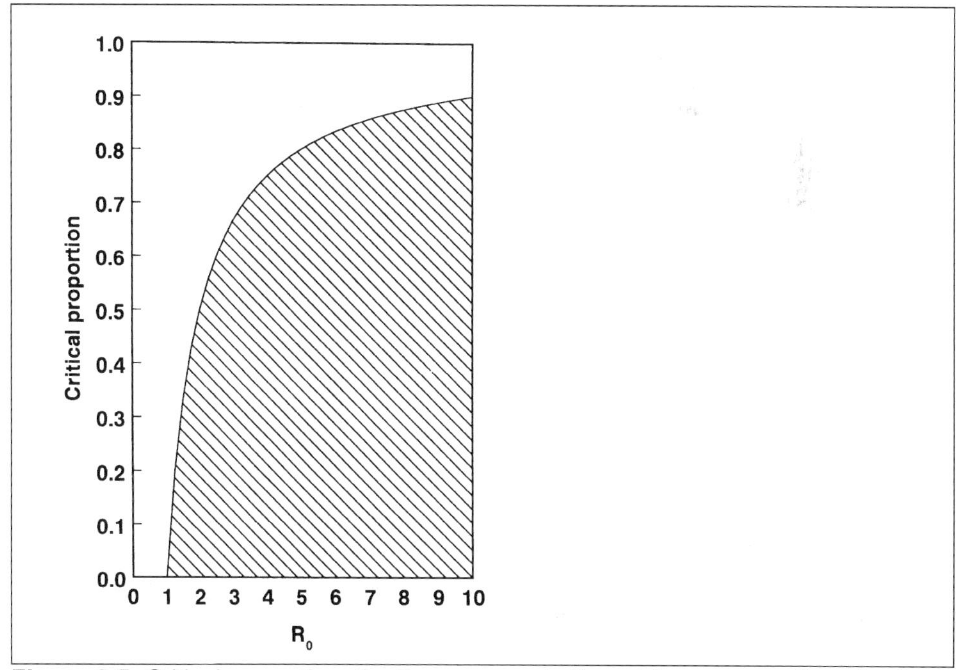

Figure 9.5. Critical proportion: the line represents the minimum proportion of animals that need to be immune in order to prevent transmission of the infectious agent (the white area is the safe area).

However, vaccine efficacy is seldom 100% and R might be used to estimate its efficacy. If R in a vaccinated population is larger than one, then the vaccine cannot prevent spread of the infection totally and an eradication programme relying on vaccination only is deemed to fail. Bosch (1997) estimated the R for two IBR vaccines under field conditions as 2.4 and 1.1. It was concluded that eradication was not possible by using solely one of these two vaccines, and that additional zootechnical measures that affect the contact rate (β) were necessary.

3.5. SIR models with birth and mortality

If μ in Figure 9.4 is not equal to 0, birth and mortality (or culling and purchase which is more common in veterinary epidemiology) have an effect on the number of individuals in each of the classes, S, I and R. In the following it is assumed that birth and mortality are in balance (N is constant), although one can account for an unbalanced situation (resulting in a more complex model with μ_1 being the birth rate and μ_2 the mortality rate). It is also assumed that all newborns enter the population as susceptible, and that mortality is not affected by infection.

In absence of infection, the change in the population size of class S is described by:

$$\frac{dS_{(t)}}{dt} = \mu - \mu * S_{(t)}$$

The solution when the population is in a steady state is when $dS_{(t)}/dt = 0$. This is true when $S_{(t)} = 1$ or, in words, when the total population consists of susceptible animals. If infectious animals are present in the population, the total set of differential equations is:

$$\frac{dS_{(t)}}{dt} = \mu - \mu * S_{(t)} - \beta * S_{(t)} * I_{(t)}$$

$$\frac{dI_{(t)}}{dt} = \beta * S_{(t)} * I_{(t)} - \alpha * I_{(t)} - \mu * I_{(t)}$$

$$\frac{dR_{(t)}}{dt} = \alpha * I_{(t)} - \mu * R_{(t)}$$

The class R now consists of immune and died individuals. Equivalent to the SIR model without birth and mortality (assuming $S_{(t=0)} = 1$ and $I_{(t=0)} = 1/N$), R_0 can be calculated as:

$$R_0(\sigma) = N * \left(\beta * 1 * \frac{1}{N}\right) * \frac{1}{\alpha + \mu} = \frac{\beta}{\alpha + \mu}$$

4. Macroparasitic Infection Models

In paragraph 3.1 it was mentioned that different mathematical models exist for microparasitic and macroparasitic infections. To recall, macroparasites are characterized by the fact that hosts do not acquire (complete) immunity and therefore reinfection might occur. In macroparasitic infections, intermediate hosts might be involved in the life cycle (e.g., fascioliasis). Further, in most macroparasitic infections, production depression and development of immunity depend on the number of parasites present. In microparasitic infections, the population of hosts is mostly divided into three classes (S, I and R) while in macroparasitic infections many classes might exist. In general, the host population shows a negative Binomial distribution, i.e., just a few hosts are infected with many parasites, whereas the majority only harbour just a few parasites.

The transmission of macroparasitic infections also can be described by the basic reproduction ratio. However, in this case, R_0 is used for the population of parasites instead of the population of hosts. Roughly, Anderson and May (1991) defined this R_0 as the average number of offspring produced during the reproductive life span of a fertile female parasite. The interpretation of R_0 is the same as in microparasitic infections, i.e., when $R_0 < 1$ the infection will eventually become extinct.

Where in microparasitic models only the dynamics of the host population need to be described, macroparasitic models are more complex. This complexity consists of describing the dynamics of the parasite population as well as the contacts between the host and parasite (stages) outside the host. The interested reader is referred to Anderson and May (1991) for further modelling details.

5. Concluding Remarks

Many variations can be made in the models described. For example, a latent period can be included (SEIR model, E is exposed) or immunity might be absent (SIS models) or only be effective during a short period of time (SIRS or SEIRS models). Secondly, in the models described, $S_{(t)}$, $I_{(t)}$ and $R_{(t)}$ were fractions of the population. The contact rate β was assumed to be constant and the proportion of newly infected animals is given by $\beta * S_{(t)} * I_{(t)}$ ('mass action' principle). This indicates that the probability of infection varies with the number of infectious and susceptible individuals. However, other models do exist; e.g., with fixed probabilities (Markov chain) or probabilities that vary according to other relations (Reed-Frost models).

Models have been developed in which the incidence is described by $\beta' * S_{(t)}' * I_{(t)}'$ with $S_{(t)}'$ being the **number** of susceptible animals and $I_{(t)}'$ the **number** of infectious animals). In the notation used throughout this chapter, it would be $\beta * N * S_{(t)} * N * I_{(t)}$. The β' is equal to β/N and depends on the size of the population. Using a constant β, it is assumed that irrespective of the population size the number of contacts per individual remains constant. For diseases transmitted by direct contact this assumption is reasonable. If the number of contacts increases, e.g., due to crowding then β' is assumed to be constant and β would increase with N. An experiment showing that, at least for Aujeszky's disease in pigs, a constant β is valid, is described by Bouma *et al.* (1995).

In all models, it was assumed that sizes of class S, I and R can be regarded as continuous. However, in small populations it is more realistic to handle these variables as discrete (to prevent that half 'individuals' get infected). This can be achieved by following individuals separately in time and then the occurrence of the event 'infection' will depend on whether or not a random number will exceed a predetermined probability (this probability can be determined by, for example, $\beta * S_{(t)} * I_{(t)}$).

Though the title of this chapter is 'Introduction to Theoretical epidemiology', the outcomes of mathematical models can be useful in decision making (e.g., whether or not to start a vaccination programme), to evaluate vaccine efficacy (Bosch, 1997; Stegeman *et al.*, 1995) or they can aid to evaluate control strategies in an economic sense (Buijtels, 1997). Also, mathematical modelling might be used to estimate whether or not the free status obtained after a successful eradication programme can be preserved for longer times (i.e., if an outbreak on one farm results at average in less than one other infected farm, the free status will be maintained) (Graat *et al.*, 2000).

In first instance, mathematical modelling looks complicated and indeed it is not easy to grasp as the differential equations might become very complex, even for simple problems. However, computer software exists that handles these complex sets of differential equations (Mathematica®: Wolfram, 1991). Despite that, we recognize that this chapter is not sufficient to make you an expert in mathematical modelling and it was not meant that way. The intention was to show you the potentials of mathematical modelling by using simplistic models and we agree with De Jong (1995) that the mathematical approach needs more attention in veterinary epidemiology.

Finally, a sound decision, based on model outcomes, can only be made if the final user knows the limits of the model and the assumptions underlying the model very well.

References

Anderson, R.M.; May, R.M. (1991). Infectious Diseases of Humans. Oxford University Press, Oxford.

Bouma, A.; Jong, M.C.M. de; Kimman, T.G. (1995). Transmission of pseudorabies virus within pig populations is independent of the size of the population. Preventive Veterinary Medicine, 23, 163-172.

Bosch, J.C. (1997). Bovine Herpesvirus 1 marker vaccines: tools for eradication? PhD thesis, University of Utrecht, The Netherlands.

Buijtels, J.A.A.M. (1997). Computer simulation to support policy-making in Aujeszky's disease control. PhD thesis, Wageningen Agricultural University, The Netherlands.

Carpenter, T.E. (1988a). Stochastic epidemiologic modeling using a microcomputer spreadsheet package. Preventive Veterinary Medicine, 5, 159-168.

Carpenter, T.E. (1988b). Microcomputer programs for Markov and modified Markov chain disease models. Preventive Veterinary Medicine, 5, 169-179.

Frankena, K.; Franken, P.; Vandehoek, J.; Koskamp, G.; Kramps, J.A. (1997). Probability of detecting antibodies to bovine herpesvirus 1 in bulk milk after the introduction of a positive animal on to a negative farm. Veterinary Record, 140, 90-92.

Graat, E.A.M.; De Jong, M.C.M.; Frankena, K.; Franken, P. Modelling the effect of surveillance programmes on spread of bovine herpesvirus 1 between certified cattle herds. Veterinary Microbiology 2000, in press.

Hethcote, H.W. (1989). Three basic epidemiological models. In: Applied Mathematical Ecology. Levin, S.A.; Hallam, T.G.; Gross, L.J. (Eds.). Springer-Verlag, Berlin, pp. 119-144.

Hogeveen, H.; Schukken, Y.H.; Laporte, H.M.; Noordhuizen, J.P.T.M. (1994). Cystic ovarian disease in Dutch dairy cattle, II. A simulation model for predicting the herd-level consequences under varying management factors. Livestock Production Science, 38, 199-206.

Holling, C.S. (1978). Adaptive Environmental Assessment and Management. John Wiley & Sons, Chichester.

Jong, M.C.M. de; Diekmann, O. (1992). A method to calculate - for computer-simulated infections - the threshold value, R_0, that predicts whether or not the infection will spread. Preventive Veterinary Medicine, 12, 269-285.

Jong, M.C.M. de; Kimman, T.G. (1994). Experimental quantification of vaccine-induced reduction of virus transmission. Vaccine, 12, 761-766.

Jong, M.C.M. de (1995). Mathematical modelling in veterinary epidemiology: why model building is important. Preventive Veterinary Medicine, 25, 183-193.

Lotka, A.J. (1956). Elements of Mathematical Biology. Dover Publications, New York.

Starfield, A.M.; Bleloch, A.L. (1991). Building Models for Conservation and Wildlife Management. 2nd edn. Burgess International Group Inc., Edina.

Stegeman, J.A.; Nes, A. van; Jong de, M.C.M; Bolder, F.W.M.M. (1995). Assessment of the effectiveness of vaccination against pseudorabies in finishing pigs. American Journal of Veterinary Research, 56, 573-578.

Wolfram, S. (1991). Mathematica®, a system for doing mathematics by computer. 2nd edn. Addison-Wesley Publishing Company Inc., New York.

Chapter X

Veterinary Epidemiology and Foodborne Diseases

Part I

Food Hygiene: The Example of Salmonellosis

J.P.T.M. Noordhuizen
Department of Farm Animal Health
Faculty of Veterinary Medicine
University of Utrecht
The Netherlands

1. Introduction

Historically, eradication campaigns against highly contagious diseases of livestock, such as bovine tuberculosis and brucellosis have been primarily undertaken to benefit producers, rather than the public. Since infections of man with *M.bovis* and *B.abortus* are milkborne, and pasteurization largely reduces the risk to consumers, these eradication campaigns were not needed from a public health perspective. In contrast, the most currently relevant and common foodborne disease agents, such as *Salmonella*, *Campylobacter*, *Listeria*, *E.coli*, and *Yersinia*, in general only rarely produce serious disease problems in livestock. To combat these agents, a national control programme could not be justifiably based on their economic impact on the animal production sector. These disease agents have another disadvantage: they are ubiquitous; seldom is there overt disease, and complex ecological niches persist. This means that procedures to test, remove and eradicate do not always operate efficiently.

Are food animals then a source of infection or contamination of products for man? Should microbiological food safety start at the animal production level?

In this part I, these questions will be addressed both generally and by means of the example of salmonellosis in man and livestock.

2. General Reflections About Food Safety

There is no true consensus about the issue of whether or not food animals play an important role in microbial foodborne diseases in man. For infections such as *Salmonella*, *Campylobacter* and *E.coli* $O_{157}H_7$ however, this seems obvious as will be shown later. This kind of uncertainty points to the need for more informative studies to determine to what extent food animal groups or sectors contribute to foodborne disease. Analytical observational studies and risk assessment procedures seem most appropriate to this purpose. These studies are equally adequate to achieve a consensus among those who are involved in food safety and public health, in both livestock and public health organizations. After all, these are the ones who decide on the implementation of screening, control, eradication and/or prevention programmes. Waltner-Toews (1996) pointed to the need of integrating social, cultural and ecological issues into the search for solutions of foodborne diseases. He presented the example of an outbreak of verocytotoxin producing *E.coli* $O_{157}H_7$ in the USA (earlier reported by Bell *et al.*, 1994 in Waltner-Toews, 1996): causes could be attributed to personal eating habits, restaurant practices (quickly cooked, cheap food), food processing policies (fast lines, high technical efficiency, maximum labour efficiency), international and national market or trade policies (cheap meat from external sources).

During a workshop in Washington DC in 1992 on "Implementing Food Animal Pre-Harvest Food Safety Internationally", attended by members of regulatory bureaus, commerce and the scientific community, several issues were addressed and recommendations made which are addressed in paragraphs 2.1, 2.2 and 2.3 (Anonymous, 1992).

How can food safety be organized at the farm level? Let us observe 3 programme options.

2.1. Screening and/or eradication programmes run by government

The basis would be that all farms that transport animals to slaughter should be open for inspection, comparable to the milk quality control system on dairy farms. This would obviously require a lot of manpower. The inspection is only useful if critical risk and control points have been identified. Eradication programmes aimed at specific agents may be possible. Detailed knowledge of the microbiological and epidemiological features of foodborne agents is required. Various agents seem not to be eradicable, e.g., because of persistent niches in the environment. Cost-effectiveness should be assessed and the fact that budgetary neutral programmes are not always feasible, should be considered: public health authorities may impose very costly control programmes on the sector while the benefits are not for the sector but for the public. Major and broad developments in this area are not expected.

2.2. Producers-driven quality assurance programmes

The current quality assurance programmes organized by livestock producer groups, primarily addressing residue problems and other quality aspects, could be expanded to include foodborne agents. Authorities then could set standards for monitoring and could provide development funds. Programmes for individual farms could be supported regionally and include veterinary supervision. Risk factor analysis should be performed in order to implement quantitative methods, define parameters and set targets, such as elimination of an agent. The problems foreseen are a lack of coordination and structure, and knowledge of risk factors involved. The former can be overcome by better organisation, the latter by conducting observational-analytic epidemiological studies (see also Chapter V and part II of this chapter).

2.3. Retailer-driven, integrated quality assurance throughout the production chain

This approach has seen a strong development in several European countries. The system is also called an "Integrated Food Chain Quality Control Programme" (shortly IQC), as applied, for example, in The Netherlands and Denmark. The incentive was based on the high costs associated with some massive outbreaks of foodborne disease and/or the potentials of improving quality by feeding back information on findings at slaughter to the farm in order to improve animal health status. Among these costs are lost sales, liability problems, lost image of the product or sector. Product quality is defined in a broader sense than the traditional one of nutritional value and taste alone. Also included now are the exclusive use of approved medicines, animal welfare issues, veterinary health care methods, certification procedures (e.g., for good farming practice, for animal health, and even for veterinary practices). When farms are linked to slaughterhouses and a feed mill, and to retailer chains or export chains, such systems could be very worthwhile; all links in the food chain are covered. In export situations, this approach leads to the build up of premiums. For insurance against foodborne diseases, again there are constraints such as the level of knowledge and the extent to which epidemiological studies and risk analysis are undertaken (see also part II of this chapter).

In all three situations, it is paramount that there is a role for quantitative epidemiology, but authorities and industry should take the lead in setting up such programmes and include epidemiology.

In Table 10.1, three routes of approaching food safety at the farm level are given.

Table 10.1. Outline of routes for defining control points for food safety at the farm level (Anonymous, 1992).

Possible routes for control	Developments needed to identify control points
I. Eradication of specific agents	1. determine if agent is subject to eradication 2. gather data to calculate cost - effectiveness of eradication 3. determine natural history of the agent within/between herds 4. identify means of detecting herds and individuals harbouring the agent
II. Reduction in contamination level of specific agents among animals at slaughter	1. identify ecological factors favouring the agent over competing non-pathogenic flora 2. identify competing bacterial flora for possible use in competitive exclusion (Nurmi concept) 3. identify effects of pre-slaughter holding conditions on contamination level
III. Reduced contamination of all faecally-carried organisms among animals at slaughter	1. identify the role of coat contamination level on post-slaughter contamination level 2. identify determinants of coat contamination level for possible use in pre-slaughter preparation programmes 3. identify the role of microfloral differences of cattle on contamination with a range of pathogens 4. identify the determinants of critical microfloral differences for use in possible pre-slaughter preparation 5. design a system for routine quality assurance monitoring

Based on this Table, it seems logical that current veterinary herd health programmes (Brand *et al.*, 1996) do not provide the necessary means *per se* to cover food safety issues. The reason is that food safety would require specific, scientifically justified critical control points and cannot be based on the type of observations and the current parameters handled within common herd health programmes. A good example is the verocytotoxin - producing *E.coli* $O_{157}H_7$ phenomenon, causing disease in man (haemolytic - uraemia syndrome in children with a case-fatality rate of 3 - 5%), but not causing problems in cattle. Risk assessment procedures could possibly fill this gap.

Another aspect is diagnostic tests. Would it be necessary to have accurate, reliable and rapid tests which lead to the goal of adequate food safety checks at farm level? Or should we proceed with the best tests available sofar? And also: what gain is to be expected from even better tests with regard to food safety?

The Workshop in Washington DC, USA (Anonymous, 1992) presented several recommendations with regard to food safety, some of which are already adopted in other countries such as Denmark and The Netherlands. Among these recommendations are:

1. the need to establish a national advisory council on food safety, recommending guidelines for voluntary quality assurance programmes (including validation criteria; implementation of monitoring; educational programmes; defining areas for further research in particular segments of the food production chain);

2. implementing food safety screening at farm level:
   - establish a safe food philosophy;
   - develop a credible veterinarian-producer relationship;
   - develop training programmes on safe handling of foods for livestock;
   - develop the research base for improved detection of food safety hazards, model analysis of factors and processes involved and intervention strategies;
   - implement on-farm surveillance systems based on hazard analysis;
   - develop risk assessment models for foodborne disease outbreaks;
   - develop systems for purifying food and water of food animals;
   - design epidemiological and ecological studies of on-farm hazards;
   - develop certification programmes for animal product quality;
   - adopt a uniform animal identification system.

Ecological studies should be aimed at "niche engineering", that is scientific and technological investigations into persistent reservoirs and microhabitats at local level. Such investigations should comprise social, cultural and ecological issues (Waltner-Toews, 1996). Niche engineering also regards questions such as: what makes the *E.coli* $O_{157}H_7$ a foodborne disease agent? Is it its behaviour one week prior to slaughter or rather at slaughter? And then, by what is this difference caused? It seems appropriate that multivariate studies should be conducted which are aimed at differences in housing, nutrition, waste management etc. using some cattle herds endemically infected and others that are not. By which factors are niches formed and influenced? The result of niche engineering studies must be to identify actions that can reduce or eliminate niches and hence contamination at slaughter. In some respect these niche engineering studies are multivariate epidemiological studies (see below for such a study on *Salmonella* infections of poultry).

One of the conclusions of the Workshop was, that traditional microbiology is (no longer) able to provide solutions to foodborne disease problems. It is highly necessary that other, broader scientific disciplines are involved in the combat and prevention of these diseases.

3. Salmonellosis: General Remarks

In general, various factors contribute to the occurrence of Salmonella infections in man and livestock. Bolder (1981) has presented the outline of the infection cycle (Figure 10.1).

Most of the factors or conditions named in Figure 10.1 have been studied in the past in a monodisciplinary way and not integrated. Among these are feed, housing, cleaning and disinfection, colonization resistance, birds, rodents, surface water, transportation and cross-contamination at the slaughterhouse.

From this Figure it appears that *Salmonella* infections represent a multifactorial syndrome, involving various ecological conditions and routes. Furthermore, one should be aware of the fact that social and cultural behaviour of the consumer has a great impact on the level and severity of foodborne diseases. It is not easy to control all of these factors. Points in the food chain for successful strategic intervention to reduce human health hazards and disease risk must be chosen well. Moreover, it seems obvious that control procedures at farm level should go beyond the scope of the merely microbiological traditions.

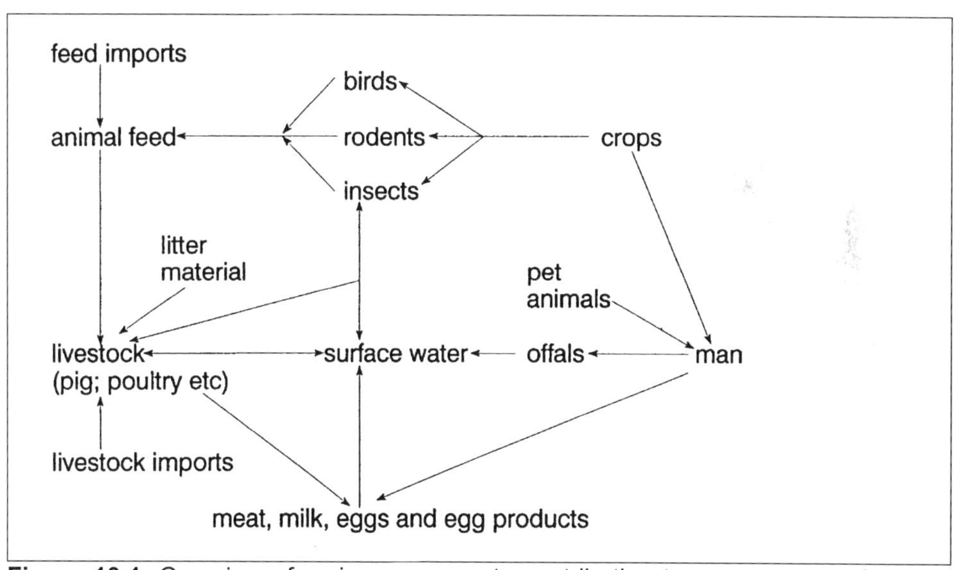

Figure 10.1. Overview of major components contributing to occurrence and spread of salmonellosis in livestock (modified after Bolder, 1981).

For diagnostic purposes, the ISO (International Standardization Organization) international standard method still can be followed (ISO-6579; ISO-6575). All strains isolated should be sent to a recognized Salmonella Reference Centre for definitive serological and biochemical typing. In that case the specificity of the detection method is

100%. The sensitivity, however, of the ISO method for faecal or caecal samples is unknown, but is estimated at 80-90%. Abundant other microflora in the sample may affect this sensitivity by overgrowing the flora of interest. The latter affects the sample size. On the other hand, not all serotypes may have equal chances of being isolated. This may be dependent on the ingredients of the culture media, hampering the growth of certain serotypes while enhancing that of others. *Salmonella spp.* are known for their vertical (transovarial) and/or their horizontal transmission; examples of the former are *S.enteritidis* and *S.pullorum*, and of the latter *S.typhimurium*, *S.dublin* and *S.enteritidis*.

4. Salmonellosis in Man

Salmonellosis is recognized worldwide as a major cause of acute human gastro-enteritis. In Germany, the number of reported cases annually amounted 214 per 100.000 inhabitants in one eastern department in 1992, while other eastern departments showed an increase to 325 cases per 100.000 inhabitants. In contrast to these figures, the western departments showed 187 cases per 100.000 inhabitants. Contributory causes to this increase have been named: the changing market movements for poultry and food, inexperience of cooks and a change in food and food preparation traditions (Kaesbohrer *et al.*, 1993).

The isolates showed a shift from *S.typhimurium* (down to 10%) to *S.enteritidis* (increase to 80% of all isolates in 1990). Age- and sexe specific incidences show particular patterns, as well as a seasonal distribution (see Figure A and B in the Appendix).

Children of 1-2 years of age were particularly at risk for *S.enteritidis*, while for *S.typhimurium* the age-group under 6 years is particularly at risk. Females were more frequently affected than males in the case of *S.enteritidis*, but for *S.typhimurium* this was the opposite. Enteritidis infections were more frequently observed during warmer, summer months (June - September). Egg products were found to be involved in 50% of the reported cases and poultry products in 30%; *S.typhimurium* was involved through meat products in 38% of the cases. *Salmonella spp.* are increasingly detected in the environment such as in garbage, surface water, drinking water, soil around feed mills and slaughterhouses (Kaesbohrer *et al.*, 1993).

The incidence rates of Salmonella infections vary widely between countries and regions. In the USA, reported incidents increased from about 25.000 in the 1950's to about 45.000 in the 1990's, pointing at 15-20 cases per 100.000 inhabitants (Waltner-Toews, 1996). Todd estimated the true incidence of salmonellosis to be 350 times higher in Canada than the reported numbers of cases; case fatality rates of 0.1 - 0.2% have been reported (Todd, 1989 in Waltner-Toews, 1996).

In The Netherlands, the incidence rate of reported cases of salmonellosis amounted to 750 cases per 1 million inhabitants per year (Hoogenboom-Verdegaal *et al.*, 1992). From an earlier study it had appeared that only 15% of persons with a *Salmonella* infection consult their doctor (Hoogenboom-Verdegaal *et al.*, 1989). This means that the true incidence of *Salmonella* infections approximates 5.000 cases per 1 million inhabitants per year. About 2000 serotypes are detected at the National Salmonella Centre annually. Results obtained over the years show that patterns of isolates changed: while *S.typhimurium* dropped, *S.enteritidis* has increased for example (Edel and Visser, 1989).

Components of economic loss directly related to the disease in man comprise disease treatment, hospitalizing costs, deaths in high risk groups such as youngsters and the elderly, extra health care, labour productivity loss, affected welfare. Some of these costs are very difficult to estimate. Roberts (1989) has estimated the national loss due to salmonellosis in humans at 50 million dollars per year in the USA.

Outbreaks of salmonellosis in man are usually limited to the high risk groups and often show seasonal patterns. The most well-known cases refer to outbreaks of salmonella infections in man after consumption of contaminated eggs or egg products.

In Figure 10.2, patterns of outbreaks of *Salmonella spp.* infections in man in relation to age are depicted; data originate from Germany (Kaesbohrer *et al.*, 1993).

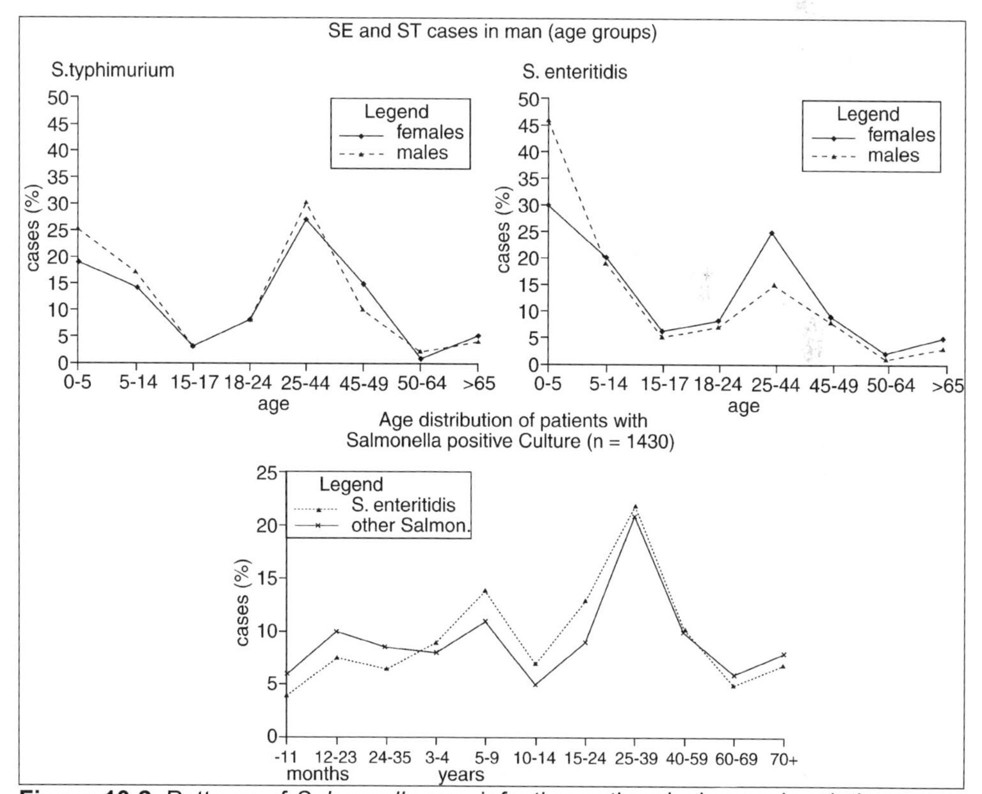

Figure 10.2. Patterns of *Salmonella spp.* infection outbreaks in man in relation to age and sex in Germany, 1992 (Kaesbohrer *et al.*, 1993).

Farm animals are generally considered to be the main source of *Salmonella* infection to man. Associations have been found between trends of serotypes in animal and in human populations. Isolates of *S.enteritidis* have increased dramatically in poultry after 1987, but the prevalence in pigs and veal calves remained low. In order to provide a better indication of the source of serotypes emerging in man and to more effectively control the transmission of these, more precise knowledge about prevalences and patterns of *Salmonella* infections in farm animals is needed; a monitoring and surveillance system could be used for that purpose (see Chapter XII). Furthermore, it seems indicated that database systems should be developed in an international setting to compare epidemiological data, not only because of the increased human mobility between countries, but also because of the increasing trade in animals and animal products, feedstuffs and commodities. The Concept Council Directive 92/117/EC of the European Union dealing with specific zoonoses and zoonotic agents, also points to the need for accurate, reliable and internationally comparable disease data.

5. Salmonellosis in the Animal Production Sector

Due to vertical and/or horizontal transmission, *Salmonella* infections can easily spread throughout the production sector along the food chain to man.

According to the outlines in Figure 10.1, there are many factors or conditions involved in the occurrence of infections. Many of these conditions have been studied during the last decades, but in a rather monodisciplinary approach, e.g., experimentally. Many *Salmonella spp.* are known as conditionally pathogenic, meaning that host defense mechanisms are hampered when environmental stressors are accumulating and affect the balance between defence and agent. Therefore, it could be worthwhile considering a multivariate epidemiological approach to the salmonellosis problem in livestock (see also Chapter VI).

As an example of this approach, we address the problem of salmonellosis in broiler breeder flocks (Henken *et al.*, 1992). In this study, covering a 5-year period and 111 broiler breeder flocks on 32 farms, data were gathered about *Salmonella* diagnosis and about the animals' environment such as location, housing, feeding, hygiene and disinfection, management, and presence of other species on the farm. The environment-related data were collected by questionnaire (see Chapter XII). The study was designed as a case-control study. See respective paper for more details on design.

Table 10.2 gives the overview of variable classes among cases and controls and the values of the crude odds ratios based on a univariate analysis. Table 10.3 presents the results of the multivariate, logistic regression analysis.

It appears that aspects such as hygiene barriers and disinfection tubs, either alone or as interaction term, play a substantial role in this type of horizontal contamination. The highest estimate of the odds ratio was obtained in situations on farms where a disinfection tub was absent, where hygiene barriers were poor, and where small feed mills delivered to the farm; the summarized OR is then $e^{-0.66-0.39+3.22+1.66} = 46$ times higher than on farms where these factors have opposite values. Small feed mills alone already increased the odds of the salmonella-positive state with a factor 5.3 ($e^{1.66}$) compared to larger feed mills. The small feed mills could comprise the phenomenon of only one production line which can easily be contaminated. Other factors featuring in the univariate analysis and disappearing in the multivariate analysis, can still be of relevance in the occurrence of infections on certain farms, although not explicitly in this study population. These include other livestock species on the premises and ventilation system.

Table 10.2. The distribution of variable classes among case and control flocks and the respective values of the crude odds ratio (OR).

Variables[1]	Percentage of exposure to the first variable class		
	Case flocks (n=86)	Control flocks (n=25)	Crude OR
Feed mill (small *versus* large)	55.8	16.0	6.63
Geographic region (northern *versus* southern)	52.3	24.0	3.48
Ventilation (natural *versus* mechanical)	53.5	44.0	1.46
Other poultry within 1 km radius (no *versus* yes)	43.0	40.0	1.13
Other species on farm (no *versus* yes)	34.9	32.0	1.14
Flock size (> 15,000 *versus* < 15,000)	36.0	12.0	4.13
Number of buildings (> 1 *versus* 1)	66.3	20.0	7.86
Number of egg collection rounds (once daily *versus* frequently)	26.2	22.7	1.21
Number of egg collection[2] rounds (minimum = 1; maximum= 6; x = 2.1)			1.04
Hygiene barriers (poor *versus* good)	52.4	28.0	2.84
Order and tidiness (poor *versus* good)	73.3	60.0	1.83
Disinfection tub present (no *versus* yes)	80.0	68.2	1.87
Age of the buildings[2] (minimum = 5; maximum = 25; x = 16.1 yr)			1.02
Farm type (litter *versus* battery)	94.2	80.0	4.05

[1] The first mentioned class of each variable is the risk class, the second one the reference class. So, 55.8% exposure in cases means that of the salmonellosis positive flocks 55.8% were served by a small feed mill *versus* 44.2% by a large feed mill

[2] As a continuous variable

Table 10.3. Results of the multivariate analysis of salmonellosis.

Source of variation	β	SE of β	Wald's chi	probability
intercept	0.59	0.86	0.46	0.50
disinfection	-0.66	1.04	0.41	0.52
hygiene	-0.39	0.91	0.19	0.67
dis * hyg	3.22	1.50	4.63	0.03
feed mill	1.66	0.62	7.07	0.0008
-2 log likelihood = 82.38				
model chi-square = 23.99				
P = 0.0001 (4 *df*)				

6. Intervention Strategy and Economics

It has been stated that effective intervention of salmonellosis in poultry should be based on slaughter of contaminated flocks as well as on the interruption of routes of contamination (Ament *et al.*, 1993). The WHO recommends the monitoring of poultry (breeder) flocks for the presence of *S.enteritidis*. Upon identification in laying flocks, the affected flocks should be slaughtered and eggs destroyed or diverted to pasteurization plants. For breeder flocks at the top of the production pyramid this procedure can be followed. For laying flocks there is an additional possibility of horizontal contamination and hence these routes have to be checked and controlled as well. Figure 10.1 describes the basic outlines of such routes.

Feasibility of interventions should be assessed economically, notwithstanding the social or political issues, but taking into account the public health relevance. An example of such an intervention is presented in Chapter XII, part II.

7. HACCP, Hazard Analysis Critical Control Points

Special attention must be given to the HACCP, the Hazard Analysis Critical Control Points, procedure with regard to the control of foodborne diseases.

This procedure is focused on the prevention of possible risks and their control at those points in a given production process where they still can be controlled. It was originally developed and implemented by the Pittsburg Company for assuring the quality and microbiological safety of food for the USA space programme (Baumann, 1993). Many disciplines and partial knowledge elements were brought together into a logical integrated concept (Buchanan, 1990). It has the name to be a universally applicable and systematic method of integrated problem approach and problem solving, e.g., in gas anaesthesia, rearing of animals, production of paint or food (Berends and Snijders, 1994). The latter authors have suggested this HACCP procedure for implementation in the modern meat quality assurance programmes. This originates from the need for scientifically valid risk analysis procedures within quality assurance programmes as pronounced by the EU in directive CEC 1990/VI/6346/90-EN and from the fact that current meat quality assurance procedures are often considered as outdated given the developments in the animal production sector and the increased speed of the processing line. The latter leads to a situation where not every carcass can be inspected and one has to be satisfied with inspection of samples of that population. It also refers to the fact that current public health hazards are related to the latent carrier state of animals with regard to zoonotic agents and the presence of residues of medicinal products or contaminants.

The applicability of HACCP to animal health care in the primary production has been addressed by Noordhuizen and Welpelo (1996). Their hypothesis is that health could be considered as a quality issue, and, hence, that health care could be approached through quality risk management procedures. Their conclusion was that HACCP was to be preferred above Good Farming Practice (GFP) or ISO-9000 series as method for a variety of described reasons (Table 10.4). HACCP is an officially approved quality management method for food processing companies within the European Union.

Table 10.4. The comparison of major features of the GXP, HACCP and NEN-ISO 9000+ approaches in quality management (n.a. = not applicable).

Field of interest	GXP process	HACCP process (+ product)	ISO-9000 system
approach	top down	bottom up	top down
demonstrable health state	-	+	+
specified corrective actions	-	+	-
documentation needed	+	+	++
suitability for certification	-	+	+
simplicity	+	+	-
farm specificity	-	+	?
labour input needed	-	-	+
degree of self-management	-	+	+
expected benefit/cost ratio	-	+	+/-
potential for developing into a quality system	-	+	n.a.
functional link with processing industries (e.g., Integrated Food Chain Quality Assurance Programmes)	-	+	+

HACCP as a potential instrument for herd health care should meet with two elementary requirements:

1. provide the farmer with clear and simple procedures for elimination and control of disease risk factors on that farm;
2. make the execution of these procedures objectively demonstrable to a third party with the goal of herd health certification and insurance.

Principles and subsequent steps in applying the HACCP concept to animal health care have been described (Noordhuizen and Welpelo, 1996). These authors stated that HACCP was well fit to be integrated into current programmes of Integrated Food Chain Quality Assurance in e.g., pig and poultry production.

HACCP comprises six major phases:

1. identification and analysis of all potential risks (of e.g., foodborne diseases) that can be related to the production, distribution, sale and use/consumption of products;
2. the identification of critical control points, CCP, in all parts of the process(es) related to the occurrence or increase of risks;
3. determination of appropriate parameters and their frequency for checking the CCP and threshold values for distinguishing normal/abnormal values;
4. monitoring of the CCP, either continuously or by sampling;

5. adjustment of deviations from the normal pattern; registration of all events including the adjustments and the treatment of products from a deviating or abnormal period;
6. verification and evaluation of the system with regard to the goals set by an external organization. This may lead to procedures of certification.

There are several primary requirements for designing a HACCP plan (see part II of this chapter).

First, a detailed description of the process(es) should be made, e.g., through flow diagrams. An example is given in Figure 10.3 for a dairy operation.

Suppose, for example, that we consider the cow and the herd as the "raw product" from the point of view of animal health care as a quality management issue. Such a cow enters the farm, e.g., after purchase, and subsequently is "processed" through the different production process units (represented in Figure 10.3 by the boxes) such as the milking parlour, the loose house with cubicles and feeding rack, the pasture. The outcome of this production process should be the healthy cow or the healthy herd as an "end product". At the same time other products (i.e., milk) are produced. In each production process unit one may distinguish different risk factors contributing to "product deviation" (i.e., disease occurrence such as salmonellosis or mastitis, or milk quality deviations). The true power of the HACCP method is in the adequate selection of the proper CCP's for each production process unit. CCP's are measuring points, conditions or process steps which are essential for eliminating or reducing risks. Criteria for selection of CCP's are that they must be related to the hazard and be measurable, target and tolerance levels be identified, corrective measures be available, and that their control should lead to decreased risk. An additional element for corrective measures is that cost-benefit calculations must have been made in order to select the best option. CCP's will originate from risk factor identification and the quantification of their contribution to "quality deviations" (e.g., expressed in odds ratios). Quantitative epidemiological methods such as in observational analytic studies should play a key role in this respect. All CCP's together are to be put in a monitoring and surveillance system, which must be able to detect loss of control. A CCP could be a bacteria count per unit of surface, or given serotitre level, or the optical cleanness of equipment etc. See further at part II of this Chapter for more details on HACCP application at farm level.

8. Monitoring and Surveillance (Risk Assessment Procedures)

As has been stated elsewhere, monitoring systems can become effectively operational if critical control points can be defined, as well as parameters covering these. The control points and parameters refer to every segment in the food production chain. Much research still has to be done before this can be defined, but in the meantime we could proceed with the first steps.

The basis of a monitoring system (see Chapter XII) is a network of sampling units in a region, chosen according to a preset protocol involving sampling procedures, diagnostic tests, data collection protocols and data analysis protocols. Throughout the whole chain, and more specifically at the level of the segment that we are aiming at, the protocols must be adopted in order to avoid misunderstanding, misinterpretation, poor communication and lack of cooperation. Training would be an essential component of the system.

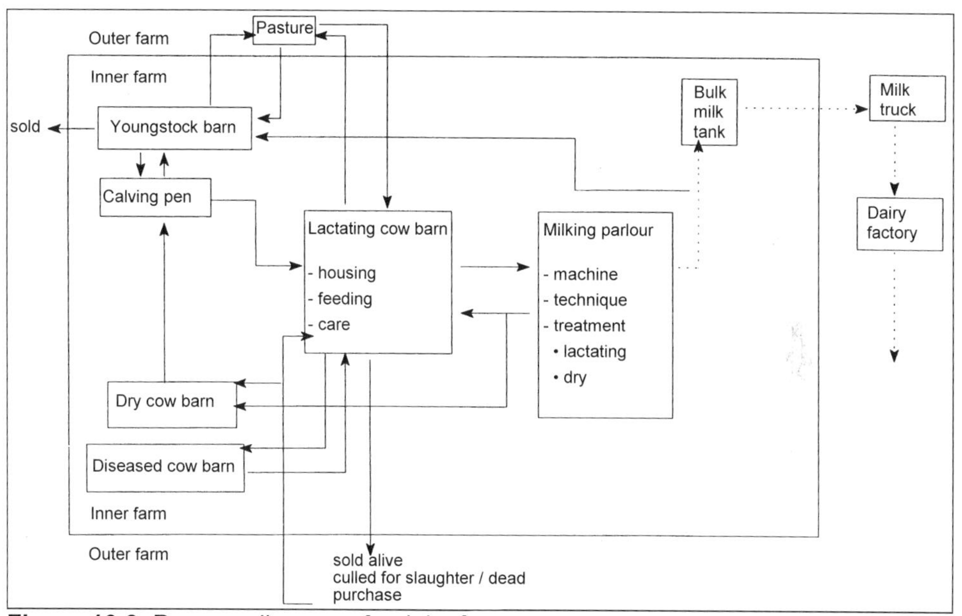

Figure 10.3. Process diagram of a dairy farm.

Monitoring involves costs, as is pointed out above. Sometimes these costs can be balanced by the higher price of a wholesome, safe product. But on the other hand it is imaginable that the primary animal production sector has to cover all the expenditures related to monitoring, for example if public opinion influences politics and it is decided that products should be free of named foodborne disease agents. In such a circumstance, the sector would be the only one that has to deal with this financial problem.

In programmes of integrated food chain quality control (IQC), farmers are already confronted with specific requirements set in the programme. With regard to the monitoring and surveillance of foodborne disease agents, it could well be worthwhile that this approach is coupled to that of integrated quality control. The other phase in this approach refers to the integration of farm certification (e.g., on animal health status, animal husbandry system and animal welfare issues) into this concept of integrated quality control. This is a development to be expected, not in the least for meat inspection and with regard to consumer demands.

In The Netherlands, several problems have been identified while implementing integrated quality control programmes in pig production. Such problems can be expected too, when monitoring, surveillance and certification become operational. Among these problems are:

- deficiencies in registration and identification;
- deficiencies in data transmission between segments of the chain.

Major causes of these problems were in the areas of communication, motivation, labour pressure and automation. It was concluded by the programme steering committee that education of all involved must have an essential position in the whole operation.

Other conclusions of a research project on integrated quality control in pig meat production were that among others the use of medicinal products was substantially lower on farms where mechanical ventilation was applied, where the herd was closed, where animal density was low, where hygiene and disinfection was high, where rodents/insects were prevented and where veterinary herd health programmes were executed.

An additional value of integrated quality control programmes comprising the monitoring of diseases and foodborne disease agents is, that with little effort data on environmental factors may become available. These data may be the start of the risk assessment procedure mentioned earlier. The basis for this procedure is the **risk chain concept** outlined in Figure 10.4, adapted after Merkhofer (1987). This concept refers to a certain disease prevalence level which may be altered through exposure to disease determinants (risk factors), provoking changes in the disease dynamics within that population. The outcomes can be provided through disease events and associated economic losses. The disease dynamics regard the changes in proportional distribution within that population of susceptible, immune and infected animals. Intervention measures, either veterinary (vaccination or medication) or zootechnical (risk factor based) are positioned within this concept. When simulation modelling techniques are being applied, it is possible to test the disease-related and economic relevance and effects of given intervention strategies. Such techniques can be of assistance to policy-makers in their decision-making process, and to researchers to detect gaps in knowledge for making the simulation run adequately and, hence, set priorities for research.

Here again, it is obvious that quantitative epidemiology (that is risk factor analysis and disease simulation), followed by animal health economic evaluation, is a most appropriate application in the area of foodborne diseases, in both the human and animal production sector.

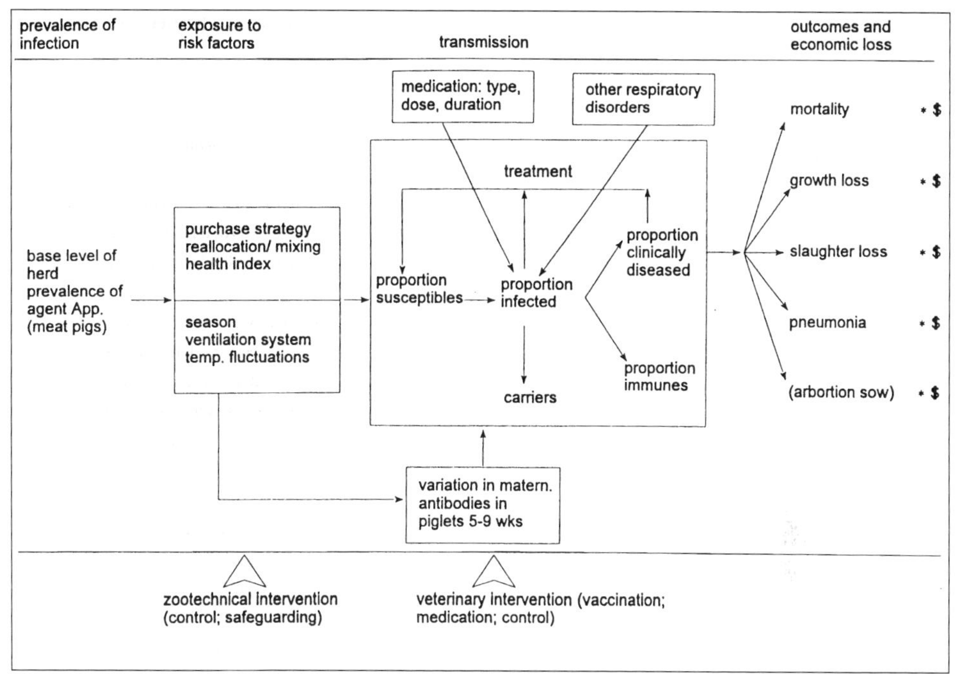

Figure 10.4. The risk chain concept after Merkhofer (1987), simplified and adapted for *Actinobacillus pleuropneumoniae* infections in pigs.

References

Ament, A.J.H.A.; Jansen, J.; Giessen, A. van der; Notermans, S. (1993). Cost benefit analysis of a screening strategy for *S.enteritidis* in poultry. Veterinary Quarterly, 15, 33-37.

Anonymous (1992). A blueprint for implementing preharvest food safety internationally. Workshop Washington D.C. The Food Animal Production Medicine Consortium.

Baumann, H. (1993). HACCP: Einführung. In: HACCP Grundlagen der Produkt- und Prozessspezifischen Risikoanalyse. Pierson; Corlett (Eds.). Behr Verlag GmbH, Hamburg.

Berends, B.; Snijders, J. (1994). Hazard Analysis Critical Control Point approach in meat production. Tijdschrift voor Diergeneeskunde, 119, 360-365.

Bolder, N.M. (1981). Mengvoeder als schakel in de *Salmonella* kringloop. Pluimveehouderij, 37, 16-18 (in Dutch).

Brand, A.; Noordhuizen, J.P.T.M.; Schukken, Y.H. (1996). Veterinary Herd Health and Production Management in Dairy Practice. Wageningen Pers, Wageningen, The Netherlands.

Buchanan, R. (1990). HACCP: a re-emerging approach to food safety. Trends in Food Science and Technology, 1, 104-106.

Edel, W.; Visser, G. (1989). *S.enteritidis* in Nederland. Tijdschrift voor Diergeneeskunde, 114, 405-410 (in Dutch).

Henken, A.M.; Frankena. K.; Goelema, J.O.; Graat, E.A.M.; Noordhuizen, J.P.T.M. (1992). Multivariate epidemiological approach to salmonellosis in broiler breeder flocks. Poultry Science, 71, 838-843.

Hoogenboom-Verdegaal, A.M.M.; During, M.; Leentvaar-Kuypers, A.; Peerbooms, P.G.H.; Kooij, W.C.M.; Van Vlerken, R.; Sobczak, H. (1989). Epidemiologisch en microbiologisch onderzoek m.b.t. gastro-enteritis bij de mens in de regio Amsterdam en Helmond in 1987. RIVM rapport 148612001, RIVM, Bilthoven, The Netherlands, (in Dutch).

Hoogenboom-Verdegaal, A.M.M.; During, M.; Engels, G.B; Hoogenveen, R.T.; Hoekstra, J.A.; Bosch, D.A. van den; Kuyvenhoven, J.V.; Mertens, P.L.J.M.; Smidt, I.R. (1992). Een bevolkingsonderzoek naar maagdarmklachten in vier regio's in Nederland uitgevoerd in 1991: Onderzoeksmethodiek en incidentie berekening gastroenterititis, RIVM report 149.101.001, RIVM, Bilthoven, The Netherlands (in Dutch).

Kaesbohrer, A.; Talaska, T.H.; Bögel, K.; Stoehr, K.; Lehmacher, W. (1993). Epidemiologische Muster von *S.enteritidis* und *S.typhimurium* beim Menschen. In: Proc. Veterinärepidemiologisches Seminar, Hannover. Lehmacher; Blaha; Kaesbohrer (Eds.).

Merkhofer, M.W. (1987). Decision Science and Social Risk Management. D. Riedel Publishing Company, The Netherlands.

Noordhuizen, J.P.T.M.; Welpelo, H.J. (1996). Sustainable improvement of animal health care by systematic quality risk management according to the HACCP concept. Veterinary Quarterly, 18, 121-126.

Roberts, T. (1989). Human illness costs of foodborne bacteria. American Journal of Agricultural Economics, 71, 936-943.

Waltner-Toews, D. (1996). An agroecosystem health perspective on foodborne illnesses. Ecosystem Health, 2, 177-185.

Appendix

Seasonal distribution of *Salmonella* cases in man (Germany).

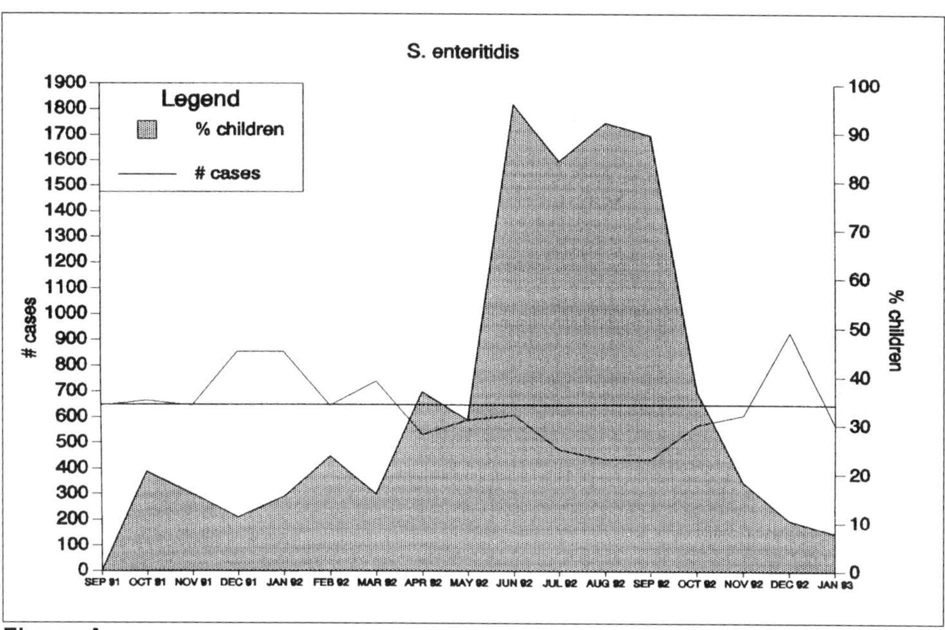

Figure A

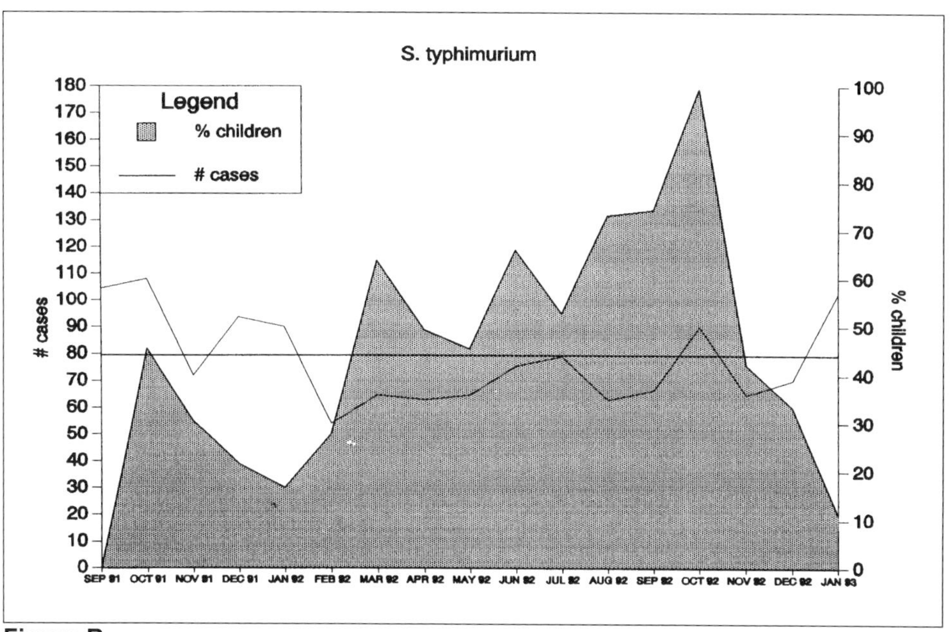

Figure B

Part II

Applying HACCP Principles to Animal Health Care at Farm Level[24]

J.P.T.M. Noordhuizen
Department of Farm Animal Health
Faculty of Veterinary Medicine
University of Utrecht
The Netherlands

K. Frankena
Wageningen University
Department of Animal Sciences
Quantitative Veterinary Epidemiology Group
The Netherlands

H.J. Welpelo
Cobroed Company
Lievelde
The Netherlands

---

[24] Paper presented at the 49th Seminar of the European Association of Agricultural Economists, February 1997, Bonn, Germany (by courtesy of Proceeding editors G. Schiefer and R. Helbig, University of Bonn).

1. Introduction

There is a growing tendency towards improvement of the animal health state in the respective memberstates of the European Union (EU). This is based on the principle of harmonization within the EU, but also on demands put forward by countries importing animals or animal products, and consumer demand with regard to health as welfare element and as part of the food animal production process.

Health impairment is the negative outcome of interactions between host and the environment, where pathogens may be part of this environment (Thrusfield, 1995). In addition to the monocausal diseases which lead to epidemics, such as foot and mouth disease or classical swine fever, many diseases of food animals are multifactorial in nature leading to an endemic disease situation on certain farms. It is the dynamic balance between the host resistance against diseases (e.g., via immune responses) and the stressors from the environment which may result in a disturbed homeostasis, leading to infection and disease. Stressors can be found in housing, climate, nutrition, management, hygiene, transport. They may alter the immune responsiveness directly or indirectly, and sensitize the animal for infection.

Health improvement is generally approached along two pathways:

1. eradication and prevention of disease;
2. reduction and control of disease.

The former applies to the highly infectious, monocausal epidemic diseases threatening large areas of the EU, or causing problems for human beings, the zoonoses or foodborne infections (e.g., brucellosis; salmonellosis). A continuous preventive surveillance to detect these diseases, and eradicate them after diagnostic confirmation of suspect cases is the primary action in this category. The second category refers to the endemic diseases with a multifactorial causality.

Given this aspect of multi-stressor related diseases and the great variation in such stressors between farms, large differences in disease prevalences exist between farms. The classical way to combat these diseases is through preventive vaccination or curative medication, and hence provoke a reduction in disease prevalence.

Recently, the EU has proclaimed the concept of reducing the application of vaccines and medicinal products in animal production, among others to meet the consumer demand with respect to product wholesomeness, safety and freedom of antimicrobial residues or pathogens. Given these new developments, it is clear that more effort has to be put to prevention than to cure alone, to disease risk management and risk control than to disease control alone.

Stressors, which are part of multifactorial disease syndromes and which contribute to their occurrence in the animal population, can be regarded as disease risks. This means that these risk factors have to be identified in the population. At the same time it should be established what the contribution of these risk factors to the disease occurrence is in a quantitative sense. These features are part of the quantitative epidemiological discipline (Martin *et al.*, 1987).

The combat and prevention of animal diseases are commonly executed along the line of managerial action. That is: in addition to diagnostic activities and curative or preventive measures, data are collected for calculating performance indices on the farm. Performance indices hence are retrospective in nature, and all action taken afterwards is based on product deviations (diseased animal, meat or milk aberrations). Applying quality control methods to animal health care could shift the attention from a retrospective to a prospective approach.

In this part II the following subjects are addressed: (1) animal health care principles, (2) position of risk analysis in aid to animal health care, and (3) potentials of quality control for prospective health improvement, certification and insurance.

2. Animal Health Care

The classical approach to disease combat is either eradication and prevention, or control and reduction. The first approach refers to highly contagious diseases endangering large areas of the EU. Upon detection and confirmation, infected herds are destroyed, other herds screened and a buffer zone installed where all animal transport is forbidden. Specific legislation covers these actions (Saatkamp *et al.*, 1996). A particular cluster of diseases in this context is represented by zoonoses and foodborne diseases (diseases or pathogens which are transferred from animals or their products to man). The relevance of all these diseases is in their macro-economic impact and their importance for public health. The second approach refers to endemic diseases which predominantly have an economic impact at sector and farm level. In certain cases export/import problems may arise, such as in the case of infectious bovine rhinotracheitis (IBR) or Aujeszky's disease in pigs. Measures to be taken for these diseases are in the area of vaccination and medication, sometimes supported by zootechnical measures such as in the area of climate control or nutrition.

The feature that applies to both approaches is that any action is taken **after** problems have been detected in the animals. Given the fact that the EU is becoming more and more reluctant to the extensive use of antimicrobial products in livestock production, and that consumer demand determines to a large extent what is named 'acceptable livestock production', new strategies for disease combat and prevention have to be developed.

Herd health programmes (Brand *et al.*, 1996), which have been under development over the past decades do not provide the proper means to such a new strategy, because they are mainly oriented to the operational side of the farm operation and not or hardly to the tactical/strategical side (Frankena *et al.*, 1994). Furthermore, they are largely based on retrospective data and performance analysis, meaning that prevention is often too late.

If health improvement should be based on proper decision-making and true preventive measures, then it becomes worthwhile to consider those factors and conditions which influence the occurrence of disease on a farm. This would mean that the focus shifts from medicated prevention to the risk prevention. This forms part of the risk analysis procedure.

3. Risk Analysis

Risk can be defined as the probability to get harmed by a hazard. Hazard in livestock production could be various, ranging from disease occurrence, impaired welfare, productivity problems to deviating product (meat, milk, eggs, wool) quality, including pathogen contamination. As has been stated before, many livestock diseases have a multifactorial aetiology where infectious micro-organisms can play a role next to animal related factors and environmental factors. An example of such factors is presented in Table 10.5.

Table 10.5. An example of animal and environment related factors contributing to atrophic rhinitis in pigs (from Sommer et al., 1991).

Transport stress in pigs	High pig density per m^2 and m^3
Purchase of carrier pigs	Climate control failures
Concurrent other diseases	Ventilation problems
High proportion of gilts	Inadequate feeding (e.g., type)

A clear disadvantage of risk factors as named in Table 10.5 is that they are qualitative in nature. There is no ranking according to importance. Furthermore, there is no indication about time-sequence, meaning that it is rather unclear which factor comes first and which next. Most of this qualitative information is based on experiments or small surveys which hampers validity. Finally, it is not clear how the different factors operate in increasing or decreasing the probability of occurrence of a disease and what the outcome in terms of animal health and economics are.

Therefore, the concept of Merkhofer (1987) about the **risk chain** is useful. An example of this risk chain concept has been given in Figure 10.4 (see in part I).

From that Figure 10.4 the sequence of the disease events can be followed. First there is a basic situation with regard to the disease. This prevalence is influenced by certain risk factors, leading to a possible disturbance in the animal population with regard to the distribution of proportions of immune, infected and susceptible animals. This on its turn results in different disease outcomes (in animals and/or man) which can be estimated in economic terms. Subsequently, it becomes possible to test the effects of defined veterinary and zootechnical intervention measures such as named in Figure 10.4.

Putting numerical values to the risk factors and calculating from there the change in probabilities that subsequent events will occur, will lead to a possible change in the

outcomes. The whole procedure can be named **risk modelling**. The most important part of risk modelling is the **risk identification** and the **risk quantification**. All are components of the **risk analysis** procedure.
In risk analysis, commonly a disease under study is sharply defined (cases and non-cases). Next, a questionnaire for field surveys is developed, based on extensive literature search for factors possibly contributing to the occurrence of that disease. Such factors are categorized into clusters. Among these clusters are: housing, nutrition, climate control, hygiene, management, animal/herd factors. Field surveys will cover a population of farms and animals, usually working with samples of the whole target population according to preset sampling procedures. The collected data are analyzed according to predefined epidemiological techniques into either univariate analysis results or e.g., multivariate analysis results (Martin *et al.*, 1987). An example is given in Table 10.6 for salmonellosis in poultry flocks.

Table 10.6. An example of results of a univariate and a multivariate analysis of factors related to salmonellosis in broiler breeder flocks (after Henken et al., 1992).

Univariate:	crude OR:
Feed mill (small *vs* large)	6.63
Geographic region (A *vs* B)	3.46
Ventilation (type 1 *vs* 2)	1.46
Other poultry (>1 km *vs* <1 km)	1.13
Other species on farm (no *vs* yes)	1.14
Flock size (>15000 *vs* <15000)	4.13
Number of houses (>1 *vs* 1)	7.86
Freq. egg collection (1x *vs* >1x)	1.21
Hygiene barriers (poor *vs* good)	2.84
Order and tidiness (poor *vs* good)	1.89
Disinfection tub present (no *vs* yes)	1.87
Age of houses	1.02
Farm type (litter *vs* battery)	4.05
Multivariate:	**adjusted OR:**
Disinfection tub present (yes *vs* no)	0.50
Hygiene barriers (good *vs* poor)	0.70
Interaction term DIS∗HYG (poor)	25.00
Feed mill (small *vs* large)	5.30

Note: for 95% confidence intervals and p-values see paper

An odds ratio (OR) of 6.6 for feed mill means that a farm that is served by a small feed mill has a more than 6 time higher odds to be among the salmonella positive group of flocks in comparison to a farm that is served by a large feed mill. When in the multivariate situation all factors are put in their worst setting, then the cumulative risk of being among the salmonella positive flocks increases dramatically to 46.

From this Table 10.6 it appears that risk factor contributions can be quantified for that population. The relative importance of each can be estimated through calculation of the attributable proportion (AP = (OR - 1)/OR, Martin *et al.*, 1987 and Chapter V). The variable factor feed mill with a AP of 85% [(5.6 - 6.6)/100] means that 85% of the salmonellosis cases can be attributed to exposure of feed delivered by small feed mills.

Hence, the risk factors can be ranked according to their relative importance. It can be determined now, on which item most emphasis has to be put for decreasing the risk, taking into account feasibility within the management scope and costs. When an economic evaluation is performed for each alternative measure proposed, it becomes even easier to make a decision.

Risk management implies all actions proposed and weighed, and subsequently taken to control or eliminate risks, hence contributing to disease control and ultimately to disease prevention. The major advantage over the approach discussed in the earlier paragraph is, that preventive measures are truly focused on prevention namely **before** calamities have occurred. This approach will strongly reduce disease losses as well as the use of antimicrobials.

Examples of the wide applicability of risk analysis are:

- analysis of welfare impairment in pigs and poultry (Willeberg, 1991);
- causes of variation in the use of antimicrobials in meat pig husbandry (Noordhuizen *et al.*, 1995);
- health risks involved in the use of BST in dairy cattle (Willeberg, 1993).

A current drawback is the fact that risk analysis studies have not (yet) largely been performed for the different disease entities. In situations, where it becomes too costly to carry out various observational-analytic studies into disease determinants, application of the methodology of conjoint analysis, CA, could be an option. CA is a method developed in marketing studies for e.g., determining consumer preferences (Vriens, 1995). CA enables the quantification of the relevance of certain attributes of a product or event, for example the relevance of disease risk factors. Experts are interviewed and they rank their scores for combination of identified risk factors, hence providing a semi-quantitative approach. An example is given by Schouten *et al.* (1997) for *S. dublin* risk factors on dairy farms.

4. Quality Control Methods

It has been hypothesized that animal health is just another feature of quality in livestock production (Noordhuizen and Welpelo, 1996). It refers to the quality of the production process as well as to the quality of the "product". Product in this context should be read as the animal or its product such as milk, meat, eggs or wool. Product quality deviations should then be read as an infected/diseased animal, or a contaminated product such as milk or meat.

Basis for their hypothesis and this comparison was the publication of a report by the Dutch Ministry of Agriculture, Nature Management and Fisheries about the developments needed in animal health care in The Netherlands in the coming decades. Core elements in this report were: disease risks, risk analysis and management, herd health certification, and animal health insurance (Julicher *et al.*, 1993). For herd health certification and herd health insurance it is absolutely necessary that a farmer is able to **demonstrate** to third parties the level of herd health at any time, the actions physically taken to control this level, and the measures foreseen in cases of deviations. Noordhuizen and Welpelo (1996) have scrutinized the potentials of different systematic quality control methods, as currently applied in various industrial fields, for application in the livestock production sector. A comparison was made between NEN ISO 9000 series, Good Manufacturing Practice codes and Hazard Analysis Critical Control Points, HACCP. The outcome of the comparison of the three quality control methods as applied to animal health care is presented briefly in Table 10.7.

At the farm level, the HACCP concept offers the best opportunities for success according to these authors. The method can be perfectly integrated with procedures of Integrated Food Chain Quality Assurance (IKB) programmes as are currently implemented in the poultry and pig production chains in The Netherlands.

HACCP is - different from the other 2 methods - specifically focused on active participation of the farmer in the production process and through this in controlling product quality, and is particularly tailor-made for his farm. HACCP is strongly oriented to prevention, requires a minimum of data collection and monitoring and documentation, is rather inexpensive, comprises economical evaluation of alternative interventions, and starts with defining hazards (e.g., animals infected with a certain pathogen), applying risk factor identification and quantification. The latter has been addressed in the previous paragraph.

Table 10.7. Comparison of 3 different quality control methods.

Field of interest	GXP process	HACCP process	ISO 9000 system
Type of approach	top-down	bottom-up	top-down
Demonstrable health	no	yes	yes
Corrective actions identified	no	yes	yes
Documentation needed	yes	yes	much
Certification fitness	no	yes	yes
Simplicity	yes?	yes	no
Farm specific	no	highly	yes?
Labour input	low	low	high
Self management	no	high	no
Expected benefits	low	high	yes
Further integration	hard	yes	n.a.
Functional link with industry (I.F.C.Q.A.)	no	yes	yes

IFCQA = integrated food chain quality assurance
n.a. = not applicable

The art of HACCP is in selecting those conditions that appear to be critical in the whole production process, the so-called Critical Control Points (CCP). Features of CCP are that they are associated with the hazard (e.g., infected animal), that these points or conditions can be measured, that they are indicative for control and potential deviations, that in case of deviations adjustment is feasible, and that preferably an economic assessment of alternative interventions is available.

Examples of potential CCP's are given in paragraph 6, while a distinction is made between CCP-1 and CCP-2. The primary CCP's (CCP-1) are those that can be controlled for 100%, such as cleaning water temperature or air velocity in barns, while the secondary CCP's (CCP-2) cannot provide full guarantee for adjustment, such as in the case of antibody titres in a herd. It is clear that in case of livestock production where live animals are involved as well as biological diagnostic tests are used, many CCP's will be of the CCP-2 nature. These CCP-2 are sometimes called Critical Management Points.

All CCP's are interconnected in a Monitoring and Surveillance System (MOSS) on the farm. It is worthwhile to notice that CCP's are not necessarily all identical on all farms. First because disease prevalences differ between farms, but also because risk factors for one or more given diseases differ between farms. It should be stressed that a minimum of CCP's must be strived for, in order to keep the system manageable for a farmer.

The 12 steps of designing a HACCP plan, including the elementary principles of HACCP and the respective areas of Risk Analysis are presented in the Appendix.

The concept for application of HACCP on animal health care at the farm level will be further addressed in the example presented in paragraph 6 of this chapter.

5. Discussion and Conclusions

The paragraphs listed above are the respective logical phases in the development of a proper herd health improvement. Originally, the starting point for animal health care was in the diagnosis and treatment of (individual) diseased animals. In the 80's and 90's this was expanded to programmes of Herd Health and Production Management (Brand *et al.*, 1996). These programmes predominantly focused on multidisciplinary management support for decision-making in terms of operational management, with an emphasis on data analysis and qualitative advice. Any quantitative basis for decision-making is lacking in general.

Risk analysis and quantitative epidemiology represent fields that can substantially support the on-farm decision-making process, because they provide a better and quantitative insight in outcomes of the production process and because they are much more focused on prospective action.

Given the fact that the livestock production market is currently consumer driven, aspects of quality become much more important. It would be erroneous to suppose that such quality feature would be applicable to the level of slaughterhouse and distribution alone. It is a primary responsibility of the livestock producer to deliver such "products" (animals, animal products) that provide the best level of safety and quality related to consumer demand. Since product quality and product acceptance are determined by both the quality of the product and the quality of the production method, these both have to be comprised in a systematic control programme. HACCP fits those goals best, and on the long term could be included in an ISO system of quality assurance. Quality control related actions should be demonstrable, that is the key word. Otherwise herd health certificates have only limited value and feature relatively short duration, and herd health risk insurance will be hard to realize. The livestock production sector should be prepared for this development, as well as those people active in that field.

As stated earlier, much effort must be put into the identification and quantification of animal disease risks. Different actions and studies are currently undertaken in e.g., The Netherlands and other countries to fill this gap.

References

Brand, A.; Noordhuizen, J.P.T.M.; Schukken, Y.H. (1996). Herd Health and Production Management in Dairy Practice. Wageningen Pers, Wageningen, The Netherlands.

Frankena, K.; Noordhuizen, J.P.T.M.; Stassen, E.N. (1994). Applied epidemiology: another tool in dairy herd health programs? Veterinary Research, 2 and 3, 234-239.

Henken, A.M.; Frankena, K.; Goelema, J.O.; Graat, E.A.M.; Noordhuizen, J.P.T.M. (1992). Multivariate epidemiological approach to salmonellosis in broiler breeder flocks. Poultry Science, 71, 838-843.

Julicher, C.H.M.; Klink, E.G.M. van; Peuter, G. de; Schumer, D.L.; Versteijlen, G.H.J.M. (1993). De toekomst van de diergezondheid: wie zal het een zorg zijn? Publication of the Ministry of Agriculture, Nature management and Fisheries, The Hague, The Netherlands, (in Dutch).

Martin, S.W.; Meek, A.H.; Willeberg, P. (1987). Veterinary Epidemiology: Principles and Methods. Iowa State University Press, Ames, Iowa.

Merkhofer, M.W. (1987). Decision Science and Social Risk Management. D. Riedel Publishing Company, The Netherlands.

Noordhuizen, J.P.T.M.; Henken, A.M.; Frankena, K.; Mocking, W.; Vrolijk, C.T.W. (1995). Causes of variation in the use of antimicrobials in meat pig husbandry. In: Proceedings of the Society for Veterinary Epidemiology and Preventive Medicine, Reading, United Kingdom. Goodall, E.A. (Ed.). pp. 11-17.

Noordhuizen, J.P.T.M.; Welpelo, H.J. (1996). Sustainable improvement of animal health care by systematic quality risk management according to the HACCP concept. Veterinary Quarterly, 18, 121-126.

Saatkamp, H.W.; Dijkhuizen, A.A.; Geers, R.; Huirne, R.B.M.; Noordhuizen, J.P.T.M.; Goedseels, V. (1996). Simulation studies on the epidemiological impact of national identification and recording systems on the control of classical swine fever in Belgium. Preventive Veterinary Medicine, 26, 119-132.

Schouten, M.; Vonk Noordegraaf, A.; Noordhuizen, J.P.T.M. (1997). The relevance of risk factors for S. dublin on dairy farms as assessed by conjoint analysis (submitted).

Sommer, H.; Greuel, E., Müller, W. (1991). Hygiene der Rinder- und Schweineproduction. 2nd edn. Verlag Eugen Ulmer, Stuttgart, Germany.

Thrusfield, M. (1995). Veterinary Epidemiology. 2nd edn. Blackwell Science, Oxford.

Vriens, M. (1995). Conjoint analysis in marketing: developments in stimulus representation and segmentation methods. PhD thesis, University of Groningen, The Netherlands.

Willeberg, P. (1991). Animal welfare studies: epidemiological considerations. In: Proceedings of the Society for Veterinary Epidemiology and Preventive Medicine, London, United Kingdom. Thrusfield, M.V. (Ed.). pp. 76-83.

Willeberg, P. (1993). Bovine somatotropin and clinical mastitis: epidemiological assessment of the welfare risk. Livestock Production Science, 36, 55-65.

Appendix

Sequential steps in applying the HACCP concept to animal health management (HACCP principles).

Steps	Examples	Specification
Step 1	Identification of persons involved	Farmer and employees if any. External experts, such as veterinarian, extensions, authorities
Step 2	Description of products	Animals, meat, milk, eggs, wool
Step 3	Identification of intended use	Refers to disease agents the herd should be free of
Step 4	Construction of a flow diagram	Description of animal production process as a communication tool Blue-print for flow diagram to be developed at sector level, tailor-made to individual farm
Step 5	On-site verification of flow diagram	To allow specific adjustments. First review of potential hazards
Step 6	Listing of hazards at each process element; preventive measures (principle 1).	Check hazards on severity and probability. Risk quantification needed Qualitative branch expertise searched
Step 7	Application of a HACCP decision tree (principle 2)	Selection of CCP for each hazard in balance with human and financial resources Avoid surplus of data on production process and products
Step 8	Establish target levels and tolerances for each CCP (principle 3)	Animal replacement free of specific disease agents Diagnostic tests: antigen-based tests have no zero-tolerance; antibody based tests have generally accepted critical level
Step 9	Establish a monitoring system (principle 4)	CCP's are linked to a monitoring system. Monitoring aims at detecting loss of control at early stage, and at providing information for corrective action. Incidently and regular measuring
Step 10	Establish corrective actions (principle 5)	Needed for each CCP selected. Correction is also needed when monitoring indicates trend toward loss of control
Step 11	Verification of the application (principle 6)	To check for correct functioning with respect to steps 6-10 Necessary for both introducing and maintaining the system
Step 12	Documentation (principle 7)	Of relevant process characteristics. Basis for demonstrable process control, health certification and insurance. Refers to products, flow diagram, hazards, CCP's, preventive measures, tolerance levels and targets, monitoring system. Process deviations, corrections performed
Managerial action	{	Risk Assessment: principle 1 Risk Management: principle 2-6 Documentation: principle 7

6. Example

In this example we elaborate the application of HACCP to a dairy farm. The domains of *Salmonella dublin* infection together with that of dairy quality deviations are chosen for this application, because they have a relationship with both the farm itself and public health.

S.dublin which is a zoonotic agent can be transmitted to man by milk. Hence, the elimination and control of this agent is relevant with respect to public health and to the public image of the dairy sector. Additionally, it may cause disease problems in calves and adult cattle leading to economic losses for the farmer. Dairy quality deviations are represented by e.g., a high level of somatic cells, milk containing antimicrobials and/or bacteria, and poor hygiene as expressed by dirt on the milk filter.

First, we have to distinguish the different steps in the production process on the dairy farm. This is shown in Figure 10.3 where the different locations within the farm where cattle pass through are identified as process steps.

The next stage is that we address the respective risk factors related to *S.dublin* infection and quality deviations.

We pay attention to the major putative factors associated with the **introduction** of *S.dublin* **into** a dairy herd. Based on literature search the following list of putative and qualitative factors can be drawn (Table 10.8):

In a further stage, a differentiation will be made between GXP-like factors and CCP-like conditions; these are suggested in the Tables 10.8 and 10.9 with the symbol "G" and "*" respectively. The selection process itself is discussed in a later paragraph.

Table 10.8. Overview of factors potentially related to the introduction of S. dublin into the dairy farm.

contact of cattle with carriers	*
feed delivered by a feed mill	G
surface water	*
pasture	*
sewage sludge on pasture	*
manure supply on pasture	*
pets, vermin, birds	G
people and attributes	G
purchase of cattle	*

(Frik, 1969; Jones, 1976; Losinger *et al.*, 1995; Richardson, 1975; Tannock and Smith, 1971; Visser *et al.*, 1992; Wray, 1994)

Subsequently, the major risk factors for the **transmission** of *S.dublin* **within** a herd are listed, based on literature search as well (Table 10.9):

Table 10.9. Overview of factors potentially related to the transmission of S.dublin within a dairy farm.

people and attributes	G
transfer of cattle between groups/pens	*
availability of a sick pen	G
pets, vermins, birds	G
feed and feed storage	*
manure storage and application	*
pasture exploitation	G
milking procedure	G
animal care and hygiene practices	G

(Bender, 1994; Frik, 1969; Jones, 1976; Losinger *et al.*, 1995; Tannock and Smith, 1971; Visser *et al.*, 1992; Wray, 1994)

Deviating milk quality originates in many cases from certain management and hygiene practices, as well as from udder infections. The latter may directly or indirectly lead to antibiotics in milk, bacteria in milk and/or elevated somatic cell counts.

The following Figure 10.5 shows the simplified relational diagram of clusters of factors related to the occurrence of milk quality deviations.

The most relevant risk factors for the occurrence of milk quality deviations are listed in the next Table 10.10, following the clusters mentioned in Figure 10.5. These also originate from literature analysis.

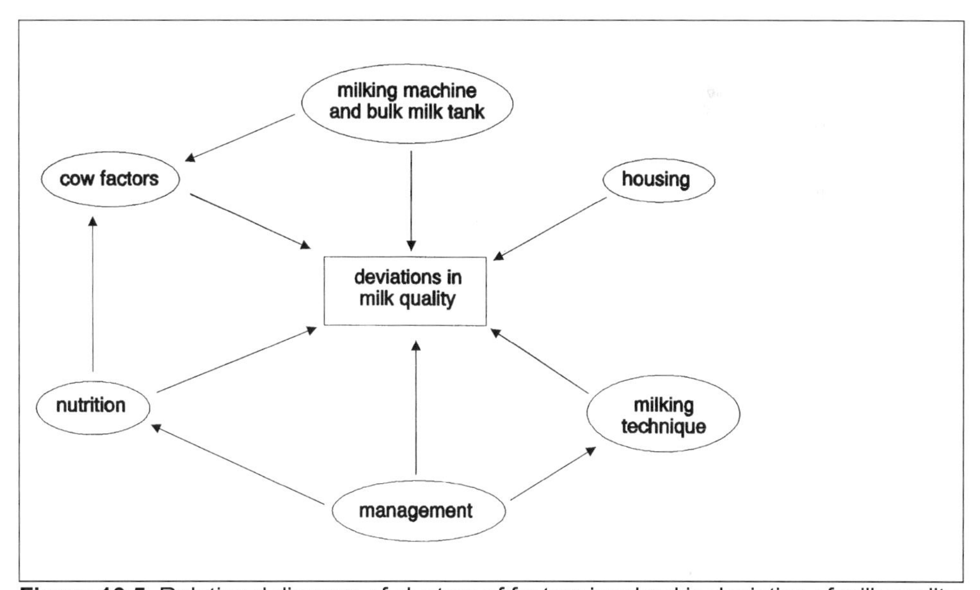

Figure 10.5. Relational diagram of clusters of factors involved in deviation of milk quality.

For the factors related to milk quality deviations a distinction has to be made between GXP-like factors and CCP-like conditions. This distinction is made for several items in Table 10.10 by adding respectively the symbol "G" and "*".

Table 10.10. Overview of factors related to milk quality deviations.

milking machine:	function and maintenance	G
	teat cup liners	*
	pulsator function, cleanliness	G*
	regulator function, cleanliness	G*
	machine cleaning guard system	*
	cluster take-off equipment maintenance	G
	bulk milk tank: cooling	*
	cleaning, disinfection	*
	tank guard system	*
milking technique:	premilking sanitation and stimulation	G*
	cluster attachment method	G*
	checks during milking	G
	cluster adjustment during milking	G*
	application of dip/spray	G
	floor cleaning during milking	G
hygiene and management:	cleaning of the milking parlour	G
	cleaning of the waiting room	G
	fixating cows at feedrack after milking	G
	milking intervals	G
	milk filter status	*
	milking of mastitic cows	G
	occurrence of rest milk	G
	hygiene of milker	G*
	dry cow and mastitis treatment	G*
	cleaning/disinfection of the barns	G
	cleaning and drying of slats	G
	visitors' hygiene	G
housing conditions:	climatic conditions (T, RH)	G
	hygiene practices	G*
	manure handling in the barns	G*
	cubicle cleanliness and disinfection	G
	cubicle floor type	G
	cubicle size and shoulder rail level	G
nutritional factors:	milk production groups	G
	normative feeding	G
	ration composition, ration changes	G
	level of concentrate supply	G
	quality drinking water	G*
	pasture (soil type; climate; contacts)	G*
animal factors:	size and average age of lactating herd	
	number of lactating heifers	
	breed	
	body condition score	
	milk leakage	G*
	udder and teat disorders	*
	claw condition and hair condition	
	other diseases	
	behaviourial aspects	
	separation of healthy/diseased cows	

(Goodger *et al.*, 1984; Dargent-Molina *et al.*, 1988; Bendixen and Astrand, 1989; Schukken *et al.*, 1990; Nelson *et al.*, 1991; Schukken *et al.*, 1991; Woolford, 1995; Blowey and Edmondson, 1996; Smith and Hogan, 1996)

All factors in Tables 10.8, 10.9 and 10.10 are qualitative in nature: it is not known what the quantitative contribution of each factor to the occurrence of a *S.dublin* infection or quality deviations is. Which factor would be more relevant than an other? Or, in other words, it is not known what their relative risk (or odds ratio) and attributable proportion is. Specific intervention measures are difficult to design because they are not specifically focused on the location where the risk is highest. Therefore, the risk conditions should be assigned to the respective process steps, where they belong to (see Figure 10.3). In other words, where these factors exert their risk-increasing (or decreasing) action with respect to *S.dublin* infection or quality deviations. Then, we may design appropriate intervention measures.

Largely seen, the production process on the dairy farm can be divided into several process steps which are depicted in Figure 10.3. The calving pen, young stock housing, adult cows barn, milking parlour, bulk milk tank house, dry cow house, sick pen and pasture are the most important process steps and process locations the animals will pass through on their way to "become a healthy cow and to produce high quality milk".

Once the risk factors have been assigned to the different process steps, the next stage can be passed: the selection of conditions which can be reallocated to Good Farming Practice or Good Animal-health and Quality Practice codes, and the selection of factors and conditions according to a CCP selection protocol. The former are more general in nature and are related to an attitude, while the latter are much more specific for health and dairy quality.

The selection procedure for determining CCPs is comprised of the following criteria:

- it should have a relationship with the hazard (i.e., the *S.dublin* infection and milk quality deviation);
- it should be measurable;
- target level and accepted tolerance levels must be known;
- corrective measures must be available and cost-effective;
- correction must lead to restoration of lost control.

Because we are dealing with animals and the variation between these animals, it is not always possible to guarantee control through a CCP for 100%. The latter is feasible for physical parameters such as temperature and humidity. Therefore, we distinguish the CCP-1 and CCP-2 categories. The former are related to the 100% control, the latter to a lesser degree of control but at least reduction of risks.
On the basis of the forenamed criteria the differentiation between GXP-like items and CCP-like items has been made in the Tables 10.8, 10.9 and 10.10. Field studies and managerial evaluation have to refine and adjust the suggested HACCP plan. These are currently under way, in various parts of the world, such as in Australia with DAIRYFIRST and PROVEN PERFECT (milk quality) and CATTLECARE (meat residue control) and in The Netherlands with salmonellosis, IBR and milk quality in dairy herds (Ryan, 1997; Noordhuizen and Frankena, 1997; Schouten *et al.*, 1997).

References

Bender, J. (1994). Reducing the risk of *Salmonella* spread and practical control measures in dairy herds. Bovine Practitioner, 28, 62-65.

Bendixen, P.H.; Astrand, D.B. (1989). Removal risks in Swedish Friesian dairy cows according to parity, stage of lactation and occurrence of clinical mastitis. Acta Veterinaria Scandinavia, 30, 37-42.

Blowey, R.W.; Edmondson, P. (1996). Mastitis Control in Dairy Herds. Farming Press, United Kingdom.

Dargent-Molina, P.; Scarlett, J.; Pollock, R.V.H.; Erb, H.N.; Sears, P. (1988). Herd-level risk factors for *Staphylococcus aureus* and *Streptococcus agalactiae* intramammary infections. Preventive Veterinary Medicine, 6, 127-142.

Frik, J.F. (1969). *Salmonella dublin* infections in cattle in The Netherlands. PhD thesis, University of Utrecht, The Netherlands.

Goodger, W.J.; Ruppanner, R.; Slenning, B.D.; Kushman, J.E. (1984). An approach to scoring dairy management on large-scale dairies. Journal of Dairy Science, 67, 675-685.

Jones, P.W. (1976). The effect of temperature, solid content and pH on the survival of salmonellas in cattle slurry. British Veterinary Journal, 132, 284-291.

Losinger, W.C.; Wells, S.J.; Garber, L.P.; Hurd, H.S.; Thomas, L.A. (1995). Management factors related to Salmonella shedding by dairy heifers. Journal of Dairy Science, 78, 2464-2472.

Nelson, W.; Philpot, Ph.D.; Stephen, C.; Nickerson, Ph.D. (1991). Mastitis: Counter Attack. Babson Bros. Company, USA.

Noordhuizen, J.P.T.M.; Frankena, K. (1997). Epidemiology and Quality Assurance: applications at farm level. Paper presented at the International Society for Veterinary Epidemiology and Economics, July 1997, Paris France (to be published in Preventive Veterinary Medicine 1997/1998).

Richardson, A. (1975). Salmonellosis in cattle. Veterinary Record, 96, 329-331.

Ryan, D. (1997). Three HACCP-based programmes for quality management in cattle in Australia. Dairy Extension, NSW Australia, through the Dairy Discussion list:"Dairy-L@UMDD.UMD.EDU"

Schouten, M.; Vonk Noordegraaf, A.; Noordhuizen, J.P.T.M. (1997). The relevance of risk factors for S. dublin on dairy farms as assessed by conjoint analysis (submitted).

Schukken, Y.H.; Grommers, F.J.; Geer, D. van de; Brand, A. (1990). Risk factors for clinical mastitis in herds with a low bulk milk somatic cell count: 1. Data and risk factors for all cases. Journal of Dairy Science, 73, 3463-3471.

Schukken, Y.H.; Grommers, F.J.; Geer, D. van de; Erb, H.N.; Brand, A. (1991). Risk factors for clinical mastitis in herds with a low bulk milk somatic cell count: 2. Risk factors for *E.coli* and *Staphylococcus aureus*. Journal of Dairy Science, 74, 826-832.

Smith, K.L.; Hogan, J.S. (1996). Future prospects for mastitis control. In: Proceedings of the XIX World Buiatrics Congress, Vol.1, Edinburgh, UK. pp. 263-268.

Tannock, G.W.; Smith, J.M.B. (1971). Studies on the survival of *Salmonella typhimurium* and *Salmonella bovismorbificans* on pasture and in water. Australian Veterinary Journal, 47, 557-560.

Visser, J.R.; Veen, M.; Giessen, J.W.B. van der (1992). *Salmonella dublin* infections in cattle, a review. Tijdschrift voor Diergeneeskunde, 117, 730-735 (in Dutch with English summary).

Vriens, M. (1995). Conjoint analysis in marketing: developments in stimulus representation and segmentation methods. PhD thesis, University of Groningen, The Netherlands.

Woolford, M.W. (1995). Milking machine effects on mastitis: progress 1985-1995. In: Proceedings of the 3rd International Mastitis Seminar of the International Dairy Federation, Tel Aviv, s-6, 3-12.

Wray, C. (1994). Salmonellosis in dairy cattle in the United Kingdom. In: Proceedings of the Symposium on Salmonellosis in dairy cattle and small ruminants. Animal Health Service, Drachten, The Netherlands, pp. 13-17 (in Dutch).

Part III

Developments in Meat Inspection Systems[25]

J.M.A. Snijders
Department of the Science of Food of Animal Origin
Faculty of Veterinary Medicine
Utrecht University
The Netherlands

B. Berends
Department of the Science of Food of Animal Origin
Faculty of Veterinary Medicine
Utrecht University
The Netherlands

[25] Adapted from the proceedings of the 40th ICoMST, 1994, The Hague, The Netherlands.

1. Introduction

In the preceding parts I en II of this chapter emphasis was on implementation of epidemiological concepts at farm level. The current part III addresses the next link in the food production chain: the slaughterhouse and meat inspection. It is elaborated why meat inspection has to change and how epidemiological concepts should be involved.

Although the quality of products, production systems and animal welfare may not be neglected, ensuring the safety and wholesomeness of meat may be considered as the main objective of meat inspection. Western European meat inspection procedures are thereby aimed at the detection and exclusion of animals and parts of animals with:

1. pathological anatomical abnormalities (e.g., *B.anthrax*, *M.tuberculosis*);
2. pathogens (e.g., *M.tuberculosis*; but how about possibilities to detect *Salmonella spp.* or *Campylobacter spp.*);
3. residues of veterinary drugs;
4. residues of environmental contaminants (MOSS needed);
5. contamination during processing.

However, the efficiency, cost effectiveness and scientific validity of current *ante* and *post mortem* meat inspection procedures in the industrialized countries are nowadays seriously being doubted (Snijders *et al.*, 1989; 1993a; b; Hathaway and McKenzie, 1991; 1993; Berends *et al.*, 1993).

Furthermore, the responsibility for the quality and the safety of meat cannot entirely lie with the meat inspection service. With respect to this, the suppliers of the animals have a certain responsibility.

This part III of the chapter discusses the main reasons for these doubts and tries to point out along which lines revisions of the current system of meat inspection should take place. It also points out how suppliers and producers should acquire more responsibility with respect to the safety and quality of animals and meat produced.

2. Why a Revision of the Current System

The current meat inspection system can be divided in an *ante mortem* and a *post mortem* inspection. The *ante mortem* inspection is, in fact, a simple clinical examination. *Post mortem* inspection is a simple pathological-anatomical examination. Because of its laborious nature, it is currently also the most expensive part of meat inspection.

In the industrialized countries, improvements in technology, animal husbandry and animal health care have led to a significant rise in the numbers of animals kept for animal production, while this production has also become more and more concentrated in large production units and in certain regions. Thus, the slaughter of a few animals, originating from the same farm, has evolved into the slaughter of large numbers of uniform, relatively young and healthy animals, often with a common genetic background (Berends *et al.*, 1993).

Furthermore, zoonotic diseases that lead to characteristical pathological-anatomical changes in slaughter animals, such as tuberculosis and anthrax, have also become sporadic in such countries. Current zoonotic public health hazards in the industrialized countries are agents that can be carried by animals without symptoms, such as *Salmonella*, *Campylobacter* and *Yersinia spp.* (Berends *et al.*, 1993). Modern animal husbandry seems to facilitate the presence of these bacterial zoonotic agents. Meat inspection, however, was not designed and equipped to detect these agents. Some inspection procedures, i.e., the incision of lymph-nodes, can even have a negative effect on the safety and quality of meat.

In addition, it is doubtful whether on-line inspection, palpation and incision are sensitive enough methods to detect all abnormalities that are present in an animal. Reported observations show relatively low sensitivities that vary from less than 20% for the detection of *Cysticercus bovis* to 41 % for the detection of cysts of *Taenia ovis* in lambs. Also, abnormalities with a low prevalence are more often missed by meat inspectors than abnormalities with a high prevalence (Berends *et al.*, 1993; Harbers, 1991; Harbers *et al.*, 1992a).

Veterinary drugs are administered "on purpose" in animals. The owner knows, or should know, that his animals were treated. Checking and controlling whether animals have been treated is possible, but this is very costly and time consuming. The current system gives no absolute guarantee that virtually all delivered animals will be free of residues. That is why it is necessary to develop a system that can "guarantee" the absence of residues. In this system the producer should bear the responsibility for this, and profitability should be the main incentive for voluntary cooperation (bonus-malus principle).

Regarding the presence of environmental contaminants, the farmer can mostly not be blamed. Therefore, countrywide surveillance programmes are necessary to obtain insight in these matters. Based on the results of the surveillance programmes, direct action can be undertaken and intervention strategies designed.

On the grounds of the number of foodborne infections in human populations, it must be concluded that meat inspection services should pay considerably more attention to hygiene control during slaughtering, dressing and further processing than they do now. This, however, needs a highly developed safety and control system.

Regarding the development in safety and control systems during production and processing of meat, four stages can be distinguished (Gerats, 1990):

a. **Passive control stage**
   At this stage, there is no specific system for controlling the end product. If there is something wrong with the end product, the buyer will complain and, as a result of this, the seller will probably lower his price and promise that it will not happen again. The consequences are that production costs a lot of money and improvements in safety and quality will fail to appear.

b. **End product control stage**
Hereby, every individual product is checked and will be rejected if abnormalities are detected. The failure costs in this system are high, and if there is no feedback to prevent the diagnosed abnormalities, nearly the same percentage of the next production batches will be rejected or condemned. Many production lines work in this way. In this stage the control is focused on the end product and not on the production system itself.

c. **Process control stage**
In a process control system the checking procedures are focused on the production line itself. In the food industry this approach is also known as the Hazard Analysis Critical Control Point HACCP) approach. For each critical control point Codes of Good Manufacturing Practices GMP), control procedures and criteria that have to be met are designed. Thus ensuring a production with a controlled, constant level of safety and quality. See also the preceding part II of this chapter.

d. **Integrated Quality Control (IQC) stage**
In an IQC approach attention is not only focused on the production line itself, but also to the production system as a whole: from stable to table; from conception to consumption. Each participant in this food chain has his own responsibility. The exchange of relevant data between the links of this chain enables a constant optimization of production, and thus of quality and safety.

With respect to this, it can be stated that meat inspection must be considered as a system that is working as an "end product control" of the production of slaughter animals, leading to higher failure and labour costs than are necessary. Moreover, because there is no structural feedback of relevant data, meat inspection does not contribute much to improvements in the quality and safety of the delivered animals, or, for that matter, the profitability of animal production.

Information about the presence of *post mortem* abnormalities in particular, could help farmers to improve the quality and safety of their livestock. Data obtained from the registration of post mortem abnormalities could also be used in epidemiological studies and risk analysis (Hathaway *et al.*, 1988). In The Netherlands and Denmark the experiences with integrated quality control systems, especially in pork production, have proven that such systems can lead to a better quality and safety of animals and meat produced. (Berends *et al.*, 1991; Elbers *et al.*, 1992; Harbers *et al.*, 1992a, b, c).

3. How to Revise the Current System

Based on the results of the field trials regarding the IQC approach, the following system is now applied in practice in The Netherlands (Hathaway and McKenzie, 1991; Snijders *et al.*, 1993a, b).

The Dutch Product Board for Livestock and Meat has set up general rules for Integrated Quality Control in finishing pigs, which have to be fulfilled by the participants. Those rules are supervised by an independent organisation. At the moment this is done by National Council for Applied Scientific Research (TNO) and the International Control Company (ICM). Until 1993 thirteen Dutch slaughterhouses were certified by these organisations, and approximately three million pigs have been produced with this IQC system.

The basic rules for taking part in the IQC system are:

1. Adequate identification and registration of the animals for tracing origin.

2. Only specified veterinary drugs (positive list) and feeds may be used during the fattening period and the required withholding period must be strictly obeyed.

3. Veterinary practitioners must act according to the Code of Good Veterinary Practice. This means that they may only use the specified drugs. Their signatures should also be a guarantee for their correct application. Only veterinarians who are willing to work under contract will be allowed to treat the IQC animals for these cooperatives.

4. The farmers must feed their animals only with feed manufactured by producers who fulfil the requirements of Codes of Good Manufacturing Practices in the feed industry.

5. All treatments and transactions must be registered in a health logbook.

6. All animals must be delivered with a Quality Information Card. This card contains the most important information of the logbook and can be considered as a specific guarantee certificate.

7. The meat inspection service registers relevant pathological anatomical abnormalities.

8. The slaughterhouse has to feed back the information regarding these pathological anatomical abnormalities to the farmer.

9. The slaughterhouse fulfils a central role in the IQC system and the mutual exchange of information. The slaughterhouse is responsible for ensuring that every link in the meat production chain complies with the IQC-regulations.

10. The farmer must give absolutely reliable information about his production. If the supplied information appears to be incorrect, the farmer will no longer be allowed to take part in the IQC system.

11. Twice a year both an internal and an external audit have to be carried out.

According to art. 17 of the new EU Directive Fresh Meat 91/497/EEC revision of meat inspection procedures for uniform deliveries is allowed, when this new method ensures a level of safety equivalent to that guaranteed by existing ante and post mortem inspection procedures.

A proposal for some revisions of current EU meat inspection procedures regarding pigs, has been presented to the Commission in Brussels. The proposal is based on the aforementioned rules of the IQC system with some additional recommendations. In this proposed system the producer of slaughter animals will be held responsible for the wholesomeness and quality of the whole production he delivers. Batches without guarantees require rigid meat inspection of individual carcasses, which means higher costs for the farmer (malus). If the farmer can and does guarantee that the additional requirements are met, his effort will be rewarded (bonus).

In addition to the basic IQC rules, the farmer must preselect his animals on visible abnormalities (Harbers *et al.*, 1992b). Furthermore, he has to guarantee that the pigs, when delivered, are healthy and have no visible pathological anatomical abnormalities. This should be ascertained with a meat inspection index", which is the total sum of the percentages of the registered abnormalities in a delivery. This meat inspection index has to be stored in a database so that the average quality of the deliveries of the producer can be assessed. Finally, the animals should be delivered to the slaughterhouse separately from animals that are not guaranteed, thus preventing the mixing up of IQC and non-IQC animals.

If those conditions are fulfilled, the traditional meat inspection can be replaced by a visual *post mortem* inspection without palpation or incision (Harbers *et al.*, 1992c; Berends *et al.*, 1993). Consequently, the meat inspection services can shift their attention much more towards the control of hygiene during processing. Preconditions must be that the rules of the Codes of Good Manufacturing Practices (GMP) are followed and that the production process is under control HACCP approach, Berends and Snijders, 1994). In this way it seems possible to adapt current meat inspection from (end)product control to production process control, resulting in lower costs and better guarantees for the consumer.

However, the above described changes must be seen as the first step of the modernization of meat inspection. For an effective change to the system it is necessary to undertake a quantitative risk assessment (Hathaway *et al.*, 1988). This is because the above described changes do not solve all of the systems' fundamental disadvantages (Berends *et al.*, 1993). For example, it will still not be able to be flexible and adapt to any specific demands that certain categories of slaughter animals or certain regions or countries may have. Neither will it be able to adapt itself continuously to changes in circumstances regarding animal husbandry and health, prevalent zoonoses, veterinary drugs used or environmental contaminants.

Such a system can only be designed and maintained on the basis of a (continuous) formal (quantitative) risk assessment. This risk assessment will have to include an assessment of all sorts of risks that can be associated with the production and consumption of meat; the determination of the relative magnitude of all assessed risks so that priorities can be made; the assessment of the timing and procedure by which interventions should be effective in reducing or eliminating these risks; and the design of objective criteria with which the success of the interventions made can be assessed. For this, reliable epidemiological data concerning zoonotic agents in slaughter animals, and the prevalence or incidence of human disease caused by those agents are needed.

When a formal quantitative risk assessment has taken place for every region or country involved, it will be possible to design a system of meat inspection that can adapt itself to the circumstances as they occur in these different regions. Furthermore, the system does not have to be identical for all these different regions (Hathaway and McKenzie, 1991; Berends *et al.*, 1993).

In addition, a fundamental question connected with this is how much public authorities should be involved in the inspection of matters that concern the aesthetic or technical quality of products more than public health aspects, as it appears to be the case with the inspection of pathological anatomical abnormalities in animals from healthy populations of highly developed countries.

It may well be that the results of a risk assessment will show that a majority of currently executed procedures could be omitted or carried out by the industry itself, supervised by the competent national veterinary authority. After all, many "high risk" industries, e.g., the pharmaceutical and aeronautical industries, bear the responsibility for the safety and quality of their products themselves, and the role of the authority is thereby restricted to verification of certain legal specifications.

References

Berends, B.R.; Smeets, J.F.M.; Harbers, A.H.M.; Knapen, F. van; Snijders, J.M.A. (1991). Investigations with enzyme-linked immunosorbent assays for *Trichinella spiralis* and *Toxoplasma gondii* in the Dutch 'Integrated Quality Control for finishing pigs' research project. Veterinary Quarterly, 13, 190-198.

Berends, B.R.; Snijders, J.M.A.; Logtestijn, J.G. van (1993). Efficacy of current EC meat inspection procedures and some proposed revisions with respect to microbiological safety assurance -A critical review. Veterinary Record, 133, 411-415.

Berends, B.R.; Snijders, J.M.A (1994). The Hazard Analysis Critical Control Point Approach in meat production. Tijdschrift voor Diergeneeskunde, 119, 360-365.

Elbers, A.R.W.; Tielen, M.J.M.; Snijders, J.M.A.; Cromwijk, W.A.J.; Hunneman, W.A. (1992). Epidemiological studies on lesions in finishing pigs in the Netherlands. I. Prevalence, seasonality and interrelationship. Preventive Veterinary Medicine, 14, 217-231.

Gerats, G.E.C. (1990). Working towards Quality. Aspects of quality control and hygiene in the meat industry. PhD Thesis, University of Utrecht, The Netherlands.

Harbers, A.H.M. (1991). Aspects of meat inspection in an Integrated Quality Control system for slaughter pigs. PhD Thesis, University of Utrecht, The Netherlands.

Harbers, A.H.M.; Smeets, J.F.M.; Snijders, J.M.A. (1992a). Registration on post mortem abnormalities of pigs in the slaughterline. Fleischwirtschaft, 72, 160-163.

Harbers, A.H.M.; Elbers, A.R.W.; Geelen, A.J.; Rambags, P.G.M.; Snijders, J.M.A. (1992b). Preselection of finishing pigs on the farm as an aid for meat inspection. Veterinary Quarterly, 14, 46-50.

Harbers, A.H.M.; Smeets, J.F.M.; Faber, J.A.J.; Snijders, J.M.A.; Logtestijn, J.G. van (1992c). A comparative study into procedures for post mortem inspection for finishing pigs. Journal of Food Protection, 53, 620-626.

Hathaway, S.C.; Pullen, M.M.; McKenzie, A.I. (1988). A model for Risk- Assessment of organoleptic postmortem inspection procedures for meat and poultry. Journal of American Veterinary Medical Association, 192, 960-966.

Hathaway, S.C.; McKenzie, A.I. (1991). Postmortem meat inspection programs: separating science and tradition. Journal of Food Protection, 54, 471-475.

Hathaway, S.C.; McKenzie, A.I. (1993). Risk analysis and meat hygiene. In: Proceedings of the 11th International Symposium of the World Association of Veterinary Food Hygienists, Bangkok, 24-29th October. pp. 38-45.

Snijders, J.M.A.; Smeets, J.F.M.; Harbers, A.H.M.; Logtestijn, J.G. van (1989). Towards an improved meat inspection procedure for slaughter pigs. In: Proceedings of the 10th International Symposium of the World Association of Veterinary Food Hygienists (Satellite Symposium), Stockholm, Sweden, 2-7th July. pp. 22-25.

Snijders, J.M.A.; Schouwenburg, J.N.; Logtestijn, J.G. van; Berends, B.R. (1993a). Modernization of current meat inspection procedures. In: Proceedings of the 39th International Congress of Meat Science and Technology, Calgary, Canada, 2-6th August.

Snijders, J.M.A.; Logtestijn, J.G. van; Berends, B.R. (1993b). Integrated Quality Control and HACCP as prerequisites for a new meat inspection system. In: Proceedings of the 11th International Symposium of the World Association of Veterinary Food Hygienists, Bangkok, Thailand, 24-29th October. pp. 123-127.

Chapter XI

Animal Health and Economics

Part I

An Economist's View of Animal Disease[26]

K.S. Howe
University of Exeter
Agricultural Economics Unit
United Kingdom

[26] earlier presented at the Meeting of the Society for Veterinary Epidemiology and Preventive Medicine, Reading, U.K., March 1985; published by courtesy of the author and the proceedings editor, M. Thrusfield.

1. Introduction

The importance of economic appraisal of the consequences of animal disease and its prevention or control has been recognized increasingly in recent years. Nevertheless the approaches adopted have centered on quite narrowly defined cost/benefit studies and, to a lesser extent, estimates of resource wastage through livestock mortality. There has been no comprehensive attempt to interpret animal disease from the point of view of the part it plays within the economics process. Consequently, no well-defined methodology has yet been developed for analyzing a wide range of important economic problems concerning, among others, the ways in which disease affects resource use in general for different types of livestock production, its relationship with choice of technology, how disease may influence the interpretation of the commercial efficiency of production on the long and short term,and what is the best way to deal with disease in farm livestock in an economic rather than a veterinary sense. This part I of the chapter on economics, is intended as an introduction to some of the important conceptual issues which must be explored as the basis for subsequent applied work.

2. The Role of Economics

There is a tendency for non-economists to think of economics as concerned with problems of the nation's economy, and money. National problems, which include unemployment and inflation, belong to that part of the subject which is macro-economics". Money "per se" is, in fact, only a coincidental consideration to the main purpose of economics which is concerned with decisions affecting the availability and effective use of real resources in providing for real needs. In contrast to macro-economics, micro-economics" focuses attention on the choices made by the many producers and consumers who make up the national economy. Agricultural economists, for example, are applied micro-economists, and any study of the economics of animal disease draw on the concepts and techniques of micro-economic analysis. Fortunately, micro-economics is free from the controversies which afflict macro-economics.

A particular feature of the subject, seen exceptionally well in agriculture, is that the technical relationships which are the foundation of production are always prominent. In fact, micro-economic analysis would be largely nonsensical without them. The point is stressed, however, because sometimes economics is thought to be very different from other scientific disciplines. On first encounter some ideas can be seen a little unusual, but economics is anything but a self-contained, exclusive preserve. The interpretation of animal disease from an economic's point of view should provide some justification for this argument.

3. Economics and Animal Disease

Any production process involves the transformation of inputs into outputs. The production of animal products depends on biological processes whereby inputs of feed nutrients are changed into outputs such as meat, milk, eggs and wool. Such processes are studied widely by agricultural scientists, who describe the relationships between levels of inputs and the resulting outputs as "response functions". These relationships belong to a more general category known to economists as "production functions". Whereas agricultural scientists are interested exclusively with complex biochemical relationships between technical inputs and outputs, economists often include other inputs such as labour, the use of buildings and machinery, and management skill. For the most part these other inputs "facilitate the process" rather than undergo a direct physical transformation, but they are not less important to the economic activity of production. Without the use of labour, housing and the rest, production of output for sale could not take place. That is one important example of where agricultural scientists and economists have different, but equally legitimate, frames of reference. Both interpretations are essential to the economic analysis of animal disease, as we shall see.

Suppose that we envisage a simple production process in which output is daily liveweight gain for a group of bullocks and the single variable input is the weight of concentrates fed per day. For obvious reasons it is easier to use a simple example, but it is intended that the interpretation should be perfectly general.

This implies a production function of the form

$$G = f * \left(\frac{C}{F}, L * E, H, \ldots \right) \quad \textbf{(11.1)}$$

where

G = liveweight gain per day	]	
C = weight of concentrates fed per day	>	variable
F = intake of forage per day	]	
L = labour use	]	
E = managerial expertise of the farmer	>	fixed
H = housing system	]	

Essentially it is the response of liveweight gain to concentrates which is under examination. For animals which are deemed "healthy" by some criteria, the response function may be described in general terms by curve "H" in Figure 11.1.

Curve H indicates that higher rates of concentrate feeding give higher growth rates, but that there are diminishing returns to successive increases in concentrate use. Leaving aside for the moment the question of economic efficiency, consider the effect of disease on the response function. In so far as disease affects the animals' biological performance, it will tend to shift the response function downwards, say to curve "U". Rather than contribute to production, disease actively works against it, i.e., disease is a "negative input". For some arbitrary level of concentrates input C1, growth is now G2 rather than G1. The mathematical expression for the function should be supplemented by another variable, say "D" for disease.

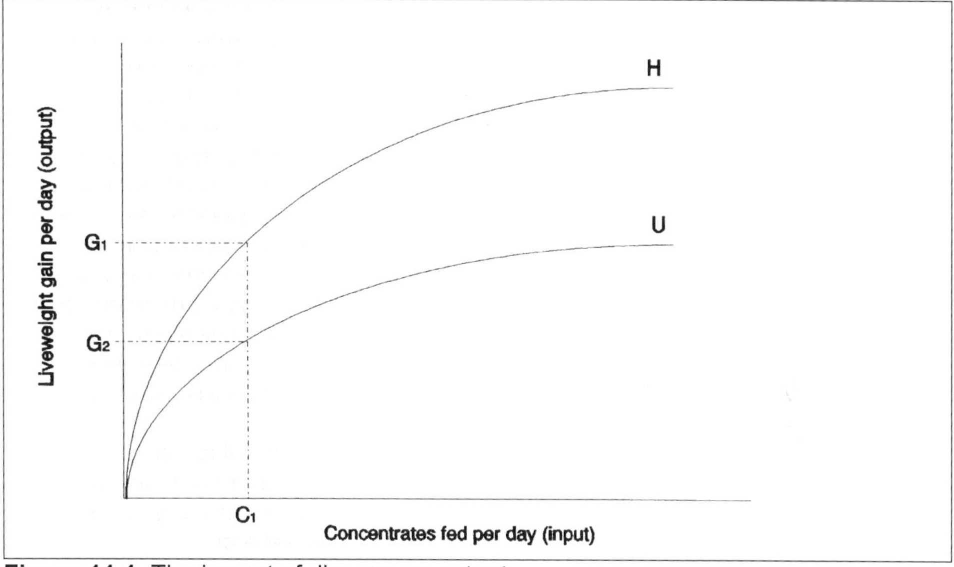

Figure 11.1. The impact of disease on output.

The crucial question is how to recover growth rate G1 having been forced back to G2 by disease. The obvious answer is to obtain the kind of veterinary inputs which are capable of restoring G1. An additional positive input" in the form of veterinary attention is necessary to offset the negative input" of disease. Often this will be the only course of action, and whether or not it is worthwhile from an economic point of view depends on the financial value of (G1 - G2). If G1 and G2 represented the finished weight of cattle for a given quantity of feed, then the difference in market value, effectively P (G1 - G2), where P is price, would be the maximum expenditure which could be justified on veterinary attention to recover the higher weight. In the model in Figure 11.1 the example is rather different, since it concerns loss of the rate of liveweight gain. The economic interpretation is made more complicated, but essentially the conclusion is the same for the reasons as follows. The loss in the rate of gain may imply the reduction in finished weight by the time it is planned to market the cattle in the sense described above. On the other hand, it can mean that the cattle will have to be kept longer to reach the same sale weight because their progress has been checked. In that case if the growth rate recovers to something like its initial level, the average rate of gain over time must have been reduced. The implications may be very significant for any farmer with limited housing facilities, for example, who is conscious of the economic importance of animal turnover in generating income from cattle. The retention of a batch of cattle for longer than is unusually necessary often will mean a delay in bringing in the next and subsequent batches, thereby reducing annual throughput. The value of P (G1 - G2) then becomes the daily revenue foregone over a period of time as a direct result of the fall in turnover.

Until now the example has been explained as if the only reaction to disease is to make use of veterinary inputs. In many instances this will be so, but not always. There are circumstances when it is feasible to substitute other inputs for veterinary attention. In justification of this statement we first reconstruct Figure 11.1 in the shape of Figure 11.2 which, though strikingly similar, has a different interpretation.

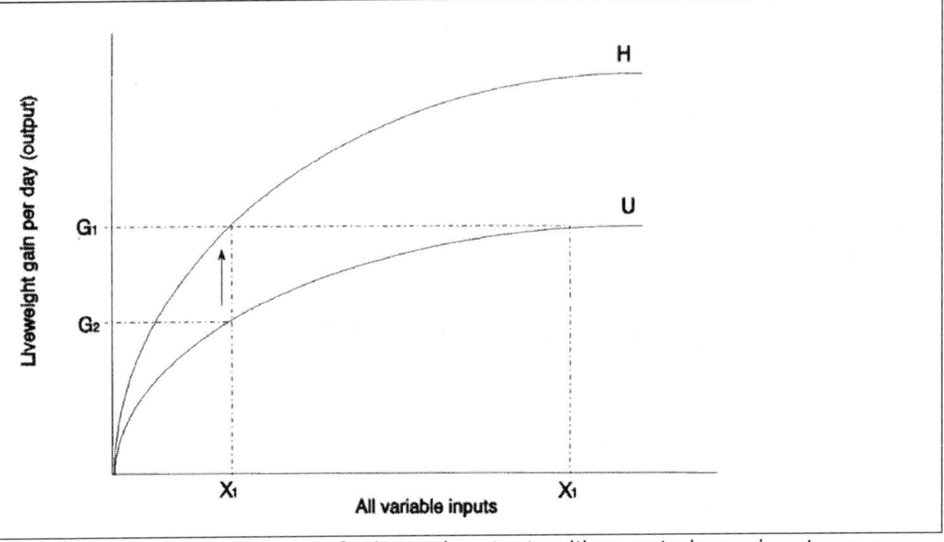

Figure 11.2. The recovery of planned output: either veterinary inputs or non-veterinary inputs.

Instead of confining attention to the response function for liveweight gain in relation to concentrates fed, now we interpret the horizontal axis to mean a measure of some "composite" input comprising a package of all relevant variable inputs.

$$G = f * \left(\frac{C}{F}, L * E, H, \ldots \right) \qquad \textbf{(11.1)} \text{ page 314}$$

$$G = g(X) \qquad \textbf{(11.2)}$$

$$X = (C, F, L * E, H, \ldots) \qquad \textbf{(11.3)}$$

This is an example of an "economic production function", which expresses the relationship between output and increasing quantities of all feed, labour use, managerial skill and other environmental variables such as lairage space. In contrast with point C1 in Figure 11.1, X1 now represents a collection of quantities of all the inputs which happens to yield growth rate G1 as before. For reasons which will become clear, veterinary inputs are presently excluded.

Again we suppose that disease causes a reduction in technical efficiency (G1 - G2) and again a question to be answered is how to recover G1. The solution may be as before, by incurring veterinary expenditures up to a maximum outlay of the value of P(G1 - G2). But there is an alternative (in fact more than one, as we shall see) which is to increase the use of other inputs from X1 to X2. The arrow in Figure 11.2 describes these two paths back to G1. However, it will clarify the explanation to state the problem in rather a different way. If a farmer wants his cattle to achieve a growth rate G1, he has to choose between the alternative production techniques which he expect will give the same result. At the two extremes, either he may devote relatively few resources to adequate nutrition, housing and supervision of his stock, while employing veterinary inputs to forestall disease, or he may take considerable care with his animal husbandry reflected in the use of more non-veterinary instead of veterinary inputs, to reach the same end. From that perspective curves H ("healthy") and U ("unhealthy") are inaptly named. Really they are simple the production functions for two different but equally valid, techniques of production, but which are differentiated in practical terms by health status of the animals. Which is chosen will depend on the relative costs of the necessary veterinary and non-veterinary inputs.

As intimated above, it is too restrictive to conceive only of two extreme alternatives. Figure 11.3 illustrates another possibility, with a more appropriate labelling of the curves and horizontal axis.

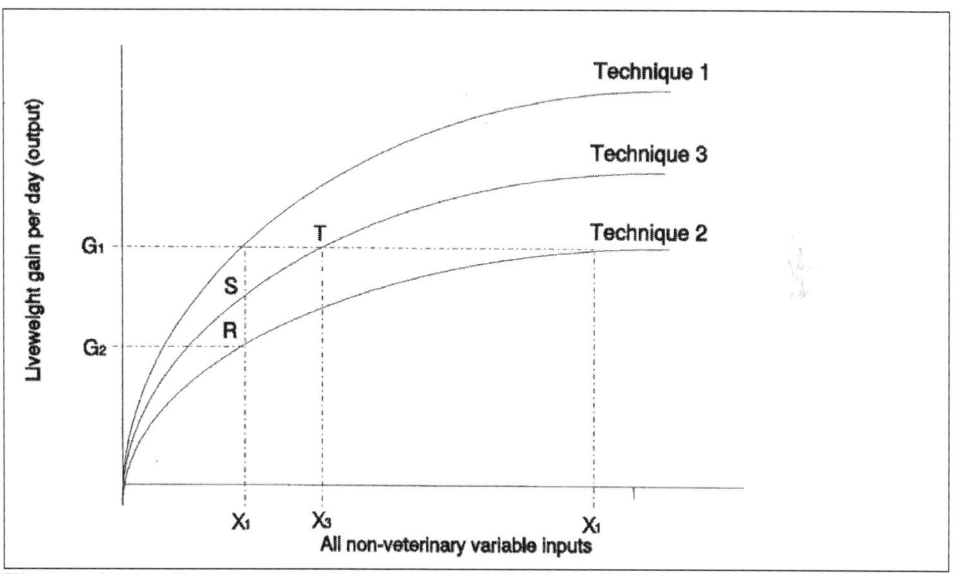

Figure 11.3. The recovery of planned output: ***both*** veterinary inputs ***and*** non-veterinary inputs.

Technique 3 introduces another possibility which may be one of any number which is available between techniques 1 and 2. It is a "middle way" which involves lifting production from G2 to G1 in two parts. That proportion of (G1 - G2) given by RS is achieved by veterinary expenditures while the remainder, equivalent to climbing from S to T, is accomplished by increasing non-veterinary inputs from X1 to X3. An important problem to an economist is the identification of the specific path corresponding to RST which enables G1 rather than G2 to be achieved most cheaply, i.e., discovering the combination of veterinary and non-veterinary inputs which meets the objective but a minimum total cost. By extension, frequently it is necessary to evaluate if the additional total outlays are at least covered by the consequent additional receipts.

4 Data Requirements

It is self-evident that data are essential to give substance to the concepts outlined above. Clearly, the precise requirements will vary with the specific disease condition or conditions to be studied. In keeping with the general perspective which has been taken here, the following is offered as a broad framework which can guide the initial steps in the economic analysis of animal disease.

4.1. Identification of the "best performance" conditions

In all circumstances it is necessary to ascertain what conditions are necessary if animals are to produce in the neighbourhood of the current technical optimum e.g., daily liveweight gain, food conversion ratio, technical optimum e.g., daily liveweight gain, food conversion ratio, lactation yield, lambing percentage etc. Such data may be provided from experimental results, but with the disadvantage that they will seldom be representative of the potential under the less controlled environment of commercial farming. Reference to the performance of "elite" herds and flocks, often identifiable from the enterprise costings conducted, for example, by universities and the Meat and Livestock Commission, is likely to be the more useful. The idea of the current technical optimum is stressed, since it is to be expected that the implementation of new scientific knowledge and husbandry practices will tend to increase potential efficiency over time. There may be occasions when it is useful to seek out expert opinion on the likely direction of future developments in the control of animal disease.

4.2. Quantification of "best performance" relationships

In essence, this activity involves using the empirical data to describe the relationships which underpin Technique 1 of Figure 11.3. Detailed case studies may suffice in some instances, while recourse to the use of more advanced statistical techniques on sample data will be helpful in others. The direct estimation of a production function using multiple regression analysis has the advantage that the relative importance of various determinants of efficiency can be measured.

4.3. Study of livestock enterprise subject to health problems

This amounts to repeating the type of analysis outlined in paragraph 4.1 and 4.2 above, but for livestock subjected to health problems i.e., defining Technique 2 of Figure 11.3, and also investigating the pathways between Techniques 1 and 2 as described and summarised with reference to Technique 3. Obviously it is seldom possible to draw a clear distinction between "healthy" and "diseased" livestock, and an important part of the exercise is to delimit the threshold points which are considered to be significant.

4.4. Economic interpretation of the technical relationships

Using the procedures which have been outlined above, it is possible to make important insights into the economic implications of animal disease. The analysis has been couched in terms of the type of problems which afflict the individual livestock enterprise. Technical and economic efficiency are seldom synonymous, and the characteristics of their interrelationship is susceptible to analysis. Moreover, farmers usually are concerned more with the profitability of their farming systems overall than with particular enterprises, it is not difficult to evaluate the economic consequences of animal health problems causing time and physical resources to be diverted from alternative uses on the farm. As an extension, knowledge of individual farm circumstances and additional epidemiological data can enable inferences to be made about the economic impact of animal disease on the national farm. By implications, the scope and direction of veterinary research and practices could be guided by reference to the kind of results forthcoming from the approach to economic appraisal which has been discussed, as well as policy with regard to disease control programmes. A prerequisite for the formulation of appropriate economic models is the classification of disease types according to their particular characteristics.

5. Conclusion

It has been argued that hitherto the application of economics to the problems of animal disease has tended to abstract from the central role of the discipline as a science choice. Economics helps with decisions about how scarce resources are to be allocated and used. Veterinary skills and medicines are no different from any other scarce resource, and it is both necessary and desirable to interpret the economic efficiency with which they are deployed in the cause of improving animal health. As part of the appraisal, the relationship between veterinary inputs and its substitutes must be studied. This part I attempted to explain some of the basic conceptual and empirical issues which should be addressed.

Part II

Economics in the Veterinary Domain: Further Dimensions[27]

J.P. McInerney
University of Exeter
Agricultural Economics Unit
United Kingdom

[27] Earlier presented at the Meeting of the Society for Veterinary Epidemiology and Preventive Medicine, Edinburgh, UK, April 1988; published by courtesy of the author and the proceedings editor, M. Thrusfield

1. Introduction

Although the economics element contained in veterinary curricula varies widely among institutions, the very fact that it always gets some mention shows (presumably) that economic considerations in animal disease are simply realizing that economics cannot be ignored and recognising precisely **why** it is important, and hence identifying what kind of economics understanding is useful for veterinarians. It is not surprising, therefore, that there seems no clear agreement over what to teach or how to teach it.

It is no criticism that the veterinary profession may not know what economics it needs, for the answer is not all self-evident. Every discipline has its own abstractions, conceptual frameworks and analytical approaches which derive from the way problems are defined within that discipline. It takes a very long time often to appreciate these fully and develop the intuitions that enable one's specialist training to be used as a mode of thinking, rather than just as a set of rules or technical methods[28].

It is unlikely that 'outsiders' can ever achieve this appreciation. Even for professional economists, crossing this intellectual divide in relation to their own subject is not easy. It has to be said that most economics graduates don't **understand** economics - they merely know, to a greater or lesser extent, what they have been taught about it (and it is sad that many never develop beyond this point).

Consequently, as non-specialists, veterinary teachers cannot be expected to know automatically, what economics content is most appropriate for inclusion in their curricula, and economists as a group have not been very evident in helping them decide. The economic issues relevant to veterinary studies seem never to have been confronted in a structured manner by either of the two interested parties, and this part of the chapter could represent a valuable step forward in this respect.

There are numerous viewpoints on economics, and therefore many contexts in which it can be taught. They vary from generalized notions concerning the creation and distribution of wealth in society, through the establishment of relationships describing the workings of major segments of the economy, to very applied techniques for assessing the financial implications of particular actions. Before any sensible planning of economics training can be conducted, it would seem necessary to decide what sort of economics might be relevant to those preparing for a career in veterinary science.

2. What Sort of Economics

It is unfortunate that the basic notions of economics are frequently summarized and purveyed as 'the economics of .... (animal disease, forestry, home ownership,

[28] Rather like learning to **think** in a foreign language, as opposed to being able to translate words into or from it.

education, etc.)'. This phrase is generally interpreted as an excuse to detail the financial aspects of the subject, setting monetary costs and returns against one another to yield some figure(s) to indicate the balance of advantage and how it is influenced by various factors. This is, perhaps, an unavoidable element of economic analysis, but is not really what economics is all about. For one thing, it implies no concepts or analytical frameworks, but reduces economic analysis to merely a series of measurements - as though expressing things in monetary terms in itself made some answer obvious.

This popular misconception confuses economics with accountancy; it is a major barrier to any functional appreciation of what economics might offer, and lies at the root of the often dismissive attitude that 'real' scientists hold towards the subject. The simple view that veterinary science is all to do with spaying cats, helping with difficult calvings, and treating sick animals is on about the same level.

Three different approaches to the teaching of economics might be considered as appropriate for adoption within the veterinary profession.

2.1. 'Pure' economics

It could be argued that everyone should be exposed to the basic principles of economics, simply because the society in which we live and work is fundamentally an economic system. Consequently, an understanding of the elements of how that system functions is an essential part of our general education, in precisely the same way as is a basic appreciation of science, history, geography, literature, etc. The social sciences are not included in the core curriculum at school level (because they require more maturity to be understood?) so they should at least be encountered by the university student, of whatever discipline. This view is common in American universities, where economics, sociology and politics are among the compulsory subjects for virtually all first year students.

However, while there are undoubted failings in the narrow specialisation to which our university students are subject, there is no reason why veterinary students in particular should be taught something to make them better informed citizens if the same principle is not applied everywhere. Because something would be beneficial is not to say that it can be justified. The time constraints on covering the scientific elements of the veterinary curriculum are perceived as severe enough, without diverting resources to teaching more general matters. And it would require a substantial resource commitment to create any self-contained understanding of economics. The selected snippets of the economist's analytical framework (such as the 'explanation' of price formation on markets, elasticity concepts, opportunity cost, discounting, etc.) which frequently gain a mention in non-specialist summaries amount merely to pointing out a few exotic shrubs in an unfamiliar garden. They yield neither specific understanding nor general appreciation of why the study of economics might be important, they make no contact with ideas in veterinary science with which the student is otherwise pre-occupied, and do not even allow him to appreciate any better the economic commentary found in newspapers. To create a workable picture of general economic principles would require emphasis on the structure of economic systems, the elements of both micro-economics and macro-economics, the major relationships that underlie economic analysis, and the way economic forces mould the development of firms, industries and societies. Everyone should know about these things - but they do not belong in the curricula of veterinary schools.

2.2. The economics of agriculture

On the basis of Keith Howe's survey it seems the dominant form in which economics finds its way into the veterinary curriculum is through association with agricultural production. This is understandable, since much veterinary practice centres on farm animals and so it is likely the economic implications of disease, and disease control, will emerge through their effects on agricultural output. In addition, livestock husbandry and farm management offer a readily identifiable context for appreciating economic issues, compared to rather more vague ideas of costs and benefits which attach to no-one in particular.

However, the focus on agricultural economics represents a very restrictive framework because it suggests that the economic aspects of animal disease are almost entirely **commercial**. In other words, the presumption seems to be that the part of the economy using the services of veterinary science (either directly in practice, or indirectly in research, the pharmaceuticals industry or the state veterinary service) is mainly farming, and so it is the economics of farming that it is most relevant to appreciate. But economics is not synonymous with commerce. Its prime concern is with how economic benefit ('value') is generated for the people who constitute society, not just with monetary revenue to businessmen. It is true that agriculture has the most obviously measurable output that can be affected by disease control, but that is not to say that therefore it is potentially the most important source of economic benefits. The non-commercial customers of the veterinary service - the private individuals whose livestock are companion animals - are just as much a part of the economy, and just as much recipients of genuine economic value[29]. Indeed, it is arguable in a society such as ours that, overall, people would be made worse off by a reduced availability of veterinary services to the companion animal sector than by an equivalent reduction in services to the farm sector. This statement may or may not be precisely true, but it is designed to highlight the validity of the non-agricultural sector in considering the economic aspects of animal disease.

Thus, an emphasis on costings and margins for farm enterprises, accountancy and farm planning procedures, management variables and their effects on farm incomes, etc., seems a limited addition to the veterinary curriculum. It may constitute no more than an isolated cameo on another world, and unlikely to assist the student in appreciating his training in any wider context. It is only if the vet becomes fully integrated into the farm management decision making process - which occurs in some intensive pig enterprises but nowhere else - that his analytical capabilities need to develop down this pathway. Otherwise, the only 'commercial' decisions he is likely to confront are those connected with the running of a veterinary practice - and conventional agricultural economics has little to offer in this respect.

[29] And many veterinary practices recognize this when they look at where their fee income comes from.

From a strictly economic point of view it would be more relevant to consider the implications of livestock disease from the standpoint of the overall agricultural sector, rather than detail on the farm-level situation. But this is difficult to illuminate very clearly, and is still a limited perception of the economic issues. It is certainly not approximated by summary explanations of the CAP or other aspects of agricultural support policy, which are mostly just administrative and political interventions in the economy's functioning that obscure the underlying economic reality.

2.3. Veterinary economics

The above comments lead one to conclude that, if veterinary students and professionals are to make any useful contact with economics, then what they are taught should link as far as possible with their own starting perceptions and not be presented as some apparently arbitrary statement of things that are 'important'. This implies there could exist a distinct area of study, which we shall call 'veterinary economics', linked conceptually to the wider frame of economics but sufficiently self-contained to be applicable within the context of animal disease. To define it, we must seek to establish and illustrate a series of concepts and propositions that demonstrate how veterinary science and practice can be seen as part of the workings of the economy.

This may seem slightly odd, because at first sight veterinary studies are built upon the natural sciences, biological and biochemical processes, clinical diagnosis and treatment, and the objectives of enhancing the welfare of animals. However, it is no less illogical than accepting 'agricultural economics' as an identifiable and valid branch of economics. The science and practice of agriculture is the manipulation of technical processes involving plants and animals; as an area of knowledge it is basic science linked with a few organisational procedures. However, it is because these are conducted solely in order to benefit human beings that agriculture gains its economic connotations, so ultimately some understanding of agriculture as an economic process becomes necessary. If agriculture students need to know aspects of economics that relate particularly to their realm of study, and if a set of economic principles can be defined and packaged in a way that makes them directly applicable, then exactly the same can be said for veterinary students.

Vets never need to function as economists, so there is no purpose in insisting students should be capable of applying the standard concepts and analytical methods that constitute the typical elementary introduction to economics. However, as professionals, they will be operating within an environment that is governed (if not dominated) by economic considerations. This is true whether they go into private practice, research, the pharmaceuticals industry, the state veterinary service, or even university teaching. It is a defensible presumption, therefore, that every veterinarian ought to understand what 'economic considerations' are if they are to condition his lifestyle. Furthermore, if he appreciates how veterinary science fits in the spectrum of scientific knowledge and endeavour (as he must), then equally he should appreciate how the science of animal disease control fits into the spectrum of economic activity that constitutes 'the real world' in which all this takes place.

It is not practical here to set out in detail the appropriate components of a veterinary economics course. However, it is suggested that to gain any useful insight into economics the student of veterinary science should appreciate four general propositions. Each of these is considered in turn.

3. Livestock Disease is an Economic Process

The conventional view of disease sees it as a biological phenomenon which affects adversely the health status of an individual animal or animal population. From an economic standpoint, however, the important thing about livestock disease is that it adversely affects **people**, not animals. This statement is true not just for zoonoses but any disease condition about which society is sufficiently interested to do something - that-is, in which there is an economic interest. If a disease condition affects only livestock of no direct or indirect economic concern (wild shrews?) then for all practical purposes it is not a disease. Except in purely scientific terms, therefore, what we define as a disease depends on an implicit assumption that people may be in some way less well off as a result of it.

To place animal disease in its economic context, we first need the concept of an 'economic process' which lies at the core of the economist's model of the world. This is simply any activity in which basic resources are utilised to produce goods and services designed to be of benefit to people. All economic activity, in all forms and at all levels in all societies, is a collection of such basic processes. 'Resources' may be divided into natural resources (land, livestock, etc.), human resources, and capital resources (which are themselves the product of an economic process). The "goods and services" are the whole diverse array of things that satisfy the needs of human society. And the 'people' for whom this economic activity takes place means society collectively, rather than any particular person or group - though the model can be applied with equal validity at any level of aggregation referring to the people who make up a firm, a village, an industry, a region, a country, or the world (see Figure 11.4).

The central economic ideas of 'value' benefit to people) and 'cost' resources used up) emerge directly from this simple model, without any need to include the element of 'money'[30]. In addition, the guiding concept of economic efficiency (gaining maximum benefit from the collection of resources used) can be distinguished from the limited but more common notion of technical efficiency (the ratio of output to just one of the resources used - yield per cow, output per man, return on capital, etc.). In an ideal world, this resource use system would work perfectly, so maximum economic efficiency provides the conceptual benchmark against which actual standards of achievement can be assessed (rather like the perfect gas or the frictionless plane in physics).

---

[30] Contrary to popular presumption, money is not the essential element in economics; it is merely the convenient unit for measuring the varied real components, which are positive and negative benefits.

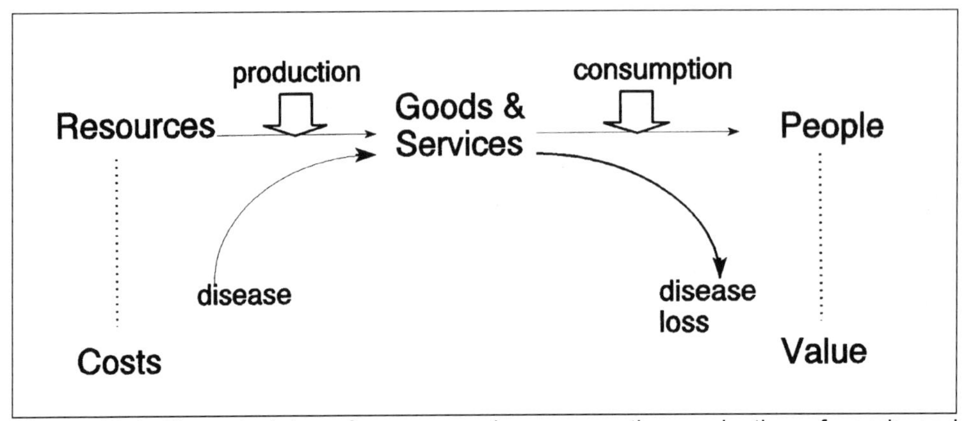

Figure 11.4. The principles of an economic process: the production of goods and services and the position of disease in this process.

The economic process of major interest to veterinary science involves transforming resources (grass, feed, labour, animals, etc.) into products (meat, milk, horserides, pet companionship, etc.) that benefit people. As a biological phenomenon, disease is an integral part of this system, disease agents being simply one natural form of influence interacting with all the others. From an economic point of view, however, disease is an intrusion into the resource transformation process. It reduces the services gained from any level of resource use, and so lowers the level of benefits available to people collectively[31]. The economic definition of a disease is then clear. It has no particular aetiological or clinical reference points. It is simply any condition affecting the health status of animals which society would prefer not to exist.

Disease can be viewed as an economic process in itself because it consumes economic resources (i.e., uses up feed or livestock), or because it generates negative benefits for society (Figure 11.4). The negative aspect of disease is not simply the directly reduced value of output or services from livestock (the commonly perceived 'disease losses'). Benefits are lost also due to an array of indirect, secondary and knock-on effects throughout the whole interconnected system of resource-using processes that constitute the total economy. Before the losses attributable to disease can be measured, their manifestation must first be identified, which implies modelling the way disease effects move through the economic system - impinging on resource use and value creation on farms, in households, via markets to all firms and individuals linked in some way with commercial and domestic livestock. Modelling livestock disease as an economic process has many similarities with epidemiology. As the epidemiologist traces the path of infection, say, from its original source out through the herd, the livestock population and perhaps to other affected livestock types, so the economist will attempt to trace all the (positive and negative) changes in value from the first manifestation of a disease in a livestock process outwards as they appear in related economic activities and processes.

[31] Although within this overall category the existence of disease may create positive benefits for some sub-groups - e.g., it generates income and employment for vets and drug companies.

4. Disease Control is an Economic Process

To the veterinarian, disease control involves the use of appropriate drugs, procedures and back-up services to lower or prevent the technical manifestations of some defined condition. In economic terms this is just another variant on the theme of transforming resources into products and services that people want. It is possible - but not particularly fruitful - to wonder whether the outcome should be defined as a negative output (less disease) or a positive one (faster liveweight gain, a happier dog owner). Either way, the basic elements of economic analysis - costs incurred, benefits gained - are an inescapable feature of what is otherwise a veterinary process.

But economic concepts have more to offer than this, because they address questions about **how best** to undertake disease control and **how far** to pursue it. The economist's model of resource use is developed from the concept of a 'production function'. This is simply a generalized statement that there is a systematic relationship between the levels of the resources used (X_i) and the level of output (Q) into which they are transformed.The importance of this relationship is not its

$$Q = f(x_1.....x_n)$$

mathematical form (the determination of which is a strictly empirical matter) but rather its embodied principle that economic resources do not have to be combined in fixed proportions[32]. A given volume of milk can be produced from countless different combinations of land, labour, feed inputs, cow numbers, capital equipment etc. - i.e., different dairying systems. Within broad limits, all inputs are substitutes for one another, and economic criteria define how the **best** (most economically efficient) combination can be determined.

In a disease control context, the production function idea highlights the fact that non-veterinary resources (feed, management practices, etc.) and direct veterinary inputs (drugs, professional services) are substitutes in reducing the impacts of disease. For example, allocating more land and labour inputs to a flock of sheep (i.e., a lower stocking rate and rotational grazing) can reduce losses due to intestinal worms in the same way as treating with anthelminthics.

Hence, no 'best' control practice can be defined for a disease - nor should one be recommended, therefore - based solely on technical criteria. The relative unit costs of veterinary and non-veterinary resources and their respective productivities in counteracting disease losses - which vary in different countries and between farming systems - will determine the best practices to adopt.

The economist's production model also considers the link between the additions to output and additional resource use. In virtually all situation this is a declining relationship (the widely misquoted 'diminishing returns') so at some point it is not worth increasing output further because the extra gains do not cover the extra costs.

[32] As compared to transformations at the biochemical level, for example, where the combination of amino acids to produce a molecule of some protein is rigidly defined.

In a disease control context this highlights the (obvious) fact that a stage will always be reached when it will not be economically worthwhile reducing disease losses further. This the introduces the (less obvious) concept that in any livestock system there is potentially 'an optimum amount of disease'.

These ideas are set out with reference to agricultural production simply because that is the easiest context to visualise. They are equally relevant to the expenditure of resources on health care in pets, wildlife or humans. Furthermore, they are applicable at all levels of aggregation - whether individual companion animal, herd or livestock sector - where decisions about disease control are made. Although not developed in detail here, they should serve to emphasise what may not easily emerge from standard veterinary considerations - that disease control is (not only, but also) an economic process[33].

5. Economic Values are not Simply 'Prices'

Disease control programmes can be conceived, designed and operated at two distinct levels - the individual animal or herd, and the overall regional, national (or international) livestock sector. Veterinary training needs to clarify the principles of action at both levels, which correspond to the individual veterinary practice and the state veterinary service. The private farmer or pet owner on the one hand, and the general public (referred to by economists as 'society') on the other, represent two quite different customers. More importantly, from an economic point of view, they imply two different contexts for the valuation (measurement) of costs and benefits. Although veterinarians are unlikely to be undertaking formal economic analyses, they should recognise this divergence - if only because it highlights the possibility, when assessing the economic merits of disease control, of conflict between the ('private') economic interests of a farmer and the wider public ('social') interest.[34]

Measurement of costs and benefits always involves applying appropriate monetary values to physical quantities of resources used and outputs gained. It is the difference in the relevant values to apply at farm and at sector level that gives rise to the divergence between 'private' and 'social' valuations of any scheme. Individual farmers (or householders) mostly buy the resources and services they use and sell their outputs through the usual market channels. To assess the net benefit of expenditures on disease control as perceived by them (whether from farm level or national schemes), it is entirely appropriate to apply observed market (commercial) prices to the elements of cost and benefit they experience. The balance between computed costs and returns captures the net effect on their personal finances, the impact as reflected in their individual bank accounts. Strictly speaking, this is an assessment of the **financial**

[33] It should also be clear that 'animal welfare' concerns are essentially part of an economic process too. The animal species for whom welfare issues are important are a matter of social choice (cats, but not rats) ; and people are prepared to forego some element of consumption benefits (cheaper pork or eggs) and incur extra resource costs in order that they feel more comfortable about how livestock live.

[34] This potential conflict of interest demonstrates that disease control is a political process too.

aspects of disease control (rather than an economic assessment), the term indicating that it is the advantage to the individuals concerned that is being measured. It is the appropriate information for deciding whether the individual should choose to participate.

An **economic** assessment, by contrast, seeks to determine the balance of gains and losses as reflected in the economy as a whole - i.e., aggregating across all groups and individuals who may be affected.[35] The use of market prices in this context may introduce major errors in valuing expenditures incurred and benefits generated. Observed prices may grossly misrepresent the real (economic) values of costs and benefits to the economy due to some main causes:

a. Taxes and subsidies raise or lower prices without in any way affecting the commodity's value to the economy. A gallon of petrol represents the same amount of real resource, and makes the same contribution to real output, regardless of whether its price includes a major or minor element of tax;
b. Other forms of market intervention distort prices so they fail to reflect real economic values. An obvious example is the intervention purchase of surplus agricultural commodities. By definition, they have a zero value to the economy because they are surplus to requirements (and so no benefit would be lost if they were not produced); yet they command a non-zero price in the market thereby creating an illusion of value.[36]

Some things representing real costs and benefits to society have no price (and so appear valueless) simply because the economic system has no markets to generate price data. The obvious examples are wildlife, human health and welfare, and farm animal welfare.

Finally, even if all prices do accurately reflect true economic values, they are sensitive to changes in the level of the commodity in question. If a disease control scheme raised the production of milk by 5 per cent this would cause the price of milk to fall, so the benefit generated cannot be captured by simply applying a price value.

Considerations such as these are complicated, frequently subtle, and always difficult to establish unambiguously. But they are also crucial. The proper measurement of economic quantities is as important to correct decision making as is the accurate measurement of drug doses in disease treatment adequate within certain limits, but potentially dangerous beyond them. Veterinary students nor professionals do not need to know how techniques of economic analysis are employed in making corrections to observed prices. But they should appreciate that this is one reason why economists have a genuine role in the analysis of animal disease issues, as distinct from just being the guys who multiply things by prices (which anyone can do).

[35] Phrases such as 'the national farm' and 'UK Ltd' are frequently used to portray interests at this level.
[36] This illusion is, of course, a reality to the individual buyer or seller.

6. The Basis of Economic Value

The formal role of the veterinarian as a member of his profession is commitment to the welfare of animals; as part of an economic process, however like everyone else his role is directed towards the welfare of people. The veterinary student deserves to be shown how these two link together. In principle, this implies some appreciation of what determines the economic value (benefit to people) placed on veterinary services.

Much of this may be thought self-evident. To the extent that the veterinarian's efforts bring about healthier and more productive farm animals, and hence increased and more secure supplies of food, therein lies his economic contribution. Its value can be traced through a potentially measurable increase in a saleable commodity that has a recognisable price. This price may need some adjusting to correct for distortions, as discussed above, but otherwise the issue seems clear. However, the core of economic thinking emphasises that the value of something is not an intrinsic characteristic like molecular weight. Rather it derives from what people want, balanced against the availability of it - and these vary according to time and place. The value of enhanced pigmeat production to people in Europe, for example, is very different as compared to people in Saudi Arabia or in Ethiopia. The important points to recognize are, first, the supremacy of **preferences** in establishing value; these are not 'scientific' but they are nevertheless real, and become the ultimate determinant of what is important in a society. Second, the value of extra food is not self-evident on the grounds that 'food is an important commodity you cannot live without'. Recognition that the real value of anything can only be measured at the **margin**, not on average, is one of the most fundamental points in economics.

Economic values as identified in commercial production have some tangible base. But what underlies the economic value of veterinary services that produce healthier hamsters or neutered fat cats? Again this varies from one situation to another because, in addition to preferences, the observed value of some good or service in an economy is determined by the willingness and ability to pay on the part of the recipient. This reinforces the point that economic values are not intrinsic measures but a function of income levels. Thus the benefit gained from eliminating fleas from dogs in the UK is apparently far greater than it would be in India, and so would justify more resources being directed towards it.

The essential point in all this is that there can be no definitive statements about how 'important' animal health issues are. The potential economic benefit derived from the availability of veterinary services, the appropriate type of services, and the level of resources that ought to be allocated to providing them are all fundamentally economic issues. In poor countries (and to poor people in rich countries) it is their contribution to more and cheaper food that underlies 'the economics of veterinary services'. In high income countries it is increasingly through the provision of health care to companion animals, rather than in agriculture, that the veterinary profession makes its economic contribution to society. Nor can one realistically specify the **need** for resources to be allocated in the veterinary field on the basis of numbers and types of livestock, etc. It is clear, however, that the **demand** for veterinary services per thousand cows in the UK is greater than it is in Bangladesh.

7. Conclusion

The four propositions set out above would neither serve nor aim to 'teach economics to veterinary students'. Rather they could provide a framework within which the linkage between veterinary science and economic activity (as opposed to its linkage with animal health, or with professional practice) might be appreciated. The purpose would be to emphasize that all information and analysis, in whatever area of study, is directed towards supporting decisions that have to be taken. Decisions are guided by objectives, and the economist would argue that it is economic objectives (i.e., relating to the benefit of people) that ultimately guide all decisions. Furthermore, those decisions always boil down in the end to some variation on a theme of what resources are to be used, and for what purpose. These decisions may be made about treatment of individual animals in commercial veterinary practices; or about allocating public resources to national disease management schemes in the state veterinary service; or about appropriate expenditures in research programmes seeking more effective drugs or a more detailed understanding of a particular disease condition. The basic principles are the same, although the complexity of issues, information and implementation are very different.

If it is insights (rather than techniques) that the veterinary student and professional should gain from the economics content of his curriculum, then perhaps the most useful of these relates to the ultimate aim of veterinary science. Since science is (apparently) free of value judgements, it says nothing about how much disease is correct or acceptable in livestock; the implicit assumption can only be that veterinary science is directed towards the minimisation - or even elimination - of disease. By emphasizing its commonality with all other resource-using processes, the economics viewpoint makes clear that veterinary scientists should be trying simply to bring about the best amount of disease in the overall livestock population. Economists may not know any more about veterinary science than vets know economics. But they must work together if the above objective is to be pursued, and so each must have some appreciation of how the other thinks.

Part III

Economic Aspects of the Animal Welfare Issue[37]

J.P. McInerney
University of Exeter
Agricultural Economics Unit
United Kingdom

---

[37] Earlier presented at the Meeting of the Society for Veterinary Epidemiology and Preventive Medicine, London UK, April 1991; published by courtesy of the author and the proceedings editor, M. Thrusfield.

1. Introduction

Human interest in the welfare of other living creatures is nothing new. Ever since man domesticated animals so as to use them for his own purposes it has been simply a matter of self-interest to ensure they were kept in a way that enabled them to best serve him. This is true in relation both to 'productive' livestock like farm animals, and those with which emotional connections develop, such as pets. Generally speaking, however, it is only with domesticated animals that such welfare interest becomes of any significance. There is little effective concern over the unsavoury manner in which hyenas terrorise a weakling Thompson's gazelle or the rather excruciating way in which rodent pests are debilitated by anticoagulant compounds. Recognition of this fact that welfare concerns are selective rather than generalised underlies the basic proposition of this part III - namely, that animal welfare is simply part of man's perception of his *own* welfare, and only indirectly to do with any objective aspects of how the animals themselves are affected by their environment. It follows that, because economics is the discipline concerned with studying how people pursue their own wellbeing, it should therefore have a central role in the debates about animal welfare.

This assertion of the social scientist's role may appear strange to those who find *much* of the formal study (as opposed to popular advocacy) about welfare lies in the literature of animal science. Certainly it is those who study animal health and behaviour who feel able to make the most specific statements about what constitutes 'good' or 'bad' welfare conditions. However, this does not make the definition of appropriate welfare standards a scientific issue, as though it were akin to specifying the appropriate dosage of a drug to correct a disease condition. Not with standing the different standpoints from which the issue can be viewed, in practical terms the appropriate way to treat animals remains strictly a matter of human preference. That preference may be informed by science-based information, but no more than it is also influenced by Walt Disney-based information, or by culture, education, experience, income, collective or personal beliefs, and a range of other factors that determine what people think and do. The failing of social scientists so far is that they have not given animal welfare issues the attention they deserve, and so there is a lack of the useful economic information that should also inform attempts to define appropriate welfare codes.

In fact, welfare codes are not 'defined' in any objective sense but rather *chosen* - and that choice is likely to change over time (as with the recent decision to ban the tethering of sows, a practice that until now has been widespread and quite accepted). Consequently we need to study the determinants and the mechanisms of welfare choices in society if we are to better identify the standards appropriate to that society. It is not easy to put those choices into a framework of scientific assessment, or to base them on scientific principles. Indeed, there appear to be so many contradictions and arbitrary assertions in the framework of welfare regulation as to make it totally inconsistent with the rigorous conceptualisation, specification and measurement that is the hallmark of science. As a result, notwithstanding the apparent definitiveness of standard welfare statements they are all disturbingly wishy-washy underneath. If 400 square centimetres is insufficient space for a battery hen what is so good about 550?

Why is it unacceptable to prevent a sow turning round by tethering it, but good practice to do the same thing using a farrowing crate? If the use of BST threatens animal welfare, what is so different about other drugs and feeding regimes that allow more of a cow's productive capacity to be captured? What makes it cruel to dock the tails of pigs but not in the case of spaniels? Why does being eaten by a Jew or a Moslem make it unnecessary to stun an animal before slaughter? The list of such awkward questions is endless, but they all share a common characteristic - the answer lies in boundaries set by social choice, not by scientific assessment.

2. Concepts of Animal Welfare

The concern humans show over animal welfare is based on their own perceptions of how animals are affected by the conditions under which they are kept. Despite studies to measure the stress that animals feel (Stott, 1981), or experiments to determine their preferences for alternative husbandry conditions, we can never actually know what they would choose for themselves. Indeed, it is not clear to what extent animals do have preferences in the considered way that we do, as opposed to largely instinctive reactions to their environment. (And anyway, even if we do recognise animal preference we then largely ignore it, because by definition the management of livestock is the imposition of our preference over theirs.) Therefore, discussions of welfare unavoidably involve a subjective human judgement on what *we* believe are appropriate conditions for animals to enjoy or suffer. In this sense it is more correct to talk in terms of 'perceived welfare' to avoid any suggestion that we are dealing with something that has been or can be objectively assessed. This distinction becomes important when we face questions of whether animal welfare should be improved, and how this might be achieved. Because the issue involves a subjective judgement there will, by definition, be no uniform basis on which that judgement can be made. Different people will have their own views as to what constitutes welfare improvement and what the target level of attainment should be. This, then, is the real source of the problem, because if welfare standards are a matter of social choice it is not clear where those standards are appropriately set - or whether logically there can be any uniform standards.

Anyone seeking to make these arbitrary specifications of welfare standards would seem to have four different reference points, each of which represents some concept of animal welfare and hence could serve as a guide for actions.

A. The first, and philosophically perhaps the most defensible of these concepts would define welfare by placing maximum emphasis on what the animal itself would choose, taking this to represent what is 'most right' for its welfare. This would offer animals the freedom to act as naturally as their innate instincts determine in terms of dietary choice, mating behaviour, rearing young, establishing and maintaining territory, aggression and imposing social dominance, etc. While the most extreme advocates of animal rights might support such a concept of natural welfare it is obviously quite inconsistent with any notion of domesticated animals, and so is hardly relevant in the context of livestock farming.

B. A rather less libertarian but nevertheless still animal-centred concept would grant to livestock the best conditions attainable in the (unnatural) environment of domestication. While some of their natural behaviour patterns have inevitably to be controlled, the emphasis would lie in making the greatest possible provision for all their other perceived needs in terms of food, shelter, space, physical comfort, health, safety, social interaction, and so forth. This concept of maximal welfare is the most anthropomorphic in its style, and would result in all domesticated animals being treated as we treat our pets (or our children) based on what we think is 'good for them'. The simple fact that animals are kept for specific human purposes, however, means that this also is an unrealistic benchmark for any action on welfare.

C. In practical terms we inevitably move on towards situations where the animal's interests have to become more subservient to human interests, and so livestock are subject to conditions that create human benefit at some perceived cost to the animal. This is clear not only because we confine them, castrate them, conjugate them and do other things they would not choose, we then in many cases kill them off when it suits us best. However, because man in general has some sensitivity towards other living creatures, particularly those he has close contact with, there exists some overall balance between human and animal interest that would define the desired welfare standards in any society. These would reflect the conditions of husbandry and treatment that leave us feeling broadly comfortable with what we impose on the animals we exploit, without losing sight of why we keep them in the first place.

D. At the furthest extreme from the natural concept of welfare is a boundary beyond which the exploitation of animals would be regarded virtually universally in society as being unacceptable. In a practical sense this concept of minimal welfare is the one most amenable to definition and specification, because it represents a lower limit rather than necessarily a norm. As a result a large proportion of the formal legislation and statutory requirements for animal welfare is recognizable in this context.

The popular concern over animal welfare has ingredients of all four of the above concepts - which is why it is worth separating them out. They are clearly mutually inconsistent, and any attempt to pursue welfare objectives which are a blend of them all will fail to yield any functional guidelines. It is worth noting that the first two welfare concepts are essentially animal-centred, being based on considerations solely concerned with what the animal wants; however, for this reason they are also irrelevant as practical targets. The last two concepts are effectively people-centred, in that they are defined in relation to what people want or will accept. They are therefore also not fixed positions, but are subject to adjustment over time or in response to changing social or economic conditions. This is yet another demonstration of the fact that animal welfare is simply a subset of human welfare.

Much of the formal discussion in this field centres on the idea of 'positive' welfare, implying a concern not simply with the avoidance of cruelty but more with the specification of whatever standards are now appropriate for livestock farming in the UK and Europe in the 1990s. In other words the focus is on what we have called 'desired' welfare. Although there is plenty of attention directed at minimal acceptable standards, these have the more negative or defensive objectives of ensuring that production practices are not cruel or inhumane. The celebrated 'five freedoms' (Webster, 1984) are not in themselves a particularly helpful guide because, although they seem to imply a specific style of animal husbandry, in reality they are so imprecise that they embrace anything between the maximal and the minimal definitions. If we are to identify what constitutes an appropriate standard of animal welfare we must explore what conditions people want associated with the food they eat, so it is a problem in socioeconomic research.

3. Animal Welfare and Economic Benefit

From a strictly economic standpoint farm animals are no more than resources that are employed in economic processes which generate benefits for people (McInerney, 1988). In this sense they are no different from the other resources, whether land, labour or capital, that are 'exploited' in economic activity. Welfare considerations arise only because a possible side-effect of gaining economically valuable output from animals can be that their well-being is to a greater or lesser extent 'used up'. There is, in effect, an additional element of cost that should be included in the accounting framework along with the other more conventional costs chargeable to livestock production. Because this cost does not appear in a monetary form and is borne by animals rather than people, however, it is excluded from all the commercial calculations and so is not reflected in the money price of the livestock product. The welfare of the animal appears in this sense as a free good; and like all other apparent free goods in the economy (air, the environment, domestic tap water) there is a tendency to use as much of it as suits the user.

However, further examination reveals that animal welfare is not at all outside the economic calculus. Quite the contrary, like many other similar phenomena that provide a basis for policy intervention it has real and complex economic connections. First, reductions in animal welfare at some stage start to represent a real economic cost to society. By definition, a cost is simply a loss of benefit experienced by people. So if we feel unease at the way our domestic animals are treated, if the thought that they are not content causes us discontent, then we gain less value benefit) than we otherwise might have from the product of those animals - we suffer an economic cost. This cost is just as real as that experienced when our holiday is spoiled by bad weather, when the filet mignon is not as tender as we would like, or any of the myriad of ways in which external factors detract from the value we enjoy from the resources we utilise. The fact that it may not be a monetary cost nor appear in any commercial computations may confuse the accountant, but is irrelevant to economic analysis (McInerney, 1991). Second, the reason we are drawn into husbandry practices that have negative effects on the welfare of animals is the pursuit of our own economic benefit - principally in the form of cheaper, better quality or more predictable food supplies. Any move to improve the welfare of animals, therefore, may involve giving up some of this benefit - i.e., impose an economic cost.

We are thus confronted by the apparently paradoxical proposition that a reduction in animal welfare, and an equivalent improvement, both result in an economic cost. (Small wonder that economics is called the dismal science.) The distinction is that, though both are real economic costs, they are different forms (in the same way as are the costs of disease and the costs of the treatment). The loss of human benefit experienced when animals are subject to suffering is not identical to the loss of human benefit experienced when food prices rise. But it is this duality that places animal welfare four square in the realm of economics. The search for appropriate welfare standards involves economic choices about whether the benefits of cheaper food compensate for the costs in terms of unease over the animals' welfare. Alternatively they are choices between the benefits we gain from feeling more comfortable about 'kinder' livestock husbandry methods and the cost this implies in terms of more expensive food. This is the standard stuff of consumer choice, of course, on which the every day workings of the economy are built. It is entirely analogous to the assessments we make about whether the benefit we will get from changing the TV for a better one will be worth the money we have to pay to do it.

4. A Simple Economic Model

The current concerns over the welfare of farm animals stem from the way in which developments in livestock farming over the years have introduced production methods which many now view as involving unacceptable conditions for the animals. The prospect that further new developments on or over the horizon (e.g., BST) might be adopted exacerbate these concerns. The incentive for such developments to occur is the potential they bring for extending animal productivity, allowing higher output levels, greater conversion efficiencies, faster production rates, and so conferring economic benefits in terms of cheaper and better food supplies. The more this production potential is exploited, however, the greater the possible stress on the animal. All this implies a general relationship between the technical productivity of farm animals and their perceived welfare. That relationship reflects life inherent conflict between the interests of animals and humans, and lies at the heart of the choices society has to make in this area. The basic form of such a relationship is portrayed in Figure 11.5. The vertical axis indicates the level of animal welfare as we perceive it, while along the horizontal axis is measured the animals' technical productivity (eggs per bird, pigs weaned per litter, rate of liveweight gain, etc.) which is a direct reflection of our own economic benefit. Increasing animal productivity through greater control and intensity of input use is broadly synonymous with higher output and lower unit costs of production, changes we regard as the benefits of increased efficiency.

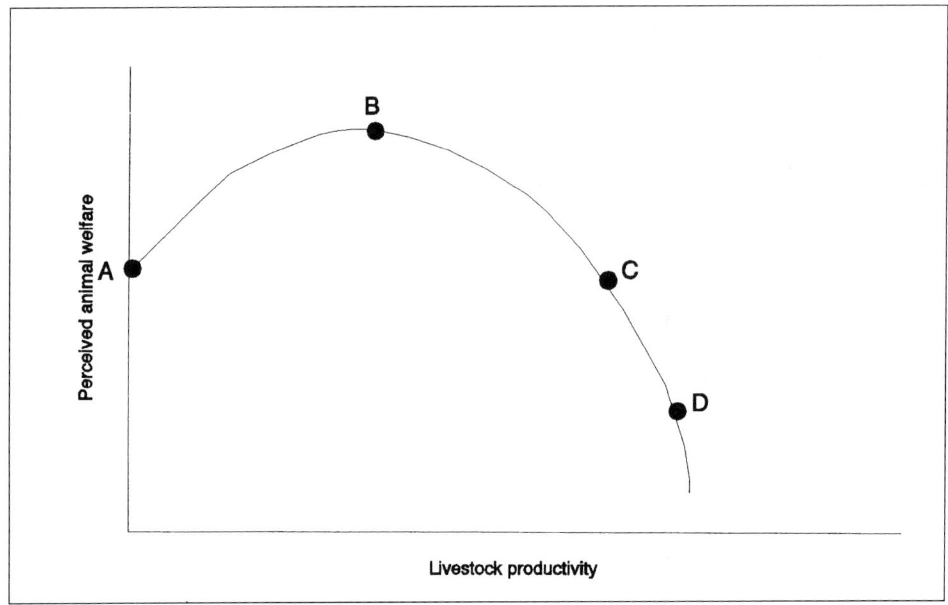

Figure 11.5. The relationship between animal welfare and livestock productivity.

The postulated relationship between these two variables is derived from simple logical reasoning, but is thought to be typical of any livestock production process. Point A is an initial reference point representing the situation where there is virtually no management or control of the animals' production processes, and approximates the concept of 'natural' welfare referred to earlier. By providing shelter, security, regular and balanced feeding, treating and preventing disease, and undertaking all the activities we associate with good husbandry we not only raise the productivity of animals to our own benefit but also believe that we raise their welfare at the same time. Such a complementary relationship may extend over quite a range of increasingly intensive management practices, ultimately reaching point B where the welfare of the animals is perceived to be as high as possible. This situation is equivalent to what we have called the 'maximal' welfare concept, and possibly represents the situation many farmers would have us believe when they assert that the welfare of their animals is obviously their primary consideration because otherwise they would not produce profitably. The fallacy in this view is evident by the fact that inevitably livestock production techniques will develop beyond this point as the commercial incentives encourage the search for greater productivity. The history of technological change in livestock farming has been to continually extend this relationship, but the gains in terms of economic productivity have come at increasing cost to animal welfare as the curve turns progressively downwards.

As long as new production techniques yield sufficient extra output to pay for the additional and increasingly expensive new inputs, however, there is an unavoidable commercial logic in favour of their adoption the welfare of the animals, not being a market commodity has no market price and so has not contributed any component to this cost calculation.

What society is now looking for is the equivalent of point C, the appropriate balance between livestock productivity and economic efficiency on the one hand, and our perception of the animals' interests on the other. This we have identified earlier as the 'desired' welfare concept. The primary questions to be resolved are whether such a balance exists as a single attainable target - and if so, where it lies and how it becomes embodied in our livestock husbandry systems. Much of the current precise specification of welfare standards which are imposed by statutory codes and regulations are equivalent to the position shown in Figure 11.5 a point D. This reflects the 'minimal' concept of welfare, the threshold of defined standards below which society would consider the conditions experienced by animals to be unacceptable, regardless of the fact that they may exploit more of the animal's production potential and so offer reductions in the cost of livestock production. The setting of these standards, too, is therefore an economic choice, but is of a slightly different nature because it defines boundary conditions rather than a norm.

5. The Costs of Improved Animal Welfare

The relationship in Figure 11.5 makes clear the conflict between animal welfare and human welfare inherent in modern livestock farming. The stresses imposed on animals have not come from man's nastiness but as an incidental side effect of the quest for higher productivity. Any improvement in welfare conditions, therefore, implies a movement back up the curve and an inevitable sacrifice of economic benefit. There is an unavoidable cost to better welfare[38]. That cost, however, although mathematically positive may be relatively insignificant in very many circumstances. This will tend to be the case, for example, with any moderate upward adjustments in the minimum welfare standards that are enforced by regulation and statutory codes. These lie by definition at the 'lower' end of the relationship (the position indicated at point D) where it would seem that quite noticeable increases in perceived welfare could be achieved with very little effect on-economic productivity. Some examples of this situation immediately spring to mind. The use of veal crates or sow tethers does offer some cost economies or they would not have been adopted in the first place, but prohibiting their use would have only marginal effects on the end price of veal or pigmeat.

The cost consequences of raising the unit space requirements for livestock in transit, limiting the maximum journey times or increasing the required period in lairage can add only very little to the overall costs of production.

The importance of such cost increases - and hence the likelihood of their being accepted as reasonable or justified - depends on three separate factors. The first is their magnitude relative to all the other costs incurred in the livestock process. The examples quoted relate to adjustments in relatively minor components of the whole

[38] There is one escape from this apparent harsh truth. If animal science research can devise new production techniques which effectively shift 'outwards' the curve in Figure 11.5, rather than simply searching for advances in achievable technical productivity, it opens the prospect of production systems which offer both higher productivity and higher animal welfare.

configuration of production activities, and so they have little significance on overall productivity or the final economic cost of the consumed food product. A second factor is the level of income of consumers, the impact of somewhat higher food prices being obviously less the higher the disposable income. Finally, the preferences and personal values in the society will greatly influence how prepared people are to accept extra costs to protect the welfare of farm animals. All these factors reflect the complexity of social choice that underlies welfare reform, They lead us to expect that far higher minimum standards are relevant to the UK, where a comparatively small component of final food price is value originating in the farm sector, and where a relatively affluent population is generally literate and increasingly aware of issues outside the environment of narrow self-interest, compared to a low-income Third World country with food products that are more basic and closer to the farm production sector, and where human living conditions inevitably engender a less liberal image of what constitutes minimal animal welfare.

When we move to consider more dramatic welfare reforms, however, the potential economic costs become more noticeable. Interpreting the appropriate animal welfare standards for a society as meaning the 'desired' welfare level, rather than simply the threshold of minimal acceptable practice, puts us higher up the curve in Figure 11.5 in the region of the point labelled as C. Here the relationship between perceived welfare gains and productivity therefore potentially more significant impacts on final food prices. It is a matter for detailed economic research to estimate the nature and magnitude of these possible production cost effects, and of course it depends on the extent of the welfare reforms under consideration. Unfortunately very little relevant empirical work has been done, despite the obvious importance of the issue. Such estimates as are available (e.g., Sandiford, 1985) suggest that in some instances the effects could be considerable, and superficial evidence of this is seen in the approximately 40 per cent price difference between 'welfare friendly' free range eggs and those produced in intensive battery systems.

While inevitably the move towards higher standards of minimal welfare will result in some additions to production costs there is nothing to say that this is 'wrong' or unacceptable. As already discussed, if higher welfare standards in livestock production is something that society genuinely wants, then it will gain a benefit if those conditions are satisfied. All of our economic activity is concerned with incurring costs in order to gain benefits, so there is no basis for characterising the outcome of our actions solely in terms of their costs. (It is unnecessary costs, or costs which are not outweighed by realised benefits, that are to be regretted.) Consequently there is no reason for livestock producers to fight against the demands for higher welfare standards on the grounds that it will raise production costs (as did the National Pig Breeders Association in January 1991 when the UK government introduced proposals to ban sow stalls and tethers). Of course it will raise costs - but if that's what consumers are demanding then economic logic asserts that it is the role of the producer to supply it. It is the *economy* that incurs higher production costs, not simply the producers, and if society does not think that cost is worth paying it will cease to demand the higher welfare product. We would be very surprised if our friendly neighbourhood electrical goods storekeeper protested when we asked for a colour TV because it was more expensive to supply than a black and white one!

6. Mechanisms for Effecting Welfare Improvements

The discussion developed here suggests there is no single concept of the welfare standards appropriate to any society. From a functional point of view there are at least two, the minimal level and the desired level - and the second of these is itself not a uniformly definable standard. This diversity is evident even if we consider only a single livestock production process, such as pig production, so it is magnified when the full range of animal farming systems are covered. The reason for this non-specificity is the fact that livestock production is a composite of numerous actions and activities, each of which has its own implications for the animal's welfare, and also because there is inevitably a diversity of view within a society as to what welfare standards are 'right'. This raises the prospect that any attempt to specify desirable welfare targets will result in a vast compendium of statements about what should, or should not, be done. It is for this reason that the primary thrust of formal animal welfare policy ends up with the rather negative orientation of setting just the lower boundaries, specifying the minimum requirements but giving little impetus to positive welfare measures. It is, however, feasible for welfare considerations to be determined by economic signals and not solely institutional regulation.

Returning to the proposition that animal welfare standards are a matter of social choice, there are two main mechanisms whereby those choices are made - by collective, or by individual decision. *Collective* choices are made in situations in which the interest of society as a whole is defined, widely accepted[39], and then imposed upon everybody. In an economic context resources are used to produce all manner of 'public goods' - things which none of us as individuals may choose to acquire or produce but which are considered to be desirable for the benefit of all - and then everyone is forced to pay the costs of provision whether they agree or not. The textbook examples are defence, law and order, health and education services, street lighting, environmental protection, libraries, etc. Many aspects of animal welfare have the characteristics of a public good because they are considered to be standards of 'service' which everyone in a civilised and humane society should be forced to purchase as part of their food supply. Hence there is a strong economic logic for the regulation and statutory of welfare codes, not only to establish the general style of livestock production but also to constrain those careless or uncaring individual livestock keepers whose personal inclinations may not be consistent with those of everyone else. However, this method of establishing animal welfare levels can never be more than a 'bottom line' approach, and involves difficult political decisions about how high to set the standards (and therefore costs) that everyone is enforced to accept. As a result, despite the vast array of legislation from the Protection of Animal Acts of 1911 onwards, the enforceable requirements are far from restrictive and tend to deal only with specific aspects of welfare. At one extreme there is a fairly horrific list of prohibited operations and practices that tend to make the eyes water just by reading them, while at the other are the legally convenient but descriptively non-specific requirements to avoid 'unnecessary' pain, suffering or distress (Baker, 1986; MAFF, 1990). While some welfare orders prevent livestock production from transgressing

[39] Never universally accepted - there are always individuals who object to even the most reasonable of propositions.

accepted notions of cruelty many others (such as requirements to inspect animals daily or provide adequate food, water and shelter) set out what to the intelligent and rational producer is merely sensible commercial practice.

Government regulation can cater for only a subset of society's preferences with respect to animal welfare. Those aspects that relate to clearly unacceptable activities and practices or insufficient provision for the animals wellbeing are obvious candidates for handling within a public good framework, and in this sense are the easy bit of the problem because they are fairly definitive. The other major characteristic of society's preferences with respect to desired animal welfare levels is that, as with everything else, they vary widely between different individuals and groups. Some people have very precise views about how they want the animals kept that provide the eggs, meat and milk they consume, views which lay great emphasis on the perceived interests of the animal and accept the consequent implications in terms of production cost. Others, while in no way being indifferent or cruel, see animals in a different context, are satisfied with lower welfare standards, and feel more concern over the food prices they have to pay. Yet others will have given no consideration to what goes on in livestock farming, either-because they have no relevant information or no particular concern anyway. If the society's attitude towards the welfare of animals is characterised by this diversity, how can there be any specific set of conditions (such as represented by point C in Figure 11.5) which reflect the 'desired' welfare standards for that society? The answer is, of course, that there cannot be any such specification of socially appropriate animal welfare levels. Nor can one assert that any one sub-group within this spectrum, whether in favour of kinder treatment of animals or more extreme exploitation of them, should determine the choices of everyone else.

Realisation of this fact leads one towards an approach to animal welfare provision based *on individual* choice. Given the safeguards of minimal standards by statutory means, there seems no reason why the array of different attitudes towards animal welfare beyond this level which characterise the overall social preference should not then be expressed through the market for livestock products, as is done elsewhere in the economy. This then makes animal welfare a 'private good', something which each individual can decide to buy more or less of according to preference. Those who wish to manifest their personal concern for the wellbeing of animals create a demand for livestock products with a 'high welfare' image. Those whose priorities are dominated more by the cost of the food product will seek the cheaper article produced from more intensive and apparently less welfare friendly systems. Provided that sufficient consumer information is available to help people identify their relevant choices, and suitable provisions for labelling and monitoring of standards is enforced, there is every prospect that the differential pattern of demands for animal welfare can be catered for in the same way as it is for newspapers, clothes, financial services, holidays abroad and all other commodity groups with recognisably different quality characteristics. Livestock producers will have the incentive to identify specific markets and cater for them, with the expectation that if there is a genuine demand for a higher cost product with higher welfare characteristics it will sell for an appropriately higher price; if not, then that demand does not exist. That this is so is already evident (Paxman, 1986) with distinct higher priced markets emerging for 'free range' eggs and poultry, 'natural' meats, and Sainsbury's recent introduction of 'traditional 'beef and 'tenderlean' lamb. The potential for greater growth and diversity has only just started to be developed.

There is a number of apparent advantages in this approach. It is probably the only way for welfare decisions which relate to different overall *systems* of production (as opposed to individual practices) to be handled. Like all market processes, it responds to the differential pattern of demands that constitute the overall social preference in a way that minimises the need for centralised decision or administrative involvements. And it avoids the undesirability of any one group - whether 'experts', civil servants, special interest advocates, or merely effective lobbyists - imposing their preferences on everyone else without reference to the implications for everyone else. In effect it transforms animal welfare into a consumer commodity like taste. music and fine art, and then treats it along with the other economic decisions in our society. People who want it will buy it if it is available and they can afford it; if they don't or can't, they won't.

References

Baker, K.B. (1986). The Ministry's role in animal welfare. In: Proceedings of the Society for Veterinary Epidemiology and Preventive Medicine, Edinburgh, pp. 97-103.

MAFF (1990). At the farmer's service: a guide to agricultural legislation 1989/90. MAFF publications, London.

McInerney, J.P. (1988). Economics in the veterinary curriculum: further dimensions. In: Proceedings of the Society for Veterinary Epidemiology and Preventive Medicine, Edinburgh, pp. 20-29.

McInerney, J.P. (1991). Assessing the benefits of farm animal welfare. In: Animal Welfare - It Pays to be Humane. Carruthers, S.P. (Ed.). CAS Paper No. 22, Centre for Agricultural Strategy, University of Reading.

Paxman, P.J. (1986). Consumer reaction to cost and health consequences of free range systems for veal and poultry production. In: Proceedings of the Society for Veterinary Epidemiology and Preventive Medicine, Edinburgh, pp. 116-121.

Sandiford, F. (1985). An Economic Analysis of the Introduction of Legislation Governing the Welfare of Animals (Bulletin 201). Department of Agricultural Economics, University of Manchester.

Stott G.H. (1981). What is animal stress and how is it measured? Journal of Animal science, 52, 150-153.

Webster, A.J.F. (1984). Calf Husbandry, Health and Welfare. Collins, London.

Part IV

Analysis Techniques Commonly Used in Economics

J.P.T.M. Noordhuizen
Department of Farm Animal Health
Faculty of Veterinary Medicine
University of Utrecht
The Netherlands

1. Introduction

As stated earlier, disease can be considered part of an economic production process (McInerney, 1988). Searching the literature related to both veterinary medicine and animal health economics provides the following short list of economic techniques frequently applied in the veterinary domain:

a. partial budgeting
b. cost-benefit analysis
c. decision tree analysis
d. Markovian chains

In addition to these, several other, more or less complex models have been developed and applied to certain disease entities. Examples of the latter are linear programming (see e.g., Jalvingh, 1993, on optimizing calving pattern in dairy herds), dynamic programming (see e.g., Kennedy, 1986; Carpenter and Howitt, 1988), expert systems and decision support systems or combinations of those (see e.g., Turban, 1988; Huirne, 1990, on Computerized management support for swine breeding farms; Buijtels, 1997, on Aujeszky's disease in pigs). These models will not be further elaborated here, but are addressed - at least in part and some of their principles - in Chapter IX on mathematical modelling in epidemiology.

Next to these complex models, combinations of techniques (a) to (d) are often applied for practical reasons, such as for calculating the financial loss occurring at farm level due to disease and possible culling afterwards. For such calculations both partial budgeting and dynamic programming can be used to include e.g., the loss of production efficiency, veterinary costs, reduced slaughter value at culling and or future income lost when culling occurs prior to the economically optimum age.

In this part IV of this chapter the first 3 of the commonly applied economic techniques will be shortly presented in general terms. At the same time specific literature references are given in the Appendix for further reading on application of these techniques. Markov chains and other, more sophisticated simulation models will not be addressed here, because they have been discussed in Chapter IX on mathematical epidemiological modelling.

2. Partial Budgeting

Partial budgeting can be defined as an activity to quantify the economic consequences of a certain change carried through at (mostly) a farm, such as a mastitis control programme, an endoparasite treatment procedure for the herd or a vaccination campaign in a herd.

The partial budget addresses 4 components:

- the returns yielded by the suggested change [A];
- the cost reduction resulting from this change [B];
- the possible lost returns due to this change [C];
- the additional costs associated with the implementation of the suggested change [D].

As reference for comparison in order to know whether the suggested change has a positive outlook, the current on-farm procedure is often used. This may for example be the current udder health programme which has to be compared to the new programme involving a new dry off treatment and additional intramuscular treatment at dry off.

The suggested change (e.g., the new programme) should be implemented if

$$(A + B) > (C + D) \text{ or expressed in another way, if}$$
$$(A + B) - (C + D) > 0$$

This technique appears to be suitable for providing rapid insight in the potentials of a suggested veterinary) intervention at the farm, and as such yields a useful indicator. Other techniques may provide more detailed and more accurate results, but these are not always needed for weighing decision alternatives on the farm.

Example: quantify the net results of a strategic, preventive whole dairy herd anti-parasitic treatment in comparison to the current curative approach.

A better milk yield in lactating heifers and cows + better growth rate in young stock (known from literature or experimentation);
B less veterinary curative costs (labour and drugs use) for concurrent diseases in the current approach;
C not known;
D costs of the treatment as such + extra labour costs + increase in probability of sudden death.

Further applications of this technique can be find in the literature (see Appendix).

3. Cost-Benefit Analysis

Cost-benefit analysis is used to assess the value of a certain action or programme over a given period of time. Due to the fact that the technique has often been applied in a rather limited way, some regard this technique as being applied too loosely resulting in a more simple accounting type of exercise (Roe, 1990). That is when planning of resource allocation is not taken into account and when the production system involved is not considered.

Three major components are addressed in cost-benefit analysis:

- specification of costs and benefits

- definition of the discount rate
- identification of a value decision criterion.

The technique is often applied at groups of farms, at sector level or national (government planning) level, and not at the level of individual farms. Problems in the calculation may occur when disease control programmes are complex and associated with a high degree of uncertainty. Another point regards the proper valuation of the benefits. In case of problems, one may calculate cost-effects or cost-effectiveness. This is specifically the case when one aims at identifying least cost actions to achieve a certain goal, or when one has to deal with intangible benefits. The latter is the case, when for example the increased public welfare has to be estimated as a benefit occurring after an effective zoonosis control programme.

Primary (or direct or internal) benefits are those that come in favour to the farmers paying for the programme. For example, by a reduced mortality, improved udder health status or milk quality, or increased weight gain in young stock. Primary costs are those , being capital and running costs, incurred by the programme participants and possible disease control authorities involved in the programme. Secondary benefits and costs are the so-called externalities of a programme. They come in favour to those people not directly responsible for the costs. For example, *Hypoderma bovis* causing cattle grub will also damage cattle hides, hence decreasing the leather value. The leather manufacturers will not pay for the control programme costs at the farms. Verocytotoxine producing *E.coli* oriented control programmes on cattle farms aim at safeguarding the consumer while the cattle are latent carriers without symptoms; farmers pay for this programme without the direct benefits. The calculations may become very complex and confusing when addressing all such indirect costs and benefits.

Costs and benefits have to be made mutually comparable when we perform the analysis over a given period of time. Therefore, we may define (Roe, 1990) the present value" PV as:

$$PV = \frac{FV}{\left(1 + \frac{r}{100}\right)^n}$$

where:

FV = the future value of the cost or benefit
r = the real annual interest rate in percent (if interest is 8% and inflation is 3% then r is 5%)
n = the number of years in the analysis

Now that costs and benefits have been valued and discounted to a common base, we have to decide about the value criterion for the cost benefit comparison. Three parameters are often handled: Net Present Value, Benefit Cost Ratio, Internal Rate of Return (Roe, 1990).

Net Present Value: if the present value of benefits exceeds the present value of costs of a programme, this programme is economically viable. This parameter does not show the relative volume of costs and benefits, but can be used to compare programmes with different scales or economic magnitude.

Benefit Cost Ratio: if the ratio of the present value of benefits to the present value of costs of a programme is greater than unity, the programme is economically viable. The relative volume of costs and benefits is included in this parameter but the magnitude of economics is however not in the ratio.

Internal Rate of Return: if the returns yielded by a programme exceed the discount rate, then the programme is economically viable. In this case, it is not necessary to select a discount rate; the parameter can be compared with interest rates in alternative options.

Applications of this technique have been described in literature (see Appendix).

4. Decision Tree Analysis

Decision tree analysis is a formal structured way to model chance events related to sometimes complex decisions; it uses a decision tree as a representation of the flow of events in a logical, time-related and structured way. Furthermore, it helps in elucidating the probabilities and the outcomes of certain decision alternatives (Marsh, 1993).

This type of analysis is not focused on the prediction of an event but rather on weighing the respective options in a relative sense. The analysis addresses several steps.

First of all, the problem has to be defined. For example, the decision-making about yes/no inseminating a sow after weaning. In order to inseminate the sow we have to detect an oestrus and when oestrus is not detected we have to decide about yes/no inject an oestrus-inducing hormone or "wait and see". When not treating, we have to know whether or not she will come into oestrus spontaneously and when after weaning that might occur. We have to know what the probabilities are that after spontaneous oestrus and after hormone treatment and subsequent oestrus and insemination a pregnancy will occur. It is obvious that the moment after weaning is related to the decision making process.

In a graphical presentation (Figure 11.6) this may - simplified - look as follows:

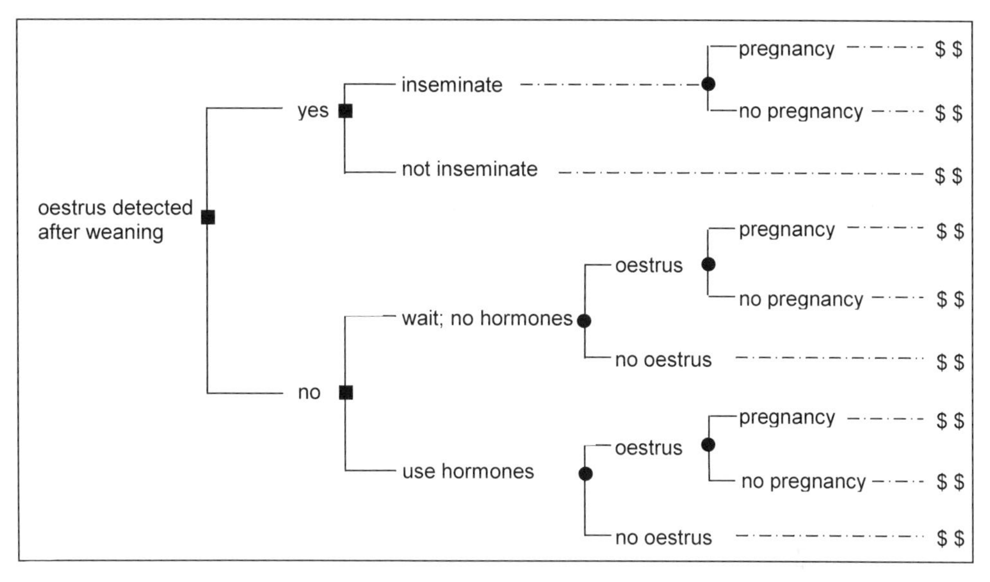

Figure 11.6. A decision tree showing the various options for oestrus detection and insemination management in a sow. (■ = decision nodes;● = chance nodes).

All decision outcomes have to be identified at each step in the process. At the same time, each outcome has a certain probability of occurring. These probabilities can be derived from literature, animal experimentation or experts in the field. The probabilities can be written in the graphic representation (Figure 11.6). It is emphasized that certain outcomes do not have any chance nodes (end of line) such as in the case that oestrus is not detected (repeatedly). Another decision tree can be built for such cases, for example the decision process about yes/no culling the sow.

At each decision step the probabilities of the outcomes have to be calculated. For example, when the decision was to treat the sow with oestrus-inducing hormones, there is a probability P_1 that oestrus will be detected afterwards and a probability $(1\text{-}P_1)$ that oestrus is not detected. The same procedure is repeated at each chance node.

Consequences of each decision and chances end in terminal nodes, such as in the case of pregnancy or non-pregnancy (Figure 11.6). These terminal nodes can be annotated with expected monetary values for that decision outcome. From this point backwards, monetary values have to be added to each preceding decision line by multiplying each probability with the monetary value at each terminal node and summing up, then take the next preceding decision line, and so on.

Ultimately, you end up with a graphic representation of decision and chance nodes, probabilities of occurrence of events, and monetary outcomes of each sequential step. That provides the basis for the final decision making. It is obvious that you may adapt the graph and the process to the particular situation of the individual farm. This may help in advising the farmer more specifically.

In certain situations where diagnostic tests are part of the decision process, for example to decide about performing testing for Johne's disease, other epidemiological principles have to be addressed. Among these are sensitivity, specificity and predictive values because these are related to probabilities of occurrence of events listed on the decision tree. Chapter IV addresses these issues in more detail.

Sensitivity analysis may be performed to detect the break-even point in this decision making process: when is it cost-effective to make a certain decision and deleting other options.

During recent years some applications of decision tree analysis have been published (see Appendix). See also paragraph 6 of this chapter for an exercise.

5. Epilogue

It is obvious that without sufficient and high quality accurate data (epidemiological and economic) modelling becomes very difficult. Since the late 70's and early 80's many developments have taken place in the domain of veterinary herd health programmes addressing both animal health, productivity, economics and quality (Noordhuizen, 1984; Brand *et al.*, 1996; Noordhuizen an Welpelo, 1996). One of the basic elements in such herd health programmes is the availability of high quality data because advice and decision-making is based on these. Advice to the farmer can be more appropriate if - in addition to the technical or veterinary technical basis - also sufficiently attention is paid to the economic justification of such advice. In that way animal health economics may be supportive in decision making and advice. The same is valid for planning and design of disease control programmes at a higher level.

> "One important principle should be followed in all analyses. This is that uncertainty in regards to the data used in conducting the analysis or in terms of the outcome of various strategies should be made explicit rather than being hidden. The limitations on the conclusions drawn from an analysis should be stated rather than a sophisticated analysis being used to give a false sense of precision" *(Roe, 1990)*

References

Brand, A.; Noordhuizen, J.P.T.M.; Schukken, Y.H. (1996). Herd Health and Production Management in Dairy Practice. Wageningen Pers, Wageningen, The Netherlands.

Buijtels, J.A.A.M. (1997). Computer simulation to support policy-making in Aujeszky's disease control. PhD thesis, Agricultural University, Wageningen, The Netherlands.

Carpenter, T.E.; Howitt, R.E. (1988). Dynamic programming approach to evaluating the economic impact of disease on production. In: Proceedings of the 5th International Symposium on Veterinary Epidemiology and Economics, Copenhagen, July 1988. Willeberg, P.; Agger, J.F.; Riemann, H. (Eds.). Acta Veterinaria Scandinavia, Supplement 84, 356-359.

Huirne, R.B.M. (1990). Computerized management support for swine breeding farms. PhD thesis, Agricultural University Wageningen, The Netherlands.

Jalvingh, A.W. (1993). Dynamic livestock modelling for on-farm decision support. PhD thesis, Agricultural University, Wageningen, The Netherlands.

Kennedy, J.O.S. (1986). Dynamic programming: applications to agriculture and national resources. Elsevier Applied Science Publishers, London.

Marsh, W.E. (1993). Decision tree analysis: drawing some of the uncertainty out of decision - making. Swine Health and Production, 1, 17-23.

McInerney, J.P. (1988). Economics in the veterinary curriculum: further dimensions. In: Proceedings of the Society for Veterinary Epidemiology and Preventive Medicine, Edinburgh, April 1988. Thrusfield, M.V. (Ed.). pp. 20-29.

Noordhuizen, J.P.T.M (1984). Veterinary herd health and production control on dairy farms. PhD thesis, University of Utrecht, The Netherlands.

Noordhuizen, J.P.T.M.; Welpelo, H.J. (1996). Sustainable improvement of animal health care by systemic quality risk management according to the HACCP concept. Veterinary Quarterly, 18, 121-126.

Roe, R.T. (1990). The social costs and benefits of animal health programmes. In: Epidemiological Skills in Animal Health. Refresher Course for Veterinarians. Proceedings 143, October 1990. Kennedy, D. (Ed.). University of Sidney, Sidney, Australia, pp. 197-204.

Turban, E. (1988). Decision support and expert systems. MacMillan Publishers, New York.

Appendix Suggestions for further reading

1. Partial Budgeting

Boehlje, M.D.; Eidman, V.R. (1984). Farm management, John Wiley and Sons, New York.
Warren, M.F. (1986). Financial management for farmers. Hutchingson, London.

2. Cost Benefit Analysis

Bech Nielsen, S.; Hugoson, G.; Wold-Troell, M. (1983). Economic evaluation of several control programmes for the cattle nematode *Parafilaria bovicola* using cost benefit analysis. Preventive Veterinary Medicine, 1, 303-320.
Berentsen, P.B.M.; Dijkhuizen, A.A.; Oskam, A.J. (1992). A dynamic model for cost benefit analysis of foot-and-mouth disease control strategies. Preventive Veterinary Medicine, 12, 229-244.
Hugoson, G.; Wold-Troell, M. (1983). Benefit cost aspects on voluntary control of bovine leucosis. Scandinavian Journal of Veterinary Science, 35, 1-17.
Mclnerney, J.P.; Turner, M.M. (1989). Assessing the economic effects of mastitis at the herd level using farm accounts data. In: Proceedings of the Society for Veterinary Epidemiology and Preventive Medicine, Exeter, April 1989. Rowlands, G.J. (Ed.). pp.46-59.
Mclnerney, J.P. (1995). Economic analysis of alternative eradication programmes. In: Proceedings of the 2nd International Symposium on Eradication of Aujeszky's disease virus, Copenhagen Denmark, August 1995. pp. 20.
Sassone, P.G.; Schaffer, W.A. (1978). Cost benefit analysis: a handbook. Academic Press, London UK.
Sugden, R.; Williams, A. (1978). The principles of practical cost benefit analysis. Oxford University Press, Oxford UK.
Taylor, A.A.; Hurnik, J.F.; Lehman, H. (1995). The application of cost-benefit dominance analysis to the assessment of farm animal quality of life. Social Indicators Research, 35, 313-329.

3. Decision Tree Analysis

Gregory, G. (1988). Decision tree analysis. Plenum, New York.
Hardaker, J.B.; Huirne, R.B.M.; Anderson, J.R. (1997). Coping with Risk in Agriculture. CAB International, Wellingford, UK.
Marsh, W.E. (1993). Decision tree analysis: drawing some of the uncertainty out of decision making. Swine Health and Production, 1, 17-23.
Ruegg, P.L.; Carpenter, T.E. (1989). Decision tree analysis of treatment alternatives for left displaced abomasum. Journal of American Veterinary Medical Association, 195, 464-467.
Scholl, D.T.; Carpenter, T.E.; Bon Durant, R.H. (1990). Economic evaluation of not treating cows with bovine cystic ovarian disease relative to gonadotropin releasing hormone therapy: a decision tree analysis approach. In: Proceedings of the Dutch Society for Veterinary Epidemiology and Economics, Wageningen, The Netherlands, 12th December. Frankena, K. (Ed.). pp. 73-85.

4. General

Dijkhuizen, A.A.; Morris, R.S. (1997). Animal Health Economics: Principles and Applications. The Postgraduate Foundation, Sydney NSW. Australia.

6. Exercise

Designed by F. Beaudeau, C. Fourichon, H. Seegers. Unit of Animal Health Management, INRA and Veterinary School, Nantes, France.

Suppose a veterinarian is called for examining and treating a sick male dairy calf born 3 days ago. This animal is expected to be sold at 15 days age. The animal is diagnosed as diseased since it was experiencing fever, diarrhoea and dehydration for 24 hours. The veterinarian warns the farmer that the treatment cost would be about US $60.

Given the current low market price of such a calf, the owner wonders about whether or not treating it. He asks the veterinarian to recommend to him the most profitable decision. The veterinarian uses decision tree analysis to give an answer.

1. What is the list of possible decisions which can be made by the farmer?

2. Once a decision is made, what are the outcomes of such a decision? Draw the corresponding decision tree.

The likelihood of survival in case of treatment is 0.7. The likelihood of death in case of no treatment is 0.8.

3. What is the likelihood of death in case of treatment?

To help the farmer to make the decision, the veterinarian needs to account for other parameters.

4. What are the parameters for which further information is needed? (multiple choices are possible)

   A. the likelihood of survival in case of no treatment
   B. the value of a dead calf
   C. the cost of treatment in case of death
   D. the price of a male dairy calf
   E. the cost of treatment in case of survival
   F. the production cost of a calf dying at 3 days
   G. the production cost of a calf living up to 15 days

The production cost of a calf dying at 3 days is considered as zero.
The production cost of a calf living up to 15 days is estimated at US $30.
The price of a male dairy calf is about US $160.

5. Finalize the decision tree. What is the most profitable decision to recommend?

7. Answers

1. The possible decisions are
   - to treat the calf
   - to let the calf untreated

2. The outcomes of treatment
   - the calf lives
   - the calf dies

   The outcomes of no treatment
   - the calf lives
   - the calf dies

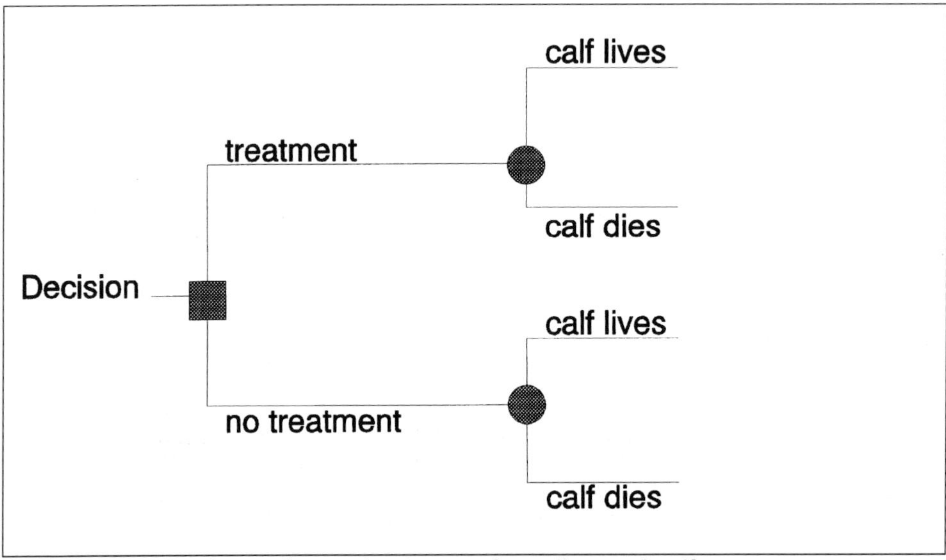

Decision tree showing option and outcomes for a diseased calf

3. The probability of death in case of treatment is (1 - 0.7) = 0.3

4. B
   D
   F
   G

   The probability of survival (choice A) in case of no treatment is already available: (1 - 0.8) = 0.2

   The cost of treatment is already available. It is the same cost (US $60), irrespective whether the calf lives or dies (choices C and E).

5.

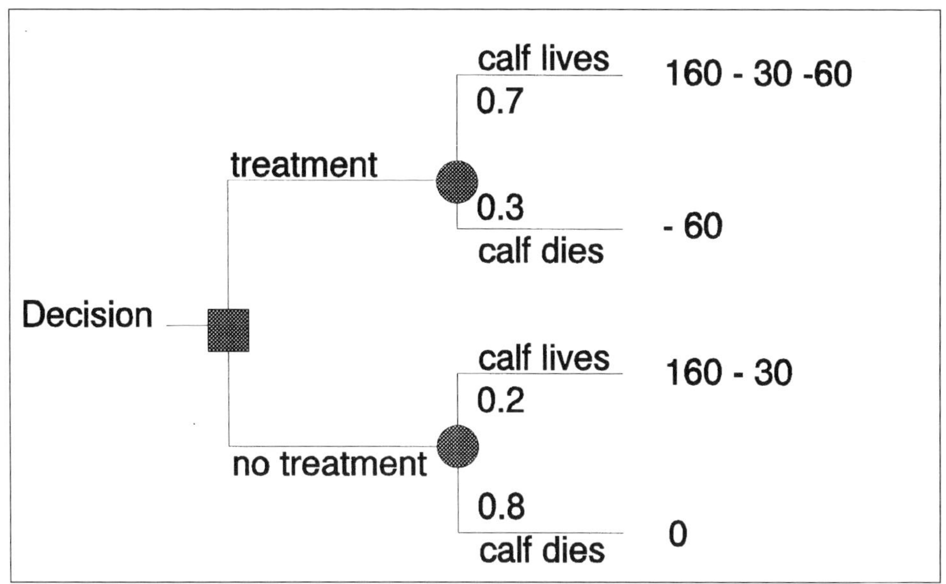

Decision tree showing probabilities and value variables for each outcome

The most profitable action, given the conditions set for this example, is to treat the calf, because

Expected value (calf treated, alive)	= 0.7∗(160-30-60)	= US $49
Expected value (treated, dead)	= 0.3∗(-60)	= US $18 -
Expected value of treating		= US $31

Chapter XII

Monitoring and Surveillance Systems (MOSS)

Part I

Design and Operationalization

J.P.T.M. Noordhuizen
Department of Farm Animal Health
Faculty of Veterinary Medicine
University of Utrecht
The Netherlands

B. Dufour
Centre National d'Etudes Vétérinaires et
Alimentaires, CNEVA
Direction Générale
Maisons-Alfort
France

1. Introduction

Current animal health care requires a proper insight in disease occurrence in a region: that means disease frequency over time and geographical distribution. That is without bias and preferably representative for the livestock production population in that region. Requirements for this insight can be based on demands put forward by a specific disease (slow or rapid), by importing countries (e.g., animals being free of described disease agents), on processes related to the improvement of the national livestock health status, or on demands put forward to livestock industry by public health authorities (e.g., animals or animal products being free of salmonella bacteria).

One of the tools to obtain this proper insight regards monitoring and surveillance systems (MOSS). Surveillance, in origin a French word dating from the Napoleonic wars, was originally referring to the "observation of potentially subversive people". In health care the term "surveillance" is related to the active observation of highly contagious diseases and their patterns, and sometimes brought into the domain of "police medicine", which has negative meaning. The current concept of MOSS was developed by A. Langmuir in the USA and is more neutral in definition. Application of MOSS can be variable and manyfold. Not in all situations a MOSS is advizable. Part I of this chapter addresses the design and operationalization of MOSS, related to technical, financial and political issues. In part II an example is given of the economic cost-benefit calculation of a MOSS for *S.enteritidis* in poultry, while in part III the investigation of disease control is addressed.

2. Definition and Objectives; Basic Applications

2.1. Definition

A monitoring and surveillance system (MOSS) is a network of locations (e.g., farms) which have been chosen according to a justified method and which are located in a region according to an order which has been determined in a justified manner. Such a MOSS should preferably be representative for the target area (e.g., a country). On the locations, the animals present or a sample of this population are being sampled following prescribed protocol directions and frequency. Such a sample should provide information about health/disease status and/or productivity, as well as about environmental risk factors.

Monitoring refers to a continuous, dynamic process of collecting data about health and disease and their determinants in a given animal population over a defined time period (descriptive epidemiology). Epidemio-vigilance is the name that sometimes is given to the process of discrimination between pathological and non-pathological phenomena.

Surveillance refers to a specific extension of monitoring where obtained information is utilized and measures are taken if certain threshold values related to disease status have been passed. It, therefore, is part of disease control programmes.

2.2. Objectives

The following objectives can be determined for operationalization of a MOSS:

a. to broaden insight in the prevalence and spread of a certain disease over time in a usually large population of animals and possibly man in a methodologically and scientifically sound manner. Subsequently, an early prediction of disease occurrence and pattern is strived for in order to make the primary production sector react adequately (e.g., by interventions, combat or export protection).

b. to broaden insight in the most relevant factors and conditions which influence the occurrence and spread of a disease in a methodologically and scientifically sound manner. Subsequently, the effect of those factors can be quantified in order to set priorities for disease combat and prevention programmes. The economic loss due to diseases can be assessed and alternative intervention measures evaluated through simulation models.

MOSS is a tool for decision-making and not a goal in itself.

A MOSS can be suitable to collect information (Staerk, 1993) about:

- disease morbidity in a certain population ("what is going on?")
- geographical distribution of diseases ("where is it going on?")
- time or season relationships ("when is it going on?")
- certain population segments ("what are high risk groups?")
- factors contributing to disease ("why is it going on?")
- economic losses related to the disease ("at what costs?")

General applications of a MOSS serve to answer basic questions such as:

- an early, quick and reliable identification of first disease cases of a highly contagious disease;
- the development or pattern of endemic diseases, trends of disease occurrence in a given population, region and time period;
- effect evaluation of disease control programmes;
- determination of the national herd health status with regard to international trade requirements, or to economic assessment of disease losses;
- herd health certification on freedom from diseases or infections.

It will be clear that MOSS for notifiable diseases will show other features than a MOSS based on a network of 1150 poultry farms and their veterinarians. The latter can be easily used for applied research in this area.

The basic principles of a MOSS are outlined in Figure 12.1.

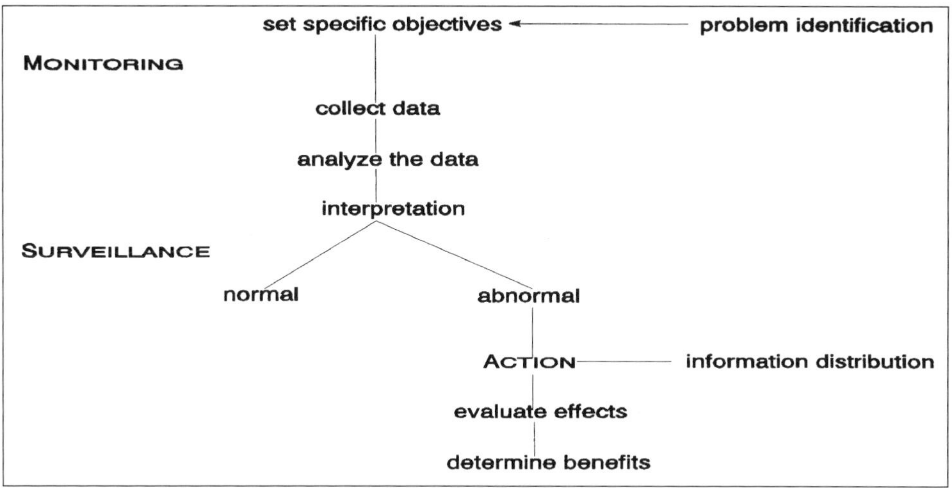

Figure 12.1. Outlines of the principles of a MOSS.

The disease situation in the population can be determined through signalling at the level of data analysis and interpretation, e.g., through comparison with previous time periods (trend analysis).

Predictions can be done on the basis of outcomes of analyses and measurements in the field.

Both simple and complex relationships between factors and disease status can be established, in both an analytical and a model approach manner (see Chapters V, VI and IX).

Surveillance can be performed on the basis of the measurements with or without being coupled to a simulation model. Measures for control and prevention are usually originating from this surveillance. Cost-benefit calculations are common elements of these activities (see Chapter XI).

3. The Design of a MOSS

3.1. Criteria for the design

At the stage of development of a MOSS, the OBJECTIVES have to be defined as specific as possible. This regards for example the question whether the MOSS is meant to detect infection levels or the presence of an infection in the population. Or, in another case, whether or not the herds in the population are free from a certain infection. Or, in yet another case, whether infection levels increase or decrease.

CRITERIA are meant to assess the functionality and feasibility of a MOSS.
Among these questions, the most relevant are:

1. can the policy questions or disease questions be answered by the built up of a MOSS? Can they not be answered otherwise?
2. is a MOSS financially justifiable for the primary production sector? (both at the herd, the sector and the national level)?
3. is a MOSS financially justifiable for the human medical sector (veterinary public health)?
4. is a MOSS technically feasible?
5. is a MOSS sufficiently reliable for decision making (e.g., with respect to sensitivity and specificity of applied diagnostic tests)?

Sometimes, questions put forward by policy makers can be more easily answered by other means such as a cross-sectional survey instead of a MOSS (e.g., what is the current prevalence of herds infected with S. *dublin*?). For the primary sector it is important to realize that, for example in the case of an exporting country, the national herd health status is highly relevant to avoid export bans. This importance for the sector is not always the same importance for an individual farmer. On the other hand, if public health requires animals or food products of animal origin to be free of certain infectious agents, it is the task and the responsibility of the producer to achieve that goal whatever that may cost!

Reliability refers to the level of confidence, at which one likes to draw conclusions. A full representative MOSS is not always needed, especially if one needs only an indication of the health status of the animals. In the case of epidemic, highly contagious infections, the European Union requires to have a 100% sample of the cattle population be examined for e.g., foot-and-mouth disease. In that case one should be sure that the diagnostic test applied does not yield too much false-negative results.

The creation of data bases which will not or not sufficiently be used should be avoided because it will lead to "data graveyards".

3.2. Operationalization steps

Several steps can be distinguished before any MOSS is to be operationalized in the field. These are listed below. Essential is that an infrastructure is created and a multidisciplinary team of people operationalized.

1. Determine which diseases or infections are relevant to public health, the livestock production sector (export) or the individual farms. Equally determine for which diseases or infections compulsory control programmes are already in action, such as in the case of notifiable diseases. Equally define the species of interest as well as the level of operation: is the MOSS planned for local, regional, national or international level. Specify the definition of a "case".
2. Determine whether the MOSS should comprise one or more diseases or infections, and whether the MOSS should operate on a temporary or continuous basis.

3. Establish the most relevant risk indicators for the occurrence and spread of the diseases after literature search, experimental research and expert interview. Define the most relevant features of the infectious agent too.
4. Estimate the size of the population at risk and define the population (e.g., regional distribution and concentration). Define the target population and the study population. Shortly, what are the numerators and what the denominators.
5. Estimate the prevalence of the disease/infection in that population.
6. Decide about the confidence level for drawing conclusions with respect to disease detection, sample size and maximum error (= accuracy).
7. Determine the size and the method of sampling. (See Chapter III)
8. Determine the operational sampling procedure and describe it in the MOSS protocol. This protocol should also comprise the diagnostic tests and the frequency of sampling within the sample. (See Chapter III and IV)
9. Design a questionnaire in order to collect standardized information about risk indicators at the herd level or regional level for the given disease, if this is part of the MOSS. Determine the timing and frequency of performing this questionnaire survey, as well as the methods for analysis.
10. Decide about the procedures in MOSS: will there be cross-sectional surveys only or also longitudinal surveys? Are there other data bases already available to answer (parts) of the questions? (See Chapter V)
11. Design a system for entering the disease related data and environment related data into the computer system. Determine the procedures for statistical analysis of data, e.g., logistic regression analysis, trend analysis, time series and survival analysis. Determine the unit of analysis: the animal, the pen, the herd or the farm. Define how the results will be transferred to participants in the MOSS and in which format. Interpretation is crucial.
12. Describe the costs and benefits of the MOSS as specific as possible, for both the preparatory and operational phases. (See Chapter XI)
13. Evaluate the effects of the MOSS with respect to both public health issues and livestock production issues in a disease related and an economic perspective. Provide suggestions for adjustment whenever indicated. Advise on intervention trials when needed. Address the media for disseminating related information. Make sure that all, potentially relevant information is passed on to parties involved and parties interested.

Many of these topics have been dealt with in preceding chapters already and will not receive further attention here. A short checklist is given in Appendix 2.

Some other topics will be addressed in more detail.

3.3. Sources of data

Currently available data sources comprise the farm/herd, the veterinary practice, a diagnostic laboratory, cattle market and livestock collection places, slaughterhouse, cheese factory, dairy plant, destruction units, or integrated food animal production chains.

Other data which are more general in nature can be found in existing livestock census, agro-economic research institutes, national statistics bureaus, pharmaceutical companies. Problems, disadvantages and advantages related to the use of such existing data bases will be addressed in another section.

Paramount prerequisite for MOSS and data collection is an adequate animal identification system (eartags, transponders, pedigree cards etc).

Next to animal identification there is the relevance of the "case definition". Animals must be assigned to the proper health categories (healthy *vs.* diseased; or, with *vs.* without disease X).

Misclassification would lead to improper conclusions. A case definition can be set on clinical, serological or pathological issues. When laboratory tests are applied, the test features like sensitivity and specificity should be known, as well as precision and validity through quality testing.

3.4. Determination of sample size

To determine the minimal size of a sample the following criteria should be considered:

- research question (disease prevalence estimation or disease detection),
- expected prevalence,
- desired level of confidence,
- accuracy (or error level).

A sample to estimate the prevalence of disease at herd level can be calculated as follows:

$$n = \left(t * \frac{SD}{L} \right)^2$$

where

n	= < 10% of the population size
t	= value of normal distribution at a certain confidence level
SD	= standard deviation of the estimated prevalence
L	= accuracy

At a confidence level of 95%, t has the value 1.96 (at 99% this is 2.58 and at 90% this is 1.64) in two-sided tests. The SD for a prevalence of 30% equals for example 0.46 ($\sqrt{P*(1-P)}$), for a prevalence P of .40 this is 0.49 and for P= .20 the SD is 0.40. Usually, the level of L is set at 0.05 or 0.01 (L= 1/2*confidence interval).

The number of herds in the sample can, for example, be 369.

In order to establish how many animals have to be sampled within herds in order to declare a herd free from infection or infected, the following formula can be used:

$$n = \left(1-(1-a)^{\frac{1}{d}}\right) * \left(N - \frac{d-1}{2}\right)$$

where

a = the desired confidence level
d = the number of expected disease cases in the population
N = the herd size
n = the sample size

From this formula it can be deduced that for example in a herd of 40 animals, there have to be 28 animals sampled for declaring a herd positive or negative (d = 1; a = 0.95).

Sample size requirements for analysis by logistic regression have been further elaborated in preceding chapters, as well as the further elaboration of the forenamed sample size calculations.

Usually, the factual sampling will be a compromise between what is scientifically needed and what is practically feasible. This is illustrated by Figure 12.2 derived from Vaillancourt (1993).

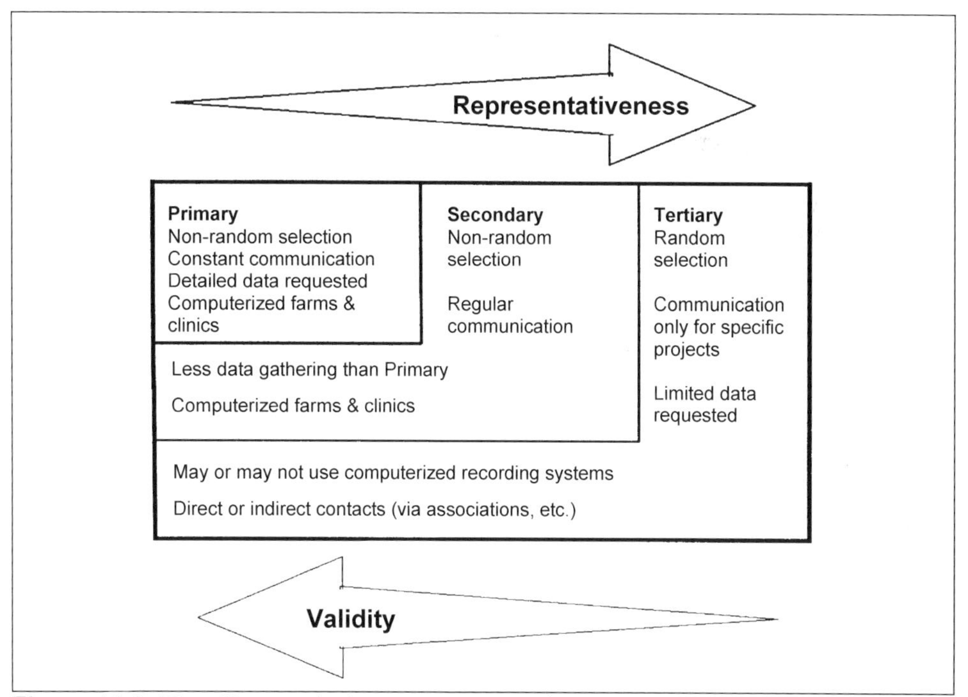

Figure 12.2. The dilemma between representativeness and validity in sampling: the search for the compromise (after Vaillancourt, 1993).

4. Diseases or Infections to Consider for a MOSS

Roughly there are 5 categories of diseases/infections to be distinguished according to the Standing Veterinary Committee of the EU (1990). These are:

Category I all notifiable diseases which are highly contagious and a potential threat to the whole territorium of the EU. Export regulations exist with respect to these infections

Category II contagious animal diseases of which the patterns are less epidemic, but which can threaten regions or groups of farms within the EU.
Export regulations exist for these infections. Several infections are of relevance for public health too. Examples are tuberculosis, brucellosis, bovine leucosis.

Category III diseases/infections which can be eradicated after formal approval of control programmes by the EU. These infections have great economic significance for export for a sector. Examples are Aujeszky's disease and bovine herpesvirus I (IBR in cattle).

Category IV Diseases/infections which can be controlled through voluntary application of control programmes in the top of the production column in order to safeguard the production farms. The programmes have to be approved by the EU too. Examples are atrophic rhinitis in pigs and *S.enteritidis* in poultry.

Category V diseases/infections in fish. No further detail will be given here.

In all situations a case definition has to be established. This may relate to clinical symptoms, serological status, pathological status or environmentally determined profile of the disease. It is sometimes even possible to establish a case definition through statistical analysis of herd performance parameters, such as in the case of PRRS, blue ears disease in pigs, at the time that the agent was still unknown (Schukken *et al.*, 1992).

4.1. Observations and measurements, existing data sources

After establishing a case definition in order to minimize misclassification, data on health and disease, and on environmental factors can be collected.

There are two major ways for collecting data for epidemiological purposes (Morris, 1990):

1. linking up to existing data bases for obtaining data which are not being used for this specific purpose, representing a rather inexpensive approach but with a limited benefit given the fact that these data were originally collected for other purposes;
2. designing a new system which is specifically designed for providing the desired information, representing a rather expensive approach.

The minimum requirements for the data are that they should comprise information about the farm identification (code name, address, locality), dates and animal identification (unique code number, breed, age/parity, sex).

Subsequently, it is determined by the objectives and the diseases under study what other information is needed and how it should be collected through observations and measurements. See also at Chapter V on Observational Studies, and part IV of this Chapter on Questionnaire Design for further information on the type of data and ways to collect them.

Existing data sources

Numerous sources of data on animal disease already exist. Usually they have been gathered for other purposes or are fragmentary in nature. The result is that their use is rather limited because of deficiencies. At that point the question is whether or not these gaps are substantially important and whether they can be filled through other sources. On the other hand, if existing data bases could be used for epidemiological research, the use of such data bases would be much more cost-efficient. Examples of existing data sources are:

- disease reports from authorities (e.g., Veterinary Service)
- reports from diagnostic laboratories
- client records from veterinary practices
- slaughterhouse information
- on-farm management information systems and records
- data bases of veterinary herd health programmes
- reports on national agronomic and farm statistics

Official reports on animal diseases can provide basic information which is objective in nature. Especially in case of reports on disease outbreaks, such as PRRS, foot-and-mouth disease or swine vesicular disease, such information could be highly valuable. An example is to investigate the temporal and spatial distribution patterns of such a disease. However, for endemic diseases these reports are not suitable at all because these diseases are usually not dealt with. The same is true for exotic diseases, newly introduced into a region.

Diagnostic laboratory records commonly comprise a quite selective population. The post-mortem information often originates from animals which died, while culturing results often are derived from animals which are disease suspected. Often these data can be related to incidences. This means that this information is biased. For on-farm use it has its value. These records could be made more valuable if these laboratories would link up with field services, practice networks or IQM (Integrated Quality Management) programmes to create a structured monitoring system.

Veterinary practice records experience the same type of features as named above. The information is commonly biased by selection. Various problems can be detected: clinical diagnoses cannot be confirmed routinely by laboratory examination; confidentiality of client records may impose a problem for broader analysis; subclinical disease/infection is not routinely investigated by practitioners. Although their relevance may be limited for epidemiological research, practices may still be involved in specific epidemiological research such as clinical trials or field surveys when they are willing to follow the preset survey protocol.

On-farm management information systems may contribute to epidemiological study if the data collected fit into the objectives. When only clinical disease data are collected, for example on cow lameness, then the major problem of subclinical lameness diagnoses will not be found (Noordhuizen *et al.*, 1992). For many surveys the on-farm recording systems can play a role and many prevalence studies have been performed at the farm level using these systems (Frankena *et al.*, 1993). These systems may become much more important in the future if they are part of a larger network and if they become more sophisticated in data collection and data handling.

National agronomic and farm statistics usually comprise census data, estimating livestock numbers and dividing them into certain categories and regions. Census data are heavily influenced by sampling procedures and timing. Census can provide the basis for sampling frames for epidemiological surveys. If census data are not available, one could look for other sources, such as cattle improvement organisations.

4.2. Data analysis and interpretation

After collection of the necessary data - often at different places - the data files have to be put together into one (mostly central) database. This central database is then used for dates analysis after preceding quality checking and correction. Data analysis procedures within the setting of MOSS may refer to:

- descriptive statistics (means, medians, tables, graphics)
- analytical studies (risk rates)
- disease or infection modelling
- risk analysis

Within MOSS the data analysis procedure should go on continuously and without time delay to be of value to participants. For interpretation of analysis results basic veterinary (patho-physiological) knowledge is required next to biostatistical experience for knowing opportunities and limitations of techniques applied. Interpretation of data in a MOSS may be used for purposes of disease pattern prediction (e.g., on BSE cases, Wilesmith *et al.*, 1988; Anderson *et al.*, 1996).

Results of analysis should be disseminated to participants in the MOSS but - when public health is involved - also to the public and the media.

5. Types of MOSS

A short overview of MOSS examples for different applications is provided in the Appendix 1. This overview is after Morris (1990). Other examples are given by Toma *et al.* (1995) with regard to a variety of MOSS in France. An outline of potential areas where MOSS could be applied for pig health monitoring is given in Figure 12.3 (after Noordhuizen, 1993).

For the notifiable diseases a MOSS in whatever format is already operational. In many countries the authorities strive for refresher campaigns for diseases which have not been detected recently. Examples of such refresher campaigns about signs and diagnostics of diseases (photo material, documentation) are: foot-and-mouth disease in The Netherlands and France, IBR in The Netherlands.

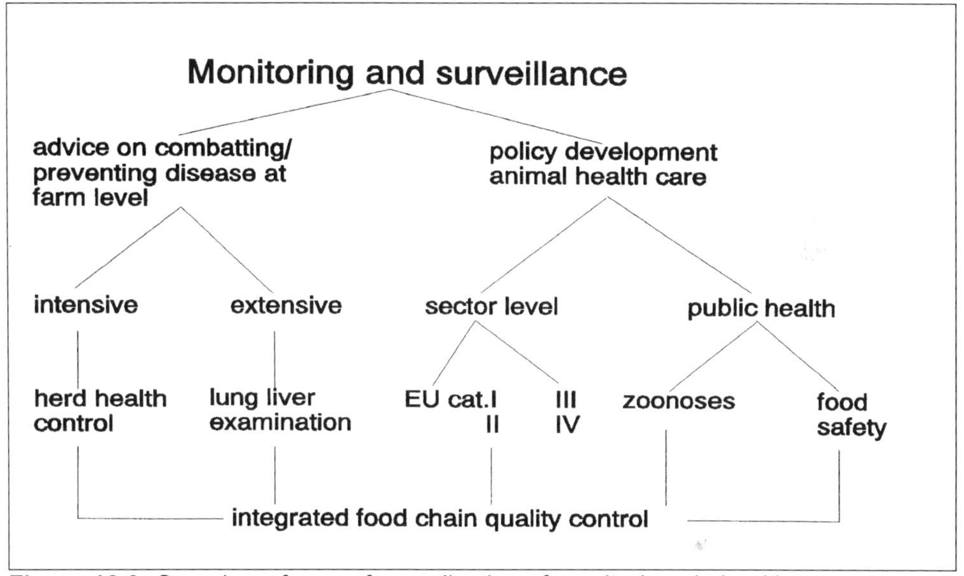

Figure 12.3. Overview of areas for application of monitoring pig health.

For the notifiable diseases a MOSS in whatever format is already operational. In many countries the authorities strive for refresher campaigns for diseases which have not been detected recently. Examples of such refresher campaigns about signs and diagnostics of diseases (photo material, documentation) are: foot-and-mouth disease in The Netherlands and France, IBR in The Netherlands.

There are "passive" and "active" MOSS. In the former situation, events are just followed and reported on a list. In the latter, events must be reported and action taken in case of outbreaks (for example tracing back). The system for notifiable diseases is, for example, an active MOSS. The same is true for lung-liver screening at the slaughterhouse and the feedback of information about pneumonia and pleurisy detected at slaughter to the pigfarmer to encourage adjustment of farm management.

Next, there are "continuous" and "periodical" MOSS, referring to the time period or frequency that monitoring is performed. Periodical could mean in a cyclic order or even incidentally (e.g., the 5-yearly survey on mastitis in dairy cows in The Netherlands). Continuous could mean at either low or high frequency of monitoring (e.g., notifiable diseases).

Intensity, detailing and specification are other features for a MOSS, depending on objectives and target population involved.

The question arises, for what other diseases a MOSS could be of substantial relevance and when.

5.1. National level

At the national level, a MOSS can be beneficial in the case of notifiable disease surveillance, mass disease campaigns, determination of the overall national herd health status (including productivity), and definition of scenario's for sudden massive disease outbreaks. MOSS at this level aim at the early detection of a notifiable disease. Upon the detection of suspect clinical cases a confirmation of the diagnosis in the laboratory is needed. After confirmation the herd will be eradicated and neighbouring herds checked; the area is blocked and movement of animals banned until the area is declared free again. It is obvious that diagnostic tests and their characteristics are playing a paramount role in this procedure.

MOSS can also be made useful for the support of mass disease - combat campaigns by increasing the efficiency of such campaigns and by evaluating the effectivity. This could mean that herds of flocks in such campaigns are sampled more frequently to detect disease or infections patterns. Although the basic relevance might be obvious, there still remain questions to be answered, and efficiency could be largely improved. Examples of systems aiming at setting priorities for combat or providing insight in overall health status of farms are NAHMS in the USA, the National Animal Health Monitoring System, and APHIN in Canada, Animal Productivity and Health Information Network.

5.2. Regional and local level

At the regional and local level, different options are possible.

Feedback of slaughterhouse findings to the primary producers can provide the latter with information which is useful for operational management. In meat pigs, this has proven to be a very adequate method, e.g., in the case of lung-liver examination at slaughter and the clinical situation on the pig farm with respect to *Actinobacillus pleuropneumoniae* infections (Willeberg *et al.*, 1984; Elbers *et al.*, 1990; Geudeke, 1992). In more modern situations this is part of a so-called Integrated Quality Management system, IQM. The IQM was originally focused on meat quality demands put forward by importing countries. Possible extensions of a basic IQM are the control of medicinal products allowed to be used on IQM approved farms, and the level of disease prevalence on those farms. In IQM whole production chains are covered: from e.g., pig breeder to multiplier to fattener farms, often involving feed mills, and slaughterhouse as well.

Slaughterhouse information could also refer to serological monitoring at slaughter. For routine herd health monitoring, serological examination on e.g., Aujeszky's disease, *Actinobacillus pleuropneumoniae*, swine vesicular disease or *Parvo-virus* infection could be useful for pig farms.

At the farm level, monitoring of endemic diseases could be regarded useful by the farmer on the basis of economic reasons. This regards multifactorial diseases with often an infectious component. Veterinary herd health programmes are examples of such monitoring systems (Brand *et al.*, 1996). Active surveillance in that case is usually limited to qualitative assessment of gathered information. This type of surveillance appeals to the farmer because farm income is directly involved. It would be highly advizable to integrate principles of quantitative epidemiology into veterinary herd health programmes in order to provide the veterinary consultant and the farmer with a list of quantified risk factors contributing to the impaired health status. Risk analysis procedures may point to "high risk groups of animals" at the farm and to conditions of increased risk in the animals' environment. Most management information systems on computers do not address this issue of environmental risk factors (yet). It is clear that MOSS at this level are not representative for a whole population and serve a specific goal.

5.3. Public health level

With regard to public health there are additional options for MOSS.

Zoonoses and foodborne diseases related to food products of animal origin are the major concern. For pigs for example, the emphasis is on brucellosis, *Salmonella spp.*, *S. suis II*, trichinellosis; in cattle: *S. dublin*, VTEC (verocytotoxin *E. coli* $O_{157}H_7$). *Campylobacter spp.* and *salmonella spp.* are primary agents in poultry. If control of these infections could be linked to existing monitoring systems, such as herd health or IQM, efficiency can be improved and costs for the sector limited. In other situations, it is imaginable that public health interest will dictate the demands for monitoring and surveillance of a certain pathogen in a given animal production sector.
An example of the latter is a formal directive from a Ministry of Public Health laid upon the animal production sector that food products of animal origin must be free of salmonella bacteria at distribution to retailers.

The relevance of the domain of food protection has increased over the recent years because of the increasing urbanisation, the related demand for special food products and innovative food, new phenomena of food preparation related to changing social structures (fast food, easy to prepare, changing eating habits) and leading to product diversification, the increased trade of commodities and mobility of man and livestock. The number and severity of foodborne diseases have increased and is usually much larger than the number of formally reported disease cases. Additionally, it is not easy to unravel this complex problem because many more issues than agrofood industry alone are involved (Waltner-Toews, 1996). The latter author proposes an ecosystem health approach to the problem area of foodborne diseases. This approach has multiscalar, ecological and cultural characteristics and is passing beyond large computer systems linear dynamics.

Milk quality control (somatic cell count, bacteria count), residue examination and trichinosis examination are other examples of monitoring systems for public health. Sometimes this monitoring is repressive (condemnation of a carcass), sometimes this monitoring is indicative (trichinosis examination in e.g., The Netherlands with an estimated yearly prevalence of 1 on 10.000).

Representativeness is apparently not always needed in a MOSS, and is related to the specific MOSS objectives, and/or financial reasons.

6. Conclusions

MOSS in animal production should only be designed and built if they can answer specific questions which cannot or only at high price be answered in another way. Indicative for the costs of a MOSS are the results presented by Ament *et al.* (1993) for a MOSS on *S.enteritidis* in poultry in The Netherlands involving 1926 layer flocks farms which were screened once every laying period of 60 weeks. Total costs for monitoring ranged between 3 and 13 million US dollar for prevalences between 1 and 10 % respectively. These authors calculated a neutral cost to benefit balance at prevalence levels lower than 10%. See also part II of this chapter.

Specific questions at the national level can sometimes be contradictory with questions at the local level. Farmers should be involved as much as possible, but then their interest should be kept in mind. It appears to be an area where authorities, production sector as a whole and individual farmers should cooperate in order to make any MOSS viable. National MOSS can be imposed, specifically for notifiable diseases and zoonoses. At the local level, farms should link to networks in order to make the best possible use of their information. IQM such as in poultry and pig production provides a sound basis for that purpose; the quality control procedure of HACCP, Hazard Analysis Critical Control Points, may be another tool of interest to health management and monitoring within IQM (Noordhuizen and Welpelo, 1996). For further details we refer to Chapter X.

The more representativeness is required, the higher are the demands put on a MOSS design (sample size; observations; diagnostic characteristics). MOSS is not a panacea for every problem, as has been explained in this chapter.

References

Ament, A.J.H.A.; Jansen, J.; Giessen, A.v.d.; Notermans, S. (1993). Cost-benefit analysis of a screening strategy for *S.enteritidis* in poultry. Veterinary Quarterly, 15, 33-37.

Anderson, R.M.; Donnelly, C.A.; Ferguson, N.M.; Woolhouse, M.E.J.; Watt, C.J.; Udy, H.J.; MaWhinney, S.; Dunstan, S.P.; Southwood, T.R.E.; Wilesmith, J.W.; Ryan, J.B.M.; Hoinville, L.J.; Hillerton, J.E.; Austin, A.R.; Wells, G.A.H. (1996). Transmission dynamics and epidemiology of BSE in British cattle. Nature, 382, 779-788.

Brand, A.; Noordhuizen, J.P.T.M.; Schukken, Y.H. (1996). Herd Health and Production Management in Dairy Practice. Wageningen Pers, Wageningen, The Netherlands.

Elbers, A.R.W.; Tielen, M.J.M.; Cromwijk, W.A.J., Hunneman, W.A. (1990). Seroepidemiological screening of pig sera collected at slaughterhouse to detect herds infected with Aujeszky's disease in the framework of an Integrated Quality Control system. Veterinary Quarterly, 12, 221-229.
Frankena, K.; Keulen, K.A.S.; Noordhuizen, J.P.; Noordhuizen-Stassen, E.N.; Gundelach, J.; Jong, D.J. de; Saedt, I. (1993). A cross-sectional study on prevalence and risk factors of *dermatitis interdigitalis* in female dairy calves in The Netherlands. Preventive Veterinary Medicine, 17, 137-144.
Geudeke, M.J. (1992). The use of slaughterhouse information in monitoring systems for herd health control in sows. PhD thesis, University Utrecht, The Netherlands (in Dutch).
Morris, R.S. (1990). Assessing regional animal health problems. In: Epidemiological Skills in Animal Health. Refresher Course for Veterinarians, proc. 143, Postgraduate Committee, D.I. Bryden (Ed.). University of Sydney, Australia.
Noordhuizen, J.P.T.M.; Frankena, K.; Stassen, E.N.; Brand, A. (1992). Applied epidemiology in aid to dairy herd health programs. In: Proceedings XVII World Buiatrics and XXV AABP Conference, St. Paul, Minnesota. William, E.I. (Ed.). pp. 6-11.
Noordhuizen, J.P.T.M. (1993). Monitoring and surveillance systems for health care in the pig production sector: sense and nonsense. Tijdschrift voor Diergeneeskunde, 118, 405-408 (in Dutch).
Noordhuizen, J.P.T.M.; Welpelo, H.J. (1996) Sustainable improvement of animal health care by systematic quality risk management according to the HACCP concept. Veterinary Quarterly, 18, 33-37.
Schukken, Y.H.; De Jong, M.C.M.; Komijn, R.E.; Braamskamp, J.; Dijkhuizen, A.A.; Noordhuizen, J.P.T.M.; Vernooy, J.C.M.; Verheijden, J.H.M. (1992). De diagnose PEARS-verdacht en onverdacht op fok- en vermeerderingsbedrijven in Nederland met behulp van statistische methoden. Tijdschrift voor Diergeneeskunde, 117, 259-264 (in Dutch).
Staerk, K.D.C. (1993). Monitoring- und Surveillance-Systeme (MOSS): Einführung und Grundlagen. I.V.I. Seminar, November 1993, Mittelhausern, Switzerland.
Toma, B.; Dufour, B.; Sanaa, M.; Benet, J.J.; Ellis, P;. Moutou, F.; Louza, A. (1995) Epidemiologie Appliquée a la lutte collective contre les maladies animales transmissibles majeures, AEEMA, Maisons Alfort, France.
Vaillancourt, J.P. (1993). The epidemiologist-practitioner relationship in research. In: Proceedings of the Society for Veterinary Epidemiology and Preventive Medicine, Exeter, 31st March-2nd April 1993. Thrusfield, M. (Ed.). pp. 180-187.
Waltner-Toews, D. (1996). An agroecosystem perspective on foodborne illnesses. Ecosystem Health, 2 (3), 177-185.
Wilesmith, J.W.; Wells, G.A.H., Cramwell, M.P.; Ryan, J.B.M. (1988). Bovine spongiform encephalopathy: epidemiological studies. Veterinary Record, 123, 638-644.
Willeberg, P.; Gerbola, M.A.; Kirkegaard, Petersen, B.; Andersen, J.B. (1984). The danish pig health scheme: nation-wide computerbased abattoir surveillance and follow-up at the herd level. Preventive Veterinary Medicine, 3, 79-91.

Appendix 1

Overview of MOSS applications (after Morris, 1990).

Level of Operation	System	Type	Species	Further Details
Individual animal	Brucellosis testing on sera collected at slaughter.	Surveillance	Cattle	To detect infected herds in eradication campaign.
	Examination for tuberculosis and contagious bovine pleuropneumonia lesions after slaughter.	Surveillance	Cattle	To detect infected herds in eradication campaign.
	Cell counts (and bacteriological examination in some cases) on quarter milk samples or bulk milk of cow.	Monitoring	Cattle	To assess infection status of individual animal and herd.
Herd or Flock	Brucellosis milk ring testing on bulk herd milk.	Surveillance	Cattle	To detect infected dairy herds in eradication campaign.
	Cell count on bulk herd milk.	Monitoring	Cattle	To evaluate current mastitis status of herd.
	Sample testing of birds and bacteriological examination of dead chickens for *Salmonella pullorum*.	Surveillance	Poultry	To detect infection in flocks during the late stages of control campaign.
	Computer-assessment of reproductive indices.	Monitoring	Pigs, cattle, sheep	To evaluate current reproductive performance in herd.
	Metabolic profile.	Monitoring	Cattle, pigs	To evaluate nutritional adequacy of diet.
Farm	Feed and production evaluation system.	Monitoring	Cattle, pigs	To evaluate balance between feed supply and nutritional requirement of animals.
Region	Spore count for fungus which causes facial eczema on selected farms.	Monitoring	Cattle, sheep	To assess likelihood of an outbreak of facial eczema in the region.
	Liver fluke risk assessment by forecast based on weather pattern.	Monitoring	Cattle, sheep	To assess likely severity of fascioliasis in region.
	Rate of reinfection of brucellosis-free herds in region.	Surveillance	Cattle	To assess breakdown rate in brucellosis eradication campaign.
Nation	Newcastle disease virus virulence testing.	Surveillance	Poultry	To detect entry of more virulent strains.

Appendix 2

Checklist of considerations and questions to be answered positively before a MOSS is considered for operationalization

1. Prevention or combat of disease is possible with the help of information from a MOSS. The MOSS is then the basis for the decision process; not for every decision a MOSS is needed; is a MOSS financially feasible and who has to make it feasible?

2. Is there really a need for a MOSS? In other words: does a MOSS add something useful and functional to existing instruments?

3. Is a diagnosis or a syndrome required for the MOSS objective and approach (for example pneumonia *versus Actinobacillus pleuropneumoniae*)?

4. What is the estimated prevalence of the disease/infection to be studied? Which guarantees are expected for obtaining results which are useful at the farm level? Is it useful to work with samples? How great is the variation between farms in the network?

5. Is sharply defined what one desires to know or to measure? Is sharply defined how one desires to measure and when? Is sharply defined how much detail is desired?

6. Can measurements be complete, accurate, reliable?

7. How simple are parameters, variables or symptoms to be observed and to record? Can these observations also be made otherwise (e.g., live animal observation *versus* carcass inspection)?

8. Has it been made clear that the MOSS observation time period is related to the objectives (incidental; periodical; continuous)?

9. How reliable and correct are sampling procedures followed?

10. Are the planned activities in the MOSS technically feasible? Against which additional labour costs and technical costs?

11. Are analysis procedures and alternatives available? Against which costs?

12. Can modules or parts of existing data bases be linked in a uniform way?

13. Which knowledge or information is available about causal relationships between selected diseases/infections and determinants?

14. Is the MOSS characterized by a prevalence or an incidence study profile, or by an exposure study profile?

15. Who will benefit from the collected and processed information? Which benefits?

16. Which precautions have been taken to reassure the cooperation of the farmers?

17. Has every partner adopted his/her responsibility with regard to e.g., implementation, conduct, maintenance, analysis, reporting and feedback of information?

18. How valuable is the ratio between study population and target population?

19. Is the MOSS adopted by all institutions and persons involved? How do you know?

20. Are participants contributing to the MOSS (design, exploitation) according to the agreement?

Part II

Cost-Benefit Analysis of a Screening Strategy for Salmonella Enteritidis in Poultry[40]

A.J.H.A. Ament
Department of Health care economics
University of Maastricht
The Netherlands

J. Jansen
Directorate of Health Protection
Rijswijk
The Netherlands

A. v.d. Giessen
National Institute for Public Health and The Environment
Bilthoven
The Netherlands

S. Notermans
National Institute for Public Health and The Environment
Bilthoven
The Netherlands

[40] Veterinary Quarterly 1993;15:33-7; reproduced with approval of the editorial board of this journal

1. Introduction

S.enteritidis infections in humans is becoming a problem in most countries (Rodrique *et al.*, 1990; WHO, 1989). It has been established that outbreaks are predominantly related to the consumption of contaminated eggs and egg products (Anonymous, 1988; St. Louis *et al.*, 1988). The 'invasive' serotype *S.enteritidis* has the potential for transovarian transmission and thus the ability to contaminate eggs (Humphrey *et al.*, 1989; Humphrey, 1991). Besides vertical transmission poultry flocks may also become contaminated by environmental factors horizontal transmission). Feed could also be a source of infection.

Several intervention strategies have been developed. It has been stated that the effective intervention strategies have to be based on slaughter of contaminated flocks and interruption of the routes of contamination. A working group of the WHO recommends monitoring poultry flocks for the presence of *S.enteritidis.* If the organism is identified in a laying flock, the flock should be slaughtered and the eggs destroyed or diverted to pasteurization plants (WHO, 1989). In The Netherlands, this strategy has been introduced successfully to eliminate *S.enteritidis* from breeder flocks. In 1991, contaminated breeder flocks were found only incidentally. Nevertheless, laying flocks have been found to be positive for *S.enteritidis.* In all probability these laying flocks are contaminated by horizontal transmission routes. Therefore an additional intervention strategy is necessary to prevent environmental contamination. We describe a cost-benefit analysis into whether an intervention strategy based on monitoring laying flocks and destroying positive flocks is feasible. The calculations made are based on the Dutch situation.

2. Intervention Strategy

The intervention strategy is based on the monitoring of poultry laying flocks for the presence of *S.enteritidis* and the subsequent slaughter of positive flocks . A bird is positive for *S.enteritidis* if the organism is cultured from faecal material. A flock is considered to be positive for *S.enteritidis* if one positive bird is found. A starting point for the cost-benefit analysis is that all *S. enteritidis* infections in humans are caused by the consumption of eggs originating from contaminated laying flocks. To analyze the cost-benefit of the above-mentioned approach, it is necessary to calculate the effectiveness of the intervention strategy. Effectiveness is defined as the percentage of eggs originating from contaminated flocks which do not become available for consumption as a result of the intervention. Effectiveness is determined by both the reliability of the detection method used and the frequency of monitoring. The costs of monitoring and the economic losses caused by premature slaughter of flocks have then to be calculated.

3. Monitoring of Laying Flocks

3.1. Sampling procedure

In Table 12.1, the probability of detecting *S.enteritidis* as function of the contamination level of a flock is presented. If, for example 10% of the birds are positive for *S.enteritidis*, at least 30 birds have to be screened for the organism to obtain a detection probability of 96%. The results presented in Table 12.1 show that at lower levels of contamination, for example 2%, more birds have to be screened. If a bird is contaminated, *S.enteritidis* will always be present in the faecal material of that bird (Giessen *et al.*, 1991). Therefore, fresh droppings are used as test material. To facilitate detection of *S.enteritidis* in a contaminated flock, use can be made of the so-called pool-sampling methodology. It is estimated that for a laying flock of 10,000 birds at least 20 pool samples, each consisting of 10-20 fresh droppings, have to be tested. However, the probability of finding positive samples also depends on whether or not the birds are free-range.

3.2. Detection method

Culture methods are used to demonstrate the presence of *S.enteritidis* in faecal samples. With this method the sample is enriched in a fluid medium, followed by plating out of the obtained culture on a suitable agar medium (ISO-method 6575). By using reference materials it has been demonstrated that the recovery of the ISO detection method is about 80-90% (In 't Veld and Notermans, 1992). Biochemical and serological identification of organisms growing on the agar plate results in a specificity of 100%.

Table 12.1. Probability of detecting S. enteritidis with varying contamination levels (adapted from ICMSF (ICMSF, 1986)).

Number of samples tested	contamination level		
	50%	10%	2%
3	87%	27%	6%
5	97%	61%	10%
10		65%	18%
20		88%	26%
30		96%	45%
60			70%
100			87%

3.3. Costs of monitoring

From the above it is clear that the probability of detecting *S.enteritidis* in a laying flock primarily depends on the number of samples analyzed and the detection technique used. If 20 pooled samples of faeces from a flock of 10,000 birds are tested, the probability of detecting *S. enteritidis* in a positive flock is estimated to be 90%. All farms with laying birds have to be visited. In 1989 there were 1926 farms in The Netherlands with more than 1,000 laying birds. An average of 1.5 flocks were present on each farm. Only these farms are included in our calculations. This means that approximately 3% of the laying flocks will not be monitored. The estimated costs of monitoring poultry flocks are presented in Table 12.2. As a starting point we proposed that laying flocks should be screened only once during their laying period of 60 weeks. Travelling expenses for visiting the 1926 farms are estimated at fl. 25.000. Laboratory costs are the major part of monitoring expenses. It costs fl. 50 to examine one faecal sample, including the cost of serotyping. If 20 samples per flock are tested, the total costs amount to 20 x fl. 50 x number of flocks (1926 x 1.5) = fl. 2,880,000. The overall cost of one screening during the active laying period is approximately fl. 3,000,000. One US dollar approximates 1.75 dutch guilder[41].

Table 12.2. Estimated costs of monitoring Dutch poultry flocks for S. enteritidis with a screening during the whole laying period of 60 weeks.

sampling	- travelling expenses	fl.	12,500
	- salary costs	--	25,000
laboratory tests		--	2 888,000
Total costs		fl.	2 917,500

4. Effectiveness and Costs of Destroying Positive Flocks

To calculate the effectiveness (% of eggs of contaminated flocks, that are not used for consumption) and the costs of destroying contaminated flocks, the average number of birds in a flock was set to be 10,000. It was also assumed that the contamination rate, as a result of horizontal transmission, would increase with time, as presented in Figure 12.4.

4.1. Effectivity

The effectiveness of the proposed strategy depends on the time of screening. If a flock is screened, for example, at week 20, contamination will not be detected since contamination by environmental factors has not occurred. The effectiveness of screening is therefore 0%. Screening of flocks at the end of the laying period will result in a high probability of detecting positive flocks. However, destroying a flock at the end of the laying period is not effective since the eggs will have been consumed. The effectiveness of screening half-way through the laying period (week 50) is 50% (Figure 12.4). Effectiveness as a function of birds is presented in Table 12.3, and was calculated with the following equation:

$$\text{Effectiveness} = \left(1-\left(\frac{1}{n}\right)^2\right)-\left(1-\frac{1}{n}\right)^2 * 100\%$$

with 1/n = 1/3 if screening is carried out at week 40 (at 1/3 of the laying cycle).

[41] this was in 1993, currently it is 2.50 (eds.)

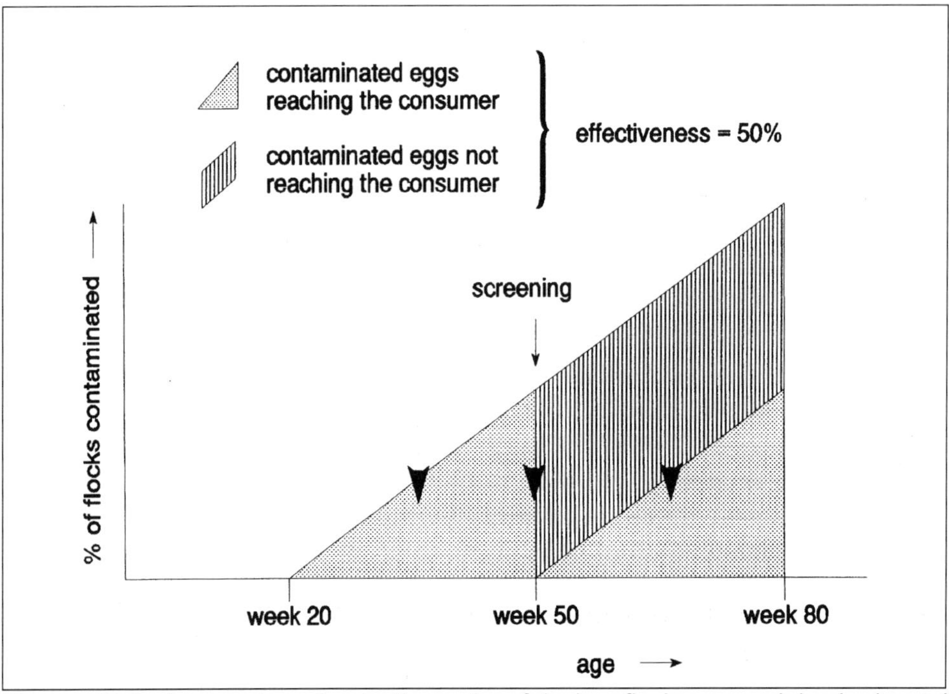

Figure 12.4. Assumed contamination rate of laying flocks caused by horizontal transmission routes and the effectiveness of screening at week 50 versus triple screening at weeks 35, 50 and 65.

The effectiveness needs to be corrected. Firstly, the sampling and laboratory test procedures have a reliability of 90%. Additionally 3% of the laying birds are not monitored. The corrected effectiveness rates are also presented in Table 12.3. Effectiveness is greatest if flocks are tested half-way through the laying season (week 50). If laying flocks are monitored randomly during the laying period, the effectiveness is only 28.3%.

Table 12.3. Effectiveness of one screening as a function of the age of birds. Effectiveness is defined as the percentage of eggs originating from positive flocks that are not available for consumption.

Time of screening (weeks)	Cumulative probability to detect positive flocks (%)	Effectiveness (%)	Effectiveness after correction*
20	0	0	0
30	16.7	27.8	24.2
40	33.3	44.4	38.7
50	50.0	50.0	43.7
60	66.7	44.4	38.7
70	83.3	27.8	24.2
80	100.0	0	0

* Sampling procedures and laboratory tests will result in a detection rate of 90%. Additionally, 3% of the birds are not monitored. Therefore, only 87.3% of the positive flocks will be detected.

It is also possible to screen flocks several times during the laying period. In Table 12.4 the overall effectiveness of multiple screening is presented. Effectiveness increases with the number of screenings, but is only 78.6% after 10 screenings.

Table 12.4. Effectiveness of multiple screening.

Number of screenings	Effectiveness (%)	Effectiveness (%) after corrections*
1 (week 50)	50	43.7
2 (week 40 and 60)	66	57.6
3 (week 35, 50 and 65)	75	65.4
-	-	-
-	-	-
10	90	78.6

* See note Table 12.3.

5. Costs of Destroying a Positive Flock

The value of a laying flock is determined by the cost of the flock and the benefits thereof. The costs include, among others, the costs of purchasing the birds, exploitation costs, and feeding costs. The benefits of a flock consists of egg production and the value of the bird at the time of slaughter. After purchase, the value of a flock will increase as egg production becomes optimal. Thereafter the value decreases slowly. If the above mentioned costs and benefits are known, the exact value of a flock at any time during the laying period can be calculated. We used the insurance value of the flock in our calculations, that is the amount of money paid by an insurance company if there is a total disaster (100% of birds killed). In Table 12.5 this value is presented. In our approach the rest value of a bird is assessed at fl. 1.50. Destroying birds at the end of the laying period seems to be attractive, but the effectivity is 0. From the results presented in Table 12.5, the total costs of destroying contaminated birds can easily be calculated. Again, it has to be taken into account that the detection rate of positive flocks is 90%. The total costs of destroying birds in week 50 (half-way the production cycle) are presented in Table 12.6, where the costs are presented as function of the percentage of flocks contaminated with *S.enteritidis* at that time.

Table 12.5. Costs of destroying a flock of 10,000 birds as function of age (based on dividend paid by insurance companies in case of a complete disaster).

Age of birds (weeks)	Cost of one bird (x fl.)	Total cost of destroying flocks* (x fl. 1,000)
17	11.5	100
20	16.5	150
30	14.5	130
40	11.6	100
50	9.1	75
60	6.5	50
70	4.0	25
80	1.5	0

* A rest value of fl. 1.50 per carcass had been subtracted

6. Benefits of the Strategy

It is relatively complex to obtain an insight into the benefits of the intervention strategy. In the last decade attempts have been made to estimate the economic impact of salmonellosis in humans (Roberts, 1989; Roberts *et al.*, 1991; Todd, 1989). On the basis of these studies, we estimated the benefit of reducing salmonellosis in humans. However, this is not easy. For example, the incidence of human salmonellosis is not known exactly. Most infected persons do not consult their general practitioners. In general, only a small part of the diseased population needs medical attention. The mortality rate is also very low and almost only those patients with other underlying conditions are at risk of dying. As a result of differences in the severity of the disease, the costs of an individual case of salmonellosis may vary considerably.

Table 12.6. Total costs of destroying contaminated poultry flocks in The Netherlands at week 50 as function of the contamination rate.

Contamination rate (%)	Total costs of destroying flocks* (x fl. 1000)
1	1.97
2	3.93
3	5.31
4	7.88
5	9.85
-	-
-	-
-	-
10	19.70

* % positive flocks x number of flocks x detection effectiveness of 90% x cost of destroying flocks elimination at week 50.

6.1. Incidence rate and costs of *S. enteritidis* infections

The incidence of *S.enteritidis* must be known to calculate the costs of infections in humans. Additionally, the proportion of people needing medical attention has to be known as well as the risk of dying. Based on research carried out in The Netherlands, it is estimated that 12,000 persons infected with a *Salmonella* organism ask for medical attention (Hoogenboom-Verdegaal *et al.*, 1989). Population studies, as carried out in several countries, have revealed that only 5-13% of infected people ask for medical attention (Hoogenboom-Verdegaal *et al.*, 1992; Krug, 1985; Roberts, 1989). Information about the death rate as a result of infection with *Salmonella* is not available for The Netherlands. The reported incidence, based on the Dutch study, reflects the number of people seeking medical attention. If the reporting rate is 5, 9 or 13% then the unreported cases, which do not need medical attention are 240,000, 133,000 and 92,300, respectively (Table 12.7). These costs cover both medical costs and decreased productivity as a consequence of absenteeism. The costs of non-reported cases only include loss of labour and are estimated to be fl. 500 (Roberts, 1989; Todd, 1989). The costs of a reported case amount to fl. 3000 (Roberts, 1989; Todd, 1989). The total cost of salmonellosis in The Netherlands as function of the reporting rate is summarized in Table 12.7. Surveillance studies carried out by the Dutch International Centre for

Salmonellosis have estimated that in 1991, 34.4% of all cases of salmonellosis in humans were caused by *S.enteritidis*. The economic impact of salmonellosis caused by *S.enteritidis* is presented on the bottom line of Table 12.7.

7. Comparison of the Costs and Benefits of the Strategy

The costs of screening week 50 (half-way through the production cycle) are presented as function of the contamination rate in the upper part of Table 12.8. The costs of monitoring are a substantial fraction of the costs of destroying positive flocks.

The benefits of the strategy are presented in the lower part of Table 12.8. The effectiveness of screening, which was estimated to be 43.7%, decreases the real benefits considerably. Comparison of the results of costs and benefits shows that the proposed screening strategy leads to a gain only if approximately less than 10% of Dutch poultry flocks are contaminated with *S.enteritidis*.

Table 12.7. Estimation of the economic benefits of screening for S.enteritidis in poultry.

	reporting rate (%)		
	5	9	13
Estimated total number of reported infections caused by *Salmonella*	12,000	12,000	12,000
Not reported cases	240,000	133,000	92,300
Total cases	252,000	145,000	104,300
Costs of reported cases (cases x fl. 3,000) x fl. 10^6	36	36	36
Costs of not reported cases (cases x fl. 500) x fl. 10^6	120	66.50	46.10
Total costs	156	102.50	82.10
35% caused by *S.enteritidis* x fl. 10^6	54.50	35.90	28.7

Table 12.8. Comparison of costs and benefits of the screening strategy if laying flocks are monitored and destroyed at week 50 (half way through the production cycle).

Costs of the strategy	Contamination rate of the Dutch flocks at week 50				
	1%	2%	3%	5%	10%
Costs of destroying flocks (See Table 12.5 x fl. 10^6	1.97	3.93	5.81	9.85	19.7
Costs of monitoring (See Table 12.2) x fl. 10^6	2.9	2.9	2.9	2.9	2.9
Total costs x fl. 10^6	4.87	6.83	8.71	12.75	22.6
Benefits of the strategy					
	Reporting rate of salmonellosis				
	5%	9%	13%		
Benefits (See Table 12.7) x fl. 10^6.	54.6	35.9	28.7		
Benefits corrected for effectiveness(43.7%) x fl. 10^6	23.9	15.9	12.5		

8. Discussion

As emphasized in the introduction, laying flocks can become contaminated with *S.enteritidis* by several routes. Owing to the invasive character of the organism, vertical transmission (from breeder to progeny) is the main route of contamination. Only if parent flocks are free of *S.enteritidis* this route of contamination is blocked. Contamination by environmental factors (horizontal transmission) plays an important role. These routes of infections also have to be interrupted. It is often emphasized that monitoring of laying flocks and the subsequent slaughter of contaminated flocks should be an effective tool to decrease contamination. Calculations, however, have shown that the effectiveness of such a strategy is relatively low. If only one screening is carried out during the whole laying cycle, a maximum 43.7% reduction in contaminated eggs will be achieved. To achieve this, screening must be carried out half way through the production cycle of laying hens. If screening is carried out randomly, the effectiveness is much lower (28.3%). Increasing the number of screenings will of course increase the effectiveness. However, a 100% effectiveness will never be obtained, and the costs of such a monitoring approach will be too high. In the proposed monitoring programme culture methods are the methods of choice to trace positive flocks. However, several immunoassays have been developed, making it relatively easy to check the presence of *S.enteritidis* in a poultry flock (McLeod and Barrow, 1991). In most assays egg yolk and/or serum is tested for the presence of antibodies directed against *S.enteritidis*. In general, immunoassays are not expensive and therefore may reduce the costs of screening. Analyses of the benefits of the strategy are still a weak point in this research. The starting point was that all human infections caused by *S.enteritidis* are caused by contaminated eggs. Several outbreaks have been reported to be caused by poultry meat contaminated with the organism. Death caused by infection was also not taken into account in the benefit analysis. Comparison of the costs and benefits indicates that the proposed screening strategy is feasible if fewer than 10% of the Dutch flocks are contaminated. It therefore seems attractive to start the proposed monitoring programme. Although the effectiveness of the screening strategy is low, it cannot be excluded that monitoring of laying flocks and subsequent slaughter of positive flocks may have a beneficial effect in the future. Because of possible losses, farmers will be stimulated to take preventive measures to avoid contamination of their poultry flocks. Such measures have to include thorough cleaning and disinfection of poultry houses, use of feed free of *Salmonella* organisms, and prevention of contamination from environmental sources, including the elimination of rodents.

References

Anonymous (1988). *Salmonella enteritidis* phage type 4: Chicken and egg. Lancet, ii, 720-722.

Giessen, A.W. van de; Peters, R.; Berkers, P.A.T.A.; Jansen, W.H.; Notermans, S.H.W. (1991). *Salmonella* contamination of poultry flocks in The Netherlands. Veterinary Quarterly, 13, 41-46.

Hoogenboom-Verdegaal, A.M.M.; During, M.; Leentvaart-Kuypers, A., Peerbooms, P.G.H; Kooij, W.C.M.; Vlerken, R. van; Sobczak, H. (1989). Epidemiologisch en microbiologisch onderzoek met betrekking tot gastro-enteritis bij de mens in de regio's Amsterdam en Helmond, in 1987. RIVM report no. 148612001, RIVM, Bilthoven, The Netherlands (in Dutch).

Hoogenboom-Verdegaal, A.M.M; During, M.; Engels, G.B.; Hoogenveen, R.T.; Hoekstra, J.A.; Bosch, D.A. van den; Kuyvenhoven, J.V.; Mertens, P.L.J.M.; Smidt, I.R. (1992). Een bevolkingsonderzoek naar maag/darmklachten in vier regio's van Nederland uitgevoerd in 1991. Deel Onderzoeksmethodiek en incidentie berekening gastro-enteritis. RIVM report 149101001, RIVM, Bilthoven, The Netherlands (in Dutch).

Humphrey, T.J.; Baskerville, A.; Mawer, S.; Rowe, B.; Hopper, S. (1989). *Salmonella enteritidis* phage type 4 from the contents of intact eggs: study involving naturally infected hens. Epidemiology and Infection, 103, 415-418.

Humphrey, T.J. (1991). Numbers of *Salmonella enteritidis* in the contents of naturally contaminated hens' eggs. Epidemiology and Infection, 106, 485-486.

ICMSF (1986). Microorganisms in Food. Part 2. Sampling for Microbiological Analysis: Principles and Specific Applications. 2nd edn. Blackwell Science, Oxford.

In 't Veld, P.H.; Notermans, S. (1992). The use of reference materials (spray dried milk artificially contaminated with *Salmonella typhimurium*) to validate detection methods for *Salmonella*. Journal of Food Production.

Krug, W. (1985). Cost benefit analysis of *Salmonella* eradication. In: Epidemiological Studies of Risks Associated with the Agricultural Use of Sewage Sludge: Knowledge and Needs. Block J.C.; Havelaar, A.H.; L'Hermite, P.L. (Eds.). Elsevier Applied Science Publishers, London/New York, pp. 34-41.

McLeod, S.; Barrow, P.A. (1991). Lipopolysaccharide specific IgG in egg-yolks from two chicken flocks infected with *Salmonella enteritidis*. Letters in Applied Microbiology, 294-297.

Roberts, T. (1989). Human illness costs of foodborne bacteria. American Journal of Agricultural Economics, 71, 468-474.

Roberts, T.; Sockett, P.N.; Sill, O.N. (1991). Economic impact of a nation wide outbreak of salmonellosis: cost -benefit of an early intervention. British Medical Journal, 298, 1227-1230.

Rodrique, D.C.; Tauxe, R.V.; Rowe, B. (1990). International increase of *S.enteritidis*: A new pandemic? Epidemiology and Infection, 105, 21-27.

St. Louis, M.E.; Morse, D.L.; Potter, M.E. (1988). The emergence of grade A eggs as a major source of *Salmonella enteritidis* infections. Journal of the American Medical Association, 259, 2103-2107.

Todd, E. (1989). Preliminary estimates of costs of foodborne diseases in the United States. Journal of Food Protection, 52, 595-601.

WHO report (1989). Report of the WHO consultation on epidemiological emergency in poultry and egg salmonellosis. WHO/CDS/VPH 89.82. WHO.

Part III

Investigation of Disease Occurrence and Disease Control

E.A.M. Graat
Wageningen University
Department of Animal Sciences
Quantitative Veterinary Epidemiology Group
The Netherlands

J.P.T.M. Noordhuizen,
Department of Farm Animal Health
Faculty of Veterinary Medicine
University of Utrecht
The Netherlands

1. Introduction

In this part III the application of epidemiological principles, as discussed in previous chapters, is outlined for the investigation and controlling of a disease outbreak and/or epidemics.

Occurrence of diseases might have considerable consequences for animal as well as human health and welfare, and economics. The importance of a disease relates to multiple dimensions. First of all, animal diseases might endanger public health. These are the zoonoses and foodborne infections (e.g., leptospirosis, salmonellosis, Campylobacter infections). In diseases, not communicable to humans, two other aspects are important: the disease might have an influence on the sector, on the individual farm or even on the individual animal. An example of the first one, influencing the sector, is classical swine fever, in which case export of pigs and pig meat is prohibited. Also, individual herds then might experience large economic losses due to destruction of the herd according to national regulations. Finally, the disease in an individual might result in decreased production, impaired welfare, or a decreased value of products of affected animals. Normally, in diseases of which the importance goes beyond that of the individual farmer, i.e., with zoonoses and diseases with export bans, (inter)national legislation exist. For diseases in which occurrence and seriousness merely act upon herd and individual level, the amount and intensity of (preventive) measures is determined by the cost benefit ratio. Thus, the extent of prevention and control of a specific disease depends on available measures, costs of the latter and benefits (e.g., increased production (efficiency)). Diseases of this latter type are not discussed in this part III, when addressing outbreak investigation.

In this part III, first different types of disease occurrence are described; outbreaks, epidemic and endemic disease occurrence. Then, factors related to disease occurrence are described. Subsequently, it is shown how to describe/display an outbreak or epidemic, which is followed by steps to be taken in the investigation process of an outbreak or epidemic, with possibilities for controlling and managing the disease.

2. Disease Occurrence

Roughly, there are three types of disease occurrence, namely endemic, epidemic and outbreaks. Thrusfield (1995) defined an outbreak as an identified occurrence of disease involving one or more animals. The terms outbreak and epidemic are often used synonymously, although an outbreak does not inevitably lead towards an epidemic. On the other hand, an outbreak can result in an epidemic and subsequently it might be possible in the end that the disease even becomes endemic. Nowadays, the term 'epidemic' is used when there is an unexpected and substantial increase in the incidence of a disease, and thus not a predictable increase. This definition implies that it can be used for endemic diseases as well, when there is a sudden increase in disease incidence of an endemic disease. Therefore, Martin *et al.* (1987) describe the term endemic as disease occurrence with a predictable pattern. An endemic disease can be prevalent at different levels of disease occurrence, e.g., low, moderate or high level.

The Office International des Epizooties (OIE, or World Organisation for Animal Health, 1996) defines outbreak as an occurrence of one of the diseases in list A or B (see Table 12.9) in an agricultural establishment, breeding establishment or premises, including all buildings and all adjoining premises where animals are present.

Table 12.9. Diseases of type A[1], a selection of B[2] diseases in cattle, pigs and birds and in the footnote an example of a C[3] disease as listed by the OIE (Office International des Epizooties).

List A	List B
Foot-and-mouth disease	Multiple Species
Vesicular stomatitis	- Aujeszky's disease
Swine vesicular disease	- Leptospirosis
Rinderpest	- Johne's disease
Peste des petits ruminants	- Rabies
Contagious bovine pleuropneumonia	Cattle
Lumpy skin disease	- Bovine brucellosis
Rift valley fever	- Infectious bovine rhinotracheitis
Bluetongue	- Bovine spongiform encephalopathy
Sheep pox and goat pox	Pigs
African horse sickness	- PEARS (mystery swine disease)
African swine fever	- Atrophic rhinitis
Classical swine fever (hog cholera)	- Transmissible gastro enteritis
Fowl plague	Birds
Newcastle disease	- Infectious bursal disease
	- Marek's disease
	- *Salmonella enteritidis*
	- *Salmonella typhimurium*

[1] Transmissible diseases which have the potential for very serious and rapid spread, irrespective of national borders, which are of serious socio-economic or public health consequence and which are of major importance in the international trade of animals and animal products.
[2] Transmissible diseases which are considered to be of socio-economic and/or public health importance within countries and which are significant in the international trade of animals and animal products.
[3] Communicable diseases with important socio-economic and/or sanitary influence at the local level, e.g., coccidiosis and bovine virus diarrhoea.

An example: When in a country, where coccidiosis is endemic, a large (usual) number of broiler flocks suffers from coccidiosis you do not call this an epidemic, whereas one case, i.e., outbreak of e.g., classical swine fever in a disease-free region is normally considered and treated as an epidemic.

3. Factors Related to Disease Occurrence

The occurrence of a disease depends on factors related to the host, the environment as well as the disease agent, and their interrelationships. These interrelations are depicted in Figure 12.5 (See also Chapter I for Evans' postulates). The three types of disease occurrence (epidemic, endemic, outbreak) are the result of the interaction between the host, agent and their environment. First, the agent of a disease might be a virus, bacteria, fungi etc., either host specific (e.g., swine vesicular disease) or not host specific at all (e.g., foot-and-mouth disease, although this disease only occurs in cloven-hooved animals). Some disease agents are very resistant to environmental conditions (e.g., *Bacillus anthrax*), whereas others are very susceptible to it (in general e.g., viruses).

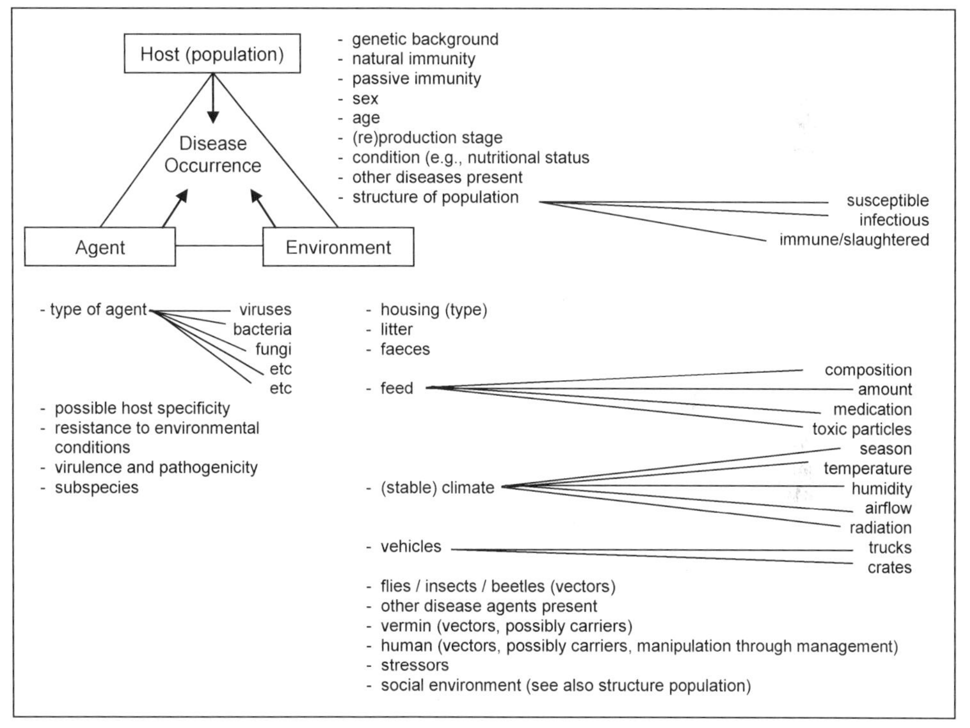

Figure 12.5. Factors of the (infectious) agent, host and environment related to occurrence of disease.

Whether or not an agent causes disease, depends amongst others on the balance between hosts (susceptibility/resistance) and agents (infection burden). The three types of disease occurrence give information about this balance (Martin *et al.*, 1987). Outbreaks are caused by the fact that the agent is suddenly present (by introduction) and infects the susceptible host, or that the infectious agent is always present but that disease occurrence is irregular and depends on other factors. For example, African swine fever is not present usually (in most developed countries), but when introduced it causes disease, whereas *E. coli* bacteria are present everywhere but only sometimes result in clinical mastitis, dependent on factors e.g., related to the environment and/or host (see Figure 12.5).

Also the structure of a population in terms of distribution of susceptible, immune and infectious (carriers) animals, is of importance with respect to spread of a disease. In a totally susceptible population, diseases will spread easily when an infectious individual is introduced. In most developed countries diseases may spread very rapidly, since animal density is relatively high and animals are fully susceptible since they do not acquire immunity during life. The introduction of disease is less likely in closed herds than in "open" herds where e.g., animals are purchased. However, in developed countries, closed populations are not truly closed, since -among other things- food, equipment and services (veterinarian, inseminators) are being introduced.

4. Describing and Displaying Disease Occurrence

As already stated in earlier chapters, epidemiology deals with the investigation of health and disease in populations. These populations can be groups of animals (e.g., litters, pens), individual farms, regions, etc. Per definition, in an epidemiological investigation of a disease it is described how many, among which groups, when and where morbidity and/or mortality occurs, always related to the population at risk. In epidemiological terms: the temporal and spatial distribution of morbidity and mortality in a defined population is described.

Measures of disease occurrence were already explained and described in Chapter IV. In disease outbreak investigation especially **incidence** and **incidence rate** are important parameters, since these make a distinction between existing and new arising cases. Incidence rate is better to use when a population is not closed and units enter or leave the population at risk; e.g., new gilts brought into a pig farrowing farm. The incidence rate is important when one wants to know the velocity of development of new cases in a certain population per time unit.

Description of disease outbreaks should be done carefully. Morbidity as well as mortality should be presented in a way that fluctuations become visible. Several methods can be used to display characteristics of the outbreak. For example, tables, histograms, graphs of cases against time, geographic maps, and geographical information systems (GIS). Tables are useful when they are transparent and give a good view on the situation. This means that only tables having only a few rows and columns are useful. Temporal patterns become clear in graphs, where cases or incidences can be displayed against time, (see e.g., Figure 12.6 for the number of farms positive for classical swine fever in The Netherlands during an outbreak period). Histograms are usually applied for displaying discrete variables or for frequency distributions of continuous data. Geographic maps and GIS can give a "birds eye view" of the situation of disease dynamics in a spatial context (Jalvingh *et al.*, 1995). It illustrates specific locations of the outbreak and gives a (quantitative) distribution of an outbreak. A GIS can also be used in the operational management of an outbreak to outline the protection, buffer and surveillance zones (Morris *et al.*, 1992).

In summary, patterns of disease can be used to generate hypotheses which give an explanation for disease occurrence (Martin *et al.*, 1987). It should, however, be done with care since occurrence may be affected by factors of the agent, host and environment (see paragraph 3). Especially with transient variables, e.g., a past environmental event, it might be difficult to find a relation between a cause and disease occurrence (see Chapters V and VI for studying relations between [causal] factors and diseases).

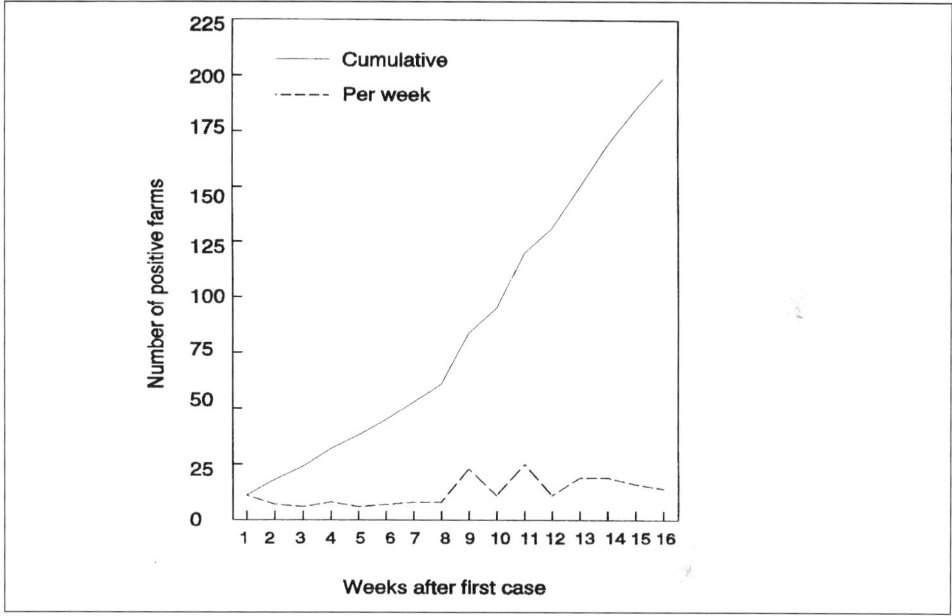

Figure 12.6. Classical swine fever: number of positive farms (per week as well as cumulative number) after the first farm diagnosed. Note: the epidemic had not yet come to an end when this figure was produced.

In summary, patterns of disease can be used to generate hypotheses which give an explanation for disease occurrence (Martin *et al.*, 1987). It should, however, be done with care since occurrence may be affected by factors of the agent, host and environment (see paragraph 3). Especially with transient variables, e.g., a past environmental event, it might be difficult to find a relation between a cause and disease occurrence (see Chapters V and VI for studying relations between [causal] factors and diseases).

5. Procedures for Investigating a Disease Outbreak

Reporting of suspected cases is the first step in the process of investigating a disease outbreak. A universally applicable outline cannot be given, since it is not valid for all disease situations. Nevertheless, it is useful to follow a standard protocol. Such a protocol comprises the different steps to be made in a logical order (see Figure 12.7) Subsequently, the occurrence of the specific disease has to be diagnosed/confirmed by laboratory examination in case of diseases with known aetiology or by statistical methods for diseases with unknown aetiology. In case of a highly contagious disease it is very important to confirm or set a diagnosis immediately in order to prevent further

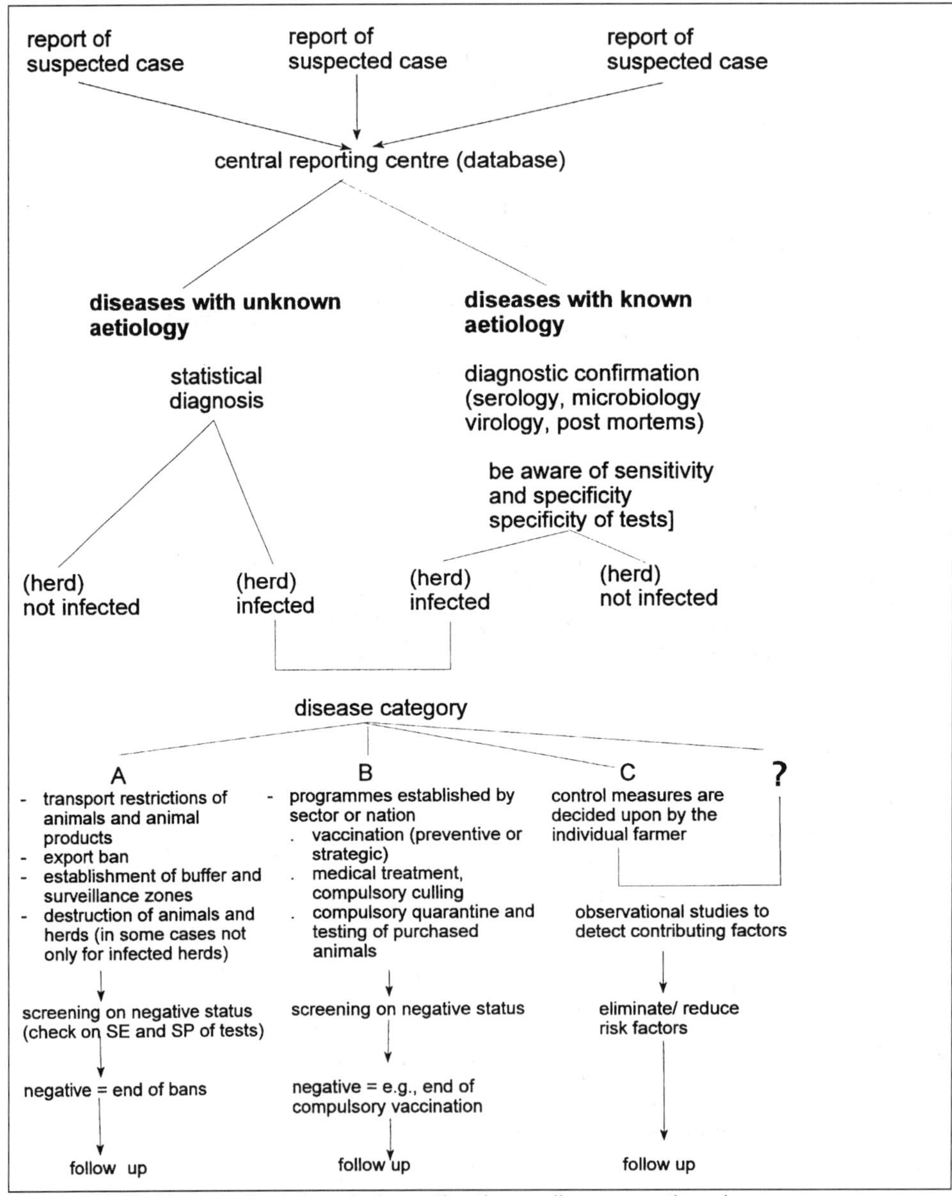

Figure 12.7. Steps to be taken in investigating a disease outbreak.

spread and to start the appropriate control measures to prevent an epidemic as soon as possible. For these two steps, it is supposed that veterinarians are capable of diagnosing the disease (which might become more and more difficult with rarely occurring diseases or diseases already being eradicated) and that reliable accurate diagnostic tests are available with sufficient laboratory capacity.

Disease reporting systems evolve increasingly, both at national and international level, mainly as a result of the rapid development of computers and computer programmes to record, analyze and exchange data. Some computer programmes can be obtained freely, and are very easily downloaded from the world wide web. E.g., WINEPISCOPE and EPI-INFO[42]. The latter guides you, amongst others in conducting an epidemiological investigation of an epidemic.

In particular diseases (e.g., foot-and-mouth disease, hog cholera) one infectious agent is the primary cause of disease. Then, factors of the host and the environment are of no or minor importance. In so-called, multifactorial diseases the interaction between host, agent, and environment is not clearly identified. Many of these multifactorial diseases are endemic, and therefore not further elaborated in this chapter.

5.1. Diseases with known aetiology

There are many diseases which can be diagnosed on the basis of clinical signs and/or laboratory tests (e.g., classical swine fever, Newcastle disease), provided that appropriate diagnostic tests are available. One should always be aware of the diagnostic methods which can result in misclassification leading to false-positives or false-negatives (see Chapter IV about sensitivity, specificity and predictive values of a diagnostic test). The reason for an outbreak might be purchase of (latently) infected materials, being food or animals (carriers), or may not be obvious at all.

5.2. Diseases with unknown aetiology

Outbreak investigation is very difficult if an infectious agent is not found, or not known. The reasoning of causation is very difficult in case of sudden drop in (re)production. In the early 90's this was the case with the so-called mystery swine disease or also named PEARS (Porcine Epidemic Abortion and Respiratory Syndrome) in The Netherlands and Germany.

The definition of a suspected farm was: A farm where in the 8 previous weeks an unusual number of spontaneous abortions or premature births in sows and death or weakness in young piglets was observed. At that time the agent was not identified, so an adequate diagnostic test was not available. Hence, the definition led towards different interpretations of "an unusual number". Therefore, it was tempting to attribute each drop in production to the mystery swine disease. Schukken *et al.* (1991) described objective criteria based on statistical methods to suspect a farm, and similar, to declare a farm free of the disease. The statistical method was based on calculated

[42] See Chapter II for references

"default" values, variance and frequency distribution of herd performance data as number of stillborn piglets per litter, the average number of live piglets per litter and piglet mortality before weaning. To classify a farm as having PEARS, 2 out of these 3 parameters should deviate from the average of the litters observed in the period before problems started. One has to observe at least 20 litters, or a maximum of one month. The authors made 3 tables on which diagnosis of PEARS can be made. One table (Table 12.10) is shown as an example. Horizontally, the average number of live born piglets per litter in the period preceding the problems, is denoted. Vertically, you can find the number of litters on which the average in the problem period is based. When the value of the parameter in the observation period is lower than the value denoted in the table, PEARS might be involved. An example: when on a farm, having a normal average of 10 piglets born alive, and 50 litters in the problem observation period, the number of piglets born alive drops under 9.04, PEARS might be involved. When 2 out of the 3 parameters deviate, then the diagnosis is "set". The authors made similar tables for farms to be declared free of the problems.

Table 12.10. PEARS decision table for the parameter "number of live born piglets before problems started (yearly average)" (Schukken et al., 1991).

No. of litters	9.00	9.25	9.50	9.75	10.00	10.25	10.50	10.75	11.00	11.25	11.50
20.0	7.49	7.74	7.99	8.24	8.49	8.74	8.99	9.24	9.49	9.74	9.99
30.0	7.77	8.02	8.27	8.52	8.77	9.02	9.27	9.52	9.77	10.02	10.27
40.0	7.93	8.18	8.43	8.68	8.93	9.18	9.43	9.68	9.93	10.18	10.43
50.0	8.04	8.29	8.54	8.79	9.04	9.29	9.54	9.79	10.04	10.29	10.54
60.0	8.13	8.38	8.63	8.88	9.13	9.38	9.63	9.88	10.13	10.38	10.63
70.0	8.19	8.44	8.69	8.94	9.19	9.44	9.69	9.94	10.19	10.44	10.69
80.0	8.24	8.49	8.74	8.99	9.24	9.49	9.74	9.99	10.24	10.49	10.74
90.0	8.29	8.54	8.79	9.04	9.29	9.54	9.79	10.04	10.29	10.54	10.79
100.0	8.32	8.57	8.82	9.07	9.32	9.57	9.82	10.07	10.32	10.57	10.82
110.0	8.36	8.61	8.86	9.11	9.36	9.61	9.86	10.11	10.36	10.61	10.86
120.0	8.38	8.63	8.88	9.13	9.38	9.63	9.88	10.13	10.38	10.63	10.88
130.0	8.41	8.66	8.91	9.16	9.41	9.66	9.91	10.16	10.41	10.66	10.91
140.0	8.43	8.68	8.93	9.18	9.43	9.68	9.93	10.18	10.43	10.68	10.93
150.0	8.45	8.70	8.95	9.20	9.45	9.70	9.95	10.20	10.45	10.70	10.95

6. Disease Control Strategies

First of all, in order to avoid introduction of diseases each country has its own import regulations. In the EU those regulations are deduced from official directives of the European Commission, such as 92/117/EC for the control of zoonoses, 64/432/EC for the control of brucellosis, 77/96/EC for the control of trichinosis, or 64/433/EC for fresh meat.

Is the disease a notifiable disease, then there are government regulations or legislation. In Table 12.9 the List A, some List B and C diseases of the OIE, the World Organisation for Animal Health are listed. The OIE informs governments of occurrence and course of animal diseases throughout the world, and of ways to control the disease. They coordinate studies involving surveillance and control of animal diseases. Thirdly, they harmonize regulations for trade in animals and animal products for their member countries (n=144 by December 1996). Notifiable diseases are characterized by the obligation to report, slaughtering of diseased and suspected herds (animals), disinfection, transport prohibition etc. These measures might apply to herds, regions, counties, as well as countries.

Control strategies usually depend on the type of disease. Below some possible actions are listed:

- doing nothing
- movement restrictions
- quarantine
- vaccination: preventive or strategic (around centre of outbreak)
- medical treatment
- zootechnical measures (improved husbandry)
- disinfection
- stamping out/slaughter/culling
- risk management
- follow up ------> monitoring and surveillance programs.

Monitoring constitutes on-going programs directed at the detection of changes in prevalence of disease in a given population and its environment, whereas surveillance means the continuous investigation of a given population to detect the occurrence of disease for active control purposes, which may involve testing of a part of the population (OIE, 1996). When monitoring and surveillance programs are used in the control or eradication of diseases we should have knowledge about the possibilities to take action, including the costs and benefits of such an action. Part I of this chapter deals with monitoring and surveillance in more detail.

An example of an investigation and controlling procedure of an outbreak of classical swine fever in a CSF-free country is the following.

To prevent the outbreak of becoming epidemic, a huge amount of resources is needed (money as well as human labour). When a farm is found positive the program starts with preventive measures to prevent spreading. In a zone of 10 kilometres around the affected herd, transportation of animals and manure is prohibited. The diseased herd is being stamped out and surveillance of farms in the surveillance zone is intensified to detect new cases (due to contacts with the primary source of infection) as soon as possible. Sometimes, preventive eradication of surrounding herds takes place. In general, vaccination strategies might be an alternative to protect all the herds in the protection zone, provided that these vaccines result in a possible discrimination between field virus and vaccine virus, and that vaccines are allowed. Furthermore, herds need to be screened on their negative status (be aware of the sensitivity and specificity of used diagnostic tests). When a complete negative status is reached all bans can be cancelled. A follow-up procedure should safeguard herds from re-introduction, or at least in detecting a re-introduction before it can be spread.

In taking control measures it is important to know which factors have an effect on disease occurrence or disease prevention.

7. Discussion

Control is not only directed towards diseases with a known cause. Control often is based on observational studies (see Chapters V and IV). This type of epidemiological studies into factors involved in disease occurrence can lead to actions to be taken, even when the causal agent is not identified. An example of this is the ban of meat and bonemeal in feed after having found an increased risk in occurrence of BSE with consumption of meat and bone meal (Wilesmith *et al.*, 1992). In case of multifactorial diseases, observational epidemiological studies might lead to the most efficient strategy to control the disease by ranking risk factors and calculate the attributable proportion (see Chapter V).

To carry out policy measures, it is a prerequisite to have an unambiguous case definition. So, whenever the diagnosis, based on biological rationales, e.g., demonstration of pathogens, antigen or antibodies, is not possible, the diagnosis might be made by statistical procedures (see paragraph 5).

In countries, with a disease-free status and without application of preventive vaccinations, any outbreak will most likely spread rapidly because the animal population is highly susceptible. Should a contagious outbreak occur, then it is of major importance to identify and eliminate all sources of the infectious agent. To react adequately, one needs to understand disease dynamics. Furthermore, during an outbreak a lot of different types of data is produced. Computerized decision support systems may help managing the data and set priorities for control measures. These systems consist of interactive computer-based systems and help decision makers to solve the problems. An example is EpiMAN, a comprehensive database, with spatial data managed by a GIS, data managed by a database management system, and epidemiological knowledge (models and expert systems) of foot-and-mouth disease (Morris *et al.*, 1992; Jalvingh *et al.*, 1995). EpiMAN can be used for operational (daily) management during the outbreak and be used by policy makers for strategic management of the outbreak by conducting "what-if" scenarios of different strategies and their effects on spread of diseases, direct costs of eradication and indirect costs of export bans. The latter one, also comprises a tool for researching and testing control strategies before an outbreak, and in case a real outbreak occurs optimize future control strategies. For these systems, however, a sound knowledge of, amongst others, pathogenesis and risk factors of specific diseases needs to be available. So, for implementing these systems still many epidemiological studies have to be done.

References

Jalvingh, A.W.; Nielen, M.; Dijkhuizen, A.A.; Morris, R.S. (1995). Review article: A computerized decision support system for contagious animal disease control. Pig News and Information, 16, 9N-12N.
Martin, S.W.; Meek, A.H.; Willeberg, P. (1987). Veterinary Epidemiology: Principles and Methods. Iowa State University Press, Ames, Iowa.
Morris, R.S.; Sanson, R.L.: Stern, M.W. (1992). EpiMAN: a decision support system for managing a foot-and-mouth disease epidemic. In: Proceedings of the Annual Meeting of the Dutch Society for Veterinary Epidemiology and Economics, December 1992, Wageningen. Frankena, K.; Hoofd, C.M. van der (Eds.). pp. 1-35.
OIE (1996). International Animal Health Code. Office International des Epizooties, 1996.
Schukken, Y.H.; Jong, M.C.M. de; Komijn, R.E.; Braamskamp, J.; Dijkhuizen, A.A.; Noordhuizen, J.P.T.M.; Vernooy, J.C.M; Verheijden, J.H.M. (1991). Diagnoses Porcine Epidemic Abortion and Respiratory Syndrome (PEARS)-positive and PEARS-negative for breeding and multiplier herds in The Netherlands using statistical methods. Tijdschrift voor Diergeneeskunde, 117, 259-264 (In Dutch).
Thrusfield, M. (1995). Veterinary Epidemiology. 2nd edn. Blackwell Science, Oxford.
Wilesmith, H.W.; Ryan, J.B.M.; Hueston, W.D. (1992). Bovine spongiform encephalopathy: case control studies of calf feeding practices and meat and bonemeal inclusion in proprietary concentrates. Research in Veterinary Science, 52, 325-331.

Part IV

Questionnaires for Field Surveys: Design and Conduct

J.P.T.M. Noordhuizen
Department of Farm Animal Health
Faculty of Veterinary Medicine
University of Utrecht
The Netherlands

1. Introduction

Field surveys are frequently applied in veterinary epidemiological research (see Chapter V). They are specifically useful to determine disease prevalence, to assess the rate of adoption of disease control programmes (see Chapter XII, part III), and to identify conditions or factors possibly contributing to disease occurrence (Edwards, 1990). Field surveys represent easy, rather cheap and rapid methodologies for achieving these objectives.

Yet, these surveys are frequently poorly designed and conducted yielding data which cannot be analyzed properly and leading to inconclusive results. The data are usually collected through questionnaires, where questions relate to the conditions or factors under study. Questionnaires appear as simple media but are usually rather complex in nature. Results of a questionnaire based survey are largely depending on the quality of the collected data. Therefore, much attention has to be paid to the design and technical features of a questionnaire.

At the same time, the animal or herd sample is a major constraint for performing proper field surveys. Theory and exercises related to determine sample size, including aspects such as population size, confidence level, expected prevalence of the disease and error, are discussed in Chapter III. This part IV deals with the design, limitations and conduct of questionnaires for field surveys.

2. Survey Objectives

Before starting a survey in the field one should clearly state the objectives. The most frequently stated objectives of a field survey are the determination of the prevalence level of a disease and/or the identification of conditions and factors possibly contributing to the disease prevalence. Each objective requires another sampling procedure (see paragraph 5 of this chapter and Chapter III).

2.1. The disease

In order to study a disease one has to establish a case definition. What is comprised in the disease diagnosis and what is not? And are there levels of severity of the disease involved? Or, what is the observational level, clinical or subclinical (e.g., serological)? And, if one is studying a disease syndrome, are there different levels of diagnosis (e.g., lameness *versus* footrot, Mortellaro disease, laminitis)? An example of cattle lameness diagnosis scoring list is given in Figure 12.8.

Assignment (1): try to establish a case definition for a field survey on PRRS (porcine respiratory and reproductive syndrome) in pigs.

Assignment (2): try to establish a case definition for a field survey on lameness in dairy calves, including different levels of severity.

Lameness Diagnosis Protocol

Date trimming:	Cow number:	Parity:
Farm code:	Pedigree number:	Breed:
Trimmer code:	Birth date:	Sire:
Observer:	Calving date:	Dry:

	Right Hind						Left Hind						Right Front						Left Front					
	outer			inner			outer			inner			outer			inner			outer			inner		
Diagnosis	1	2	3	1	2	3	1	2	3	1	2	3	1	2	3	1	2	3	1	2	3	1	2	3
Dermatitis interdig.	☐	☐	☐	☐	☐	☐	☐	☐	☐	☐	☐	☐	☐	☐	☐	☐	☐	☐	☐	☐	☐	☐	☐	☐
Laminitis	☐			☐			☐			☐			☐			☐			☐			☐		
Phlegmona interdig.	☐			☐			☐			☐			☐			☐			☐			☐		
Dermatitis digitalis	☐			☐			☐			☐			☐			☐			☐			☐		
Sole lesion WL[1]	☐	☐	☐	☐	☐	☐	☐	☐	☐	☐	☐	☐	☐	☐	☐	☐	☐	☐	☐	☐	☐	☐	☐	☐
Sole lesion TY[2]	☐	☐	☐	☐	☐	☐	☐	☐	☐	☐	☐	☐	☐	☐	☐	☐	☐	☐	☐	☐	☐	☐	☐	☐
Sole lesion SO[3]	☐	☐	☐	☐	☐	☐	☐	☐	☐	☐	☐	☐	☐	☐	☐	☐	☐	☐	☐	☐	☐	☐	☐	☐
White line process	☐	☐		☐	☐		☐	☐		☐	☐		☐	☐		☐	☐		☐	☐		☐	☐	
Sole ulcer	☐	☐		☐	☐		☐	☐		☐	☐		☐	☐		☐	☐		☐	☐		☐	☐	
White line separation	☐			☐			☐			☐			☐			☐			☐			☐		
Hyperplasia interdig.	☐			☐			☐			☐			☐			☐			☐			☐		
Bent claw	☐			☐			☐			☐			☐			☐			☐			☐		
Clinically lame	☐						☐						☐						☐					

[1] WL = White line area
[2] TY = typical sole ulcer area
[3] SO = sole area

Figure 12.8. An example of a dairy cattle lameness diagnosis scoring list.

3. The Data

3.1. Risk factors

Usually an ample literature search is carried out to collect information on the disease under study and its relationship with animal factors and environmental factors or conditions. These literature references commonly report results from experimental work. For example, the relationship between a disease in fattening pigs and climatic conditions of the houses, or the relationship between vaccination and maternal antibodies in broilers. It appears that most of these literature references deal with such conditions or factors in a rather monodisciplinary way; a multifactorial approach where interactions between factors and confounding are addressed, is hardly or not applied. Therefore, one has to be careful with naming certain factors causal in all cases. The literature search should provide the researcher with the basic information about factors to be addressed in the questionnaire. An example of such basic factors is given below for *Actinobacillus pleuropneumoniae* (App) in fattening pigs (Table 12.11).

Table 12.11. Basic factors or conditions possibly related to the occurrence of App (Actinobacillus pleuropneumoniae) in fattening pigs (literature based).

* strategy for purchasing pigs (from 1, 2 or more multipliers)
* mixing of pigs/changing pens
* frequency of input of pigs (weekly/monthly/yearly/irregular)
* strategy of input of pigs (per house/per division/per pen)
* health index of the herd (related to Aujeszky's disease and parainfluenza)
* season (winter)
* ventilation system (direct air inlet) (mechanical *versus* natural)
* aerosolization and direct contact opportunities
* temperature fluctuations in the pig house
* medication type and duration
* number of houses, herd size
* pig density per pen or m^2
* density during transportation
* other transport stressors

The animal and environment related factors can be many. For the animal factors, variables such as breed, sex, age or parity, production stage, immune status or vaccination status can be involved. For the environmental factors, variables such as housing factors, feeding factors, hygiene factors, climatic factors, management factors are comprised. These variables are usually organized in clusters. Housing factors is such a cluster; it contains several, more detailed factors such as age of the premises, ventilation system, size, number of units per house, number of pens per unit.

Another example of this combination of animal factors and environmental factors is given in Table 12.12. It has been derived from a study on salmonellosis in broiler breeder flocks (Henken *et al.*, 1992). The factors or conditions listed in the table are used for designing a relational diagram, the next step in the design process.

Table 12.12. Animal and environment related factors, possibly contributing to the occurrence of salmonellosis in broiler breeder flocks (Henken et al., 1992).

* feed mill (small *versus* large)
* geographic region (north *versus* south)
* other poultry farms around (> 1 km *versus* < 1 km)
* farm type (litter *versus* battery type)
* ventilation system (natural *versus* mechanical)
* age of the buildings
* flock size (> 15000 *versus* < 15000 birds)
* number of buildings
* number of egg collection rounds (once daily *versus* frequent)
* hygiene barriers (poor *versus* good)
* order and tidiness (poor *versus* good)
* disinfection tub present (no *versus* yes)
* other species on the premises (no *versus* yes)

4. Relational Diagram

When the literature search has been performed and, if needed, experts have been interviewed, all variables should be put into a relational diagram. In this graphical representation, the variables are positioned in such a way that their interaction and interdependence is visualized. Such a relational diagram can be useful for both the design of the questionnaire and the analysis of collected data. An example of a relational diagram is presented in Figure 12.9 on infectious bursal disease (IBD, or Gumboro disease) in poultry (Noordhuizen *et al.*, 1994) and in Figure 10.1.

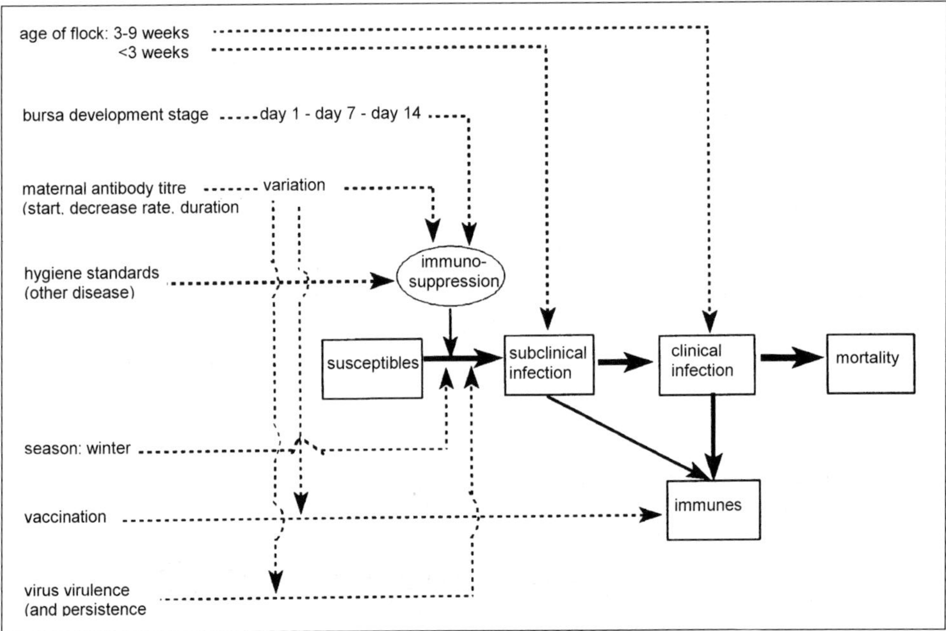

Figure 12.9. An example of a relation-diagram for factors involved in the occurrence of infectious bursal disease (IBD, or Gumboro disease) of poultry.

5. Sample of Herds/Animals

The number of herds or animals to be sampled depends on the primary objective(s) of the survey. For example, to determine the sample size for studying the prevalence of dairy herds infected with leptospirosis in a region needs another procedure than the assesment of percentage of infected animals within herds. However, for evaluation of risk factors, one needs at least 4 observations (herds/animals) for each risk factor (Greenland, 1985). Thus, for a questionnaire dealing with 50 questions, each representing a potential risk factor, 200 respondents are needed. Also the features of the diagnostic test involved may be different at the herd compared to the individual animal level. Both issues have been addressed in preceding chapters (Chapter III, IV and V).

For this part of Chapter XII, the questionnaire for prevalence estimation is not applicable; emphasis is on a questionnaire related to risk factor identification (see Chapter IV for prevalence estimation).

6. Response Rate

The primary goal for any survey should be to maximize the response rate, thus to minimize the non-response rate. If the sample size calculations have yielded a certain sample size, a high rate of non-responders can make the ultimate sample useless to the purpose of the survey, or at least not representative or inconclusive. Therefore, the proportion of responders is more important than the total sample size. Non-responders may have characteristics that are not (fully) equalized in the responders, resulting in bias.

There are several ways to increase the response rate (Edwards, 1990):

1. persistence
   For example, letters of reminding or telephone contact with the non-responders may stimulate them to cooperate.
2. personal contact
   The use of telephone questionnaires or personal interviews will usually reduce the number of non-responders.
3. ease of response
   Mail questionnaires should include at least an addressed and stamped return envelope. It is obvious that a single page form will be easier filled and returned than a 20 page questionnaire.
4. induction of response
   Farmers can be induced to return the forms if it is indicated that they may benefit from the results. Sometimes more or less attractive prizes are set on questionnaire return, e.g., for the first 50 that are returned.
5. timing of the questionnaire
   Farming activities usually show seasonal peaks. Hence, it is not advisable to send mail questionnaires during e.g., harvesting time. Furthermore, it is advised to check whether or not other surveys will take place in the same period.
6. interviewer training and planning
   The approach taken by the interviewer often strongly influences the way that questions are asked, but also the way answers are given.

Additionally, it is common practice that, above the number of farms estimated by the sample size calculations, one adds more farms or animals to serve as replacement in case of drop-outs; as a rule of thumb one may add 5 or 10% to the calculated sample.

7. Questionnaires

A questionnaire can be defined as a research method meant for collecting information about events (disease), related factors and conditions, opinions and measures. It comprises a series of questions associated with the event under study and based on given objectives. These objectives can be categorized as:

1. to describe a certain situation such as the description of disease occurrence in a region over a given time period;
2. to analyze a situation for better understanding e.g., an analysis of risk factors for leptospirosis, and;
3. to evaluate certain actions which have been taken such as interventions or education (after Dufour, 1994).

8. Pro's and Con's of Different Questionnaire Methods

Roughly spoken, there are three basic methods for questionnaire surveys: the mail questionnaire, the telephone questionnaire, the personal questionnaire. Each of these have advantages and disadvantages, which will be addressed in this paragraph. In Chapter V some additional issues related to questionnaires have been addressed (Dillman, 1978).

8.1. Mail questionnaires

Advantages:
Mail questionnaires are usually inexpensive. The format is standardized since each respondent will receive the same forms and questions. Hence, interviewer bias is avoided. The questions can be answered at the most convenient time for the respondent. On the other hand, this may cause delay in response or non-response, especially if the farmer is asked to look through his own records for information. Mail questionnaires are particularly suitable to collect factual data. It is a rapid method for obtaining information.

Disadvantages:
As pointed out above, the rate of non-response may be high, sometimes very high; depending on the interest of the farmer for the subject and the time it takes to fill in questions. If questions require a diagnosis then the answers may be unreliable. In particular those farmers who experienced a certain disease among their animals are more likely to respond than those who are not. This may cause considerable bias; even more when the response rate is low. Mail questionnaires are not suitable for collecting data on opinions and attitudes. Answers will then frequently be incomplete and often not accurate. Questions must be very simple, uniform in explanation and without need for further clarification. Those questions are often in a multiple choice format or closed question format; open questions are difficult to standardize and to code. Answers on personal questions are difficult to obtain, e.g., questions about income or personal attitude.

8.2. Personal questionnaires

Advantages:
In animal health surveys, response rates over 90% can be obtained, thus reducing the non-response rate (example: Frankena *et al.*, 1993). On the other hand, more chance of interviewer bias may occur. Questionnaires may be longer, comprising more and more complex questions than a mail questionnaire. Interviews of 1 hour are common practice. If the interview can be combined with inspection of the animals and/or the premises, considerable improvement of the diagnosis can be made. An example of such a combination is in Frankena *et al.* (1993; 1994). If needed, a further clarification of questions and answers can be given. Animals can be examined and samples taken, increasing the accuracy of the diagnosis. The personal interview is also suitable for asking questions on opinions and attitudes. Data obtained through this personal survey can be entered into a portable computer on the spot, e.g., in spread sheet programmes, checked for completeness and integrity, and entered into the central system after the visit. This reduces the error level and time for coding, writing and data entrance. At the other hand, more time is needed to prepare such a software programme for a pre-coded questionnaire. EPI-INFO provides a module on questionnaire design (see Chapter II for references).

Disadvantages:
The interviewer bias is one of the greatest disadvantages since interviewers may influence both the questions and the answers, and hence the accuracy of the response data. The number of interviewers should be restricted as much as possible. An adequate training of interviewers should be performed prior to the field survey. Personal questionnaires are often more expensive than mail or telephone questionnaires because more labour is involved as well as travel expenses.

8.3. Telephone questionnaires

Advantages:
This method is relatively cheap; it is a common method in social sciences and polls. Information is obtained rapidly and the response rate can be comparable to those of personal questionnaires. Information about opinions and attitudes can be obtained though roughly.

Disadvantages:
These questionnaires need to be shorter and the questions less complex than in the personal questionnaire. A telephone interview should last between 10 and 20 minutes at maximum. Animals cannot be examined and samples not taken.

As can be read from the listed advantages and disadvantages per method, it are the objectives of the survey which will determine which method is most appropriate. If animals need to be examined, such as in the case of the lameness study in dairy calves and cows by Smits *et al.* (1992) and Frankena *et al.* (1993; 1994), then the personal questionnaire is most appropriate. If samples need to be taken, the same is valid. If only opinions about the estimated ranking of diseases in pigs are wanted, a telephone questionnaire may be appropriate. Sometimes, additional information can be obtained through a short telephone survey after a previous personal or mail questionnaire survey, e.g., to complete the data and avoid missing values.

9. Questionnaire Design

The basic requirements for the design of a questionnaire are, that it must be easy to read, have clear instructions and be relevant. Edwards (1990) states that "a questionnaire must be treated as a delicate scientific instrument and should be calibrated, monitored and used accordingly".

The following items must be considered when designing a questionnaire:

1. size

   A questionnaire should be as short as reasonably possible without interfering with the collection of desired information. The methodology (mail, personal, telephone) will largely determine what is possible.

2. topics

   The variety of topics should be restricted as much as possible. By preference one should limit oneself to one disease-complex at the time or to the general health status.

   The questionnaire should comprise the headings of the clusters of variables (see Figure 12.8, Tables 12.11 and 12.12), and per heading the subsequent, more detailed questions on the items (see the relational diagram in Figure 10.1 and Figure 12.9).

3. appearance

   A questionnaire should be attractive and look professionally produced, especially in the case of mail questionnaires. The sequence of the questions must be easy to follow, letter type of high quality, and attractiveness increased by the use of colour pictures or drawings.

4. types of questions

   The choice of question type is depending on the kind of information desired and the type of survey conducted. Combinations of question types are also possible. The following question types can be distinguished:

   a. Open or free questions: any answer is possible; there is no restriction on length; the answer is written down and coded later; in the case that answers are pre-coded the interviewer may match the given answers with one of the pre-coded ones. This type is suitable for answers on opinions using personal questionnaires, but not in mail questionnaires. They are sometimes used as opening or closing questions to put the interviewee at ease.

   b. Closed questions: there are several types of such questions; the responder is forced to choose from a limited number of options. Dichotomous questions such as "yes/no". In this case, often an additional option must be included as well, such as "don't know".

      For example: "do you apply teatdip after milking?"

      □ yes
      □ no

or

□ always
□ sometimes □ specific cows
□ never

c. Multiple choice questions are easy to code and analyze. The range of answers is limited. Interviewer bias is reduced because the range of answers is already set. This type is very useful for mail questionnaires. When they are used in personal questionnaires the possible answers should be read aloud.

For example: "who is milking the cows?"
□ you
□ your wife/husband
□ a co-worker
□ other, i.e.; ____________________

Rating or intensity scales are used to define the strength of opinions and attitudes of the respondent. In social sciences the Thurstone's scale, Likert scale or Q-sort are often used for that purpose.

An example of an opinion question: " do you agree on the use of BST?"
□ strongly against
□ against
□ rather agree
□ agree
□ fully in favour
□ no opinion

Often questionnaires comprise mixed types of questions.

5. question construction

Questions should be short, clear and unambiguous. The interviewers should be trained to use the questions properly, that is without elaboration in proza. The meaning of a question should always be kept strictly. For that purpose Gardner (1978) has pointed out the 10 rules for question construction (Table 12.13).

Table 12.13. The 10 rules for constructing questions for surveys (Gardner, 1978).

1.	use words, phrases and style familiar to most people
2.	use simple words and simple short phrases
3.	be specific, without too much elaborate detail
4.	ask concise questions without a risk of ambiguous detail
5.	be precise and not vague
6.	aim for less than 20 words per question
7.	avoid bias and leading questions
8.	do not make presumptions
9.	be realistic and not hypothetical
10.	use common sense

6. word selection

Words should be selected carefully in order to ensure the correct meaning. For that purpose Payne (1951) proposed 6 considerations for each word to be selected:

does the word mean what we intend?
does the word have any other meaning?
does the context make the intended meaning clear?
does the word have more than one pronunciation?
is there any similar word that can be confusing?
is a simpler word or phrase available?

Edwards (1990) presents the following example of a question:

"Have you heard of heartworm disease in dogs?"

Possible answers: yes = 1; no = 2; not sure = 3.

Some people will answer "yes", because they have heard or read about it. Others will answer "yes", because they do not want to be regarded as ignorant. And again others will answer "yes", because they consider these worms to be one of the worms they regularly treat their dogs for.

This problem could have been avoided by splitting up the original question: first ask about worms in general, then follow by questions about more specific worms among which the heartworm can be included.
Another example:

"Did you vaccinate sheep against pulpy kidney?"

Some farmers will answer "no" because in their area, a sheep is considered the adult animal and does not include the lambs.
Another example:

"are the cows in good, medium or poor body condition?"

This question gives room for variable interpretation: there is no quantitative standard to refer to. The only possibility to minimize these problems is to work with one interviewer. In other situations it might be more advizable to use body condition scoring methods with a semi-quantitative scale of scoring (e.g., from 1 to 5).

7. pretesting of the questionnaire

The problems described under (6) can be largely overcome by pretesting the questionnaire among a small sample of farmers before its final use. Adjustments can then still be made. One of the questions which can be included is, for example, whether anything else to ask was forgotten. In spite of extensive literature search or expert consultation, things might be missed; on the other hand, farmers may have specific expertise in certain fields and sometimes may add relevant questions too.

10. Conduct of a Questionnaire Based Survey

All field surveys should be preceded by a letter of invitation asking for cooperation. Such a letter should explain the reasons for the survey and the expected potential benefits for the responder. Any official letter with office headings and the signature of a reputable, well-known person is likely to attract cooperation. Names and telephone numbers of contact persons should be provided. A letter which is personally addressed and signed will be more inviting than a photocopy. If external interviewers will be involved, the introductory letter should mention their names and some background information as well.

Interviewers should receive proper instructions on the conduct of the survey and on the way to complete the questionnaire. These instructions can be consulted at any time needed. Instructions are not comprised in the questionnaire itself. They refer to e.g., the time to conduct the questionnaire, to data entry methods, replacement strategies in case of drop-outs, to coding, to sampling. Interviewers should receive proper training to follow the questionnaire instructions as close as possible in order to avoid bias. Training also comprises the way not to lead the interviewees to the desired answers; any influencing of the interviewee should be avoided unless it is meant to guide the interviewee through the meaning of a certain question. Part of the training might be the pretesting of the questionnaire. For mail questionnaires, a self addressed, stamped envelope should be included for the return mail.

A new approach to identify risk factors and rank them according to perceived relevance regards the application of conjoint analysis (Steenkamp, 1985; Vriens, 1995). The conjoint analysis procedure, CAP, originates from marketing studies investigating the consumer preferences. CAP refers to a decompositional method to describe a product with a set (=conjoint) of attributes assuming certain values. Respondents are asked to assign a rank or score to a given attribute or profile of attributes. Animal disease and related risk factors can be considered as "product and attributes". Within the CAP, a disease is identified and the relevance of risk factors assessed by consulted experts through a computerized questionnaire. Standard software is on the market.[43] The answers and scores on risk factors and profiles are classified by software, after weighing consistency in answering within and between experts (= interviewers). Questions and profiles are deduced from literature search for risk factors and the associated relational diagram. An example of the application of CAP for assessing the relevance of risk factors for S. *dublin* on dairy farms is presented by Schouten *et al.* (1997).

Confidentiality should be provided and maintained as long as possible. The use of code numbers instead of owner's names must be emphasized. A "confidential" mark can be placed on the questionnaire forms.

Interviewers should strictly stick to the time set for an interview. Sometimes this is rather hard to do, since farmers often like to tell their story in full. The organization of the interview should be such that time is reserved for that, but **after** the interview.

[43] Sawtooth Software (1993) ACA system: a manual for adaptive conjoint analysis.

Good responses in future questionnaire surveys is better guaranteed, if responders receive a copy of the (summary of the) results of the survey, in plain, comprehensible text after the analysis of the survey. Together with this copy, a letter of acknowledgement should be sent to the responders, explaining the value of their contribution and the relevance of the findings.

Many different analysis procedures for survey data can be followed. Among these are the descriptive methods, such as means, standard deviations, histograms, graphs and maps, describing the features of the sampled population. The next step in the analysis is a certain series of statistical methods, meant e.g., to estimate associations between variables from the questionnaire/survey and a disease event. The statistical methods vary from bivariate to multivariate. Examples are: cross tabulations, ANOVA, simple regression analysis, multiple regression, Mantel-Haenszel, cluster analysis, logistic regression. Some of these analysis procedures are addressed in the chapters V, VI and VII.

Finally, one could check the repeatability of the answers given by respondents in order to assess validity of the questionnaire outcome, estimating measurement errors, coding and typing errors, and interpretation differences between interviewees and interviewers. An example is given by Schukken *et al.* (1989).

References

Dillman, D.A. (1978). Mail and Telephone Surveys: the Total Design Method. John Wiley and Sons, New York.

Dufour, B. (1994) Le questionnaire d'enquete. Epidemiologie et Sante Animal, Bull de l'AEEMA No., 25, 101-112, ENVA, Maisons-Alfort, France.

Edwards, J.R. (1990). Surveys and questionnaires: design, conduct and analysis. In: Epidemiological Skills in Animal Health. Refresher Course for Veterinarians. Proceedings 143, October 1990. Kennedy, D. (Ed.). University of Sydney, Sydney, Australia.

Frankena, K.; Keulen, K.A.S. van; Noordhuizen, J.P.T.M.; Noordhuizen-Stassen, E.N.; Gundelach, J.; Jong, D.J. de; Saedt, I. (1993). A cross-sectional study of prevalence and risk factors of *dermatitis interdigitalis* in female dairy calves in the Netherlands. Preventive Veterinary Medicine, 17, 137-144.

Frankena, K.; Noordhuizen J.P.T.M.; Stassen, E.N. (1994). Applied epidemiology: another tool in dairy herd health programmes? Veterinary Research, 25, 234-238.

Gardner, G. (1978). Social Surveys for Social Planners. Holt, Rinehart and Winston Publishers, Sydney Australia.

Greenland, S. (1985). Power, sample size and smallest detectable effect determination for multivariate studies. Statistics in Medicine, 4, 117-127.

Henken, A.M.; Frankena, K.; Goelema, J.O.; Graat, E.A.M.; Noordhuizen, J.P.T.M. (1992). Multivariate epidemiological approach to salmonellosis in broiler breeder flocks. Poultry Science, 71, 838-843.

Noordhuizen, J.P.T.M.; Koenen, E.P.C.; Frankena, K. (1994). Simulation modelling of poultry diseases: a preliminary report on infectious bursal disease in broiler flocks. In: Proceedings of the International Society for Veterinary Epidemiology and Economics. Rowlands, G.J.; Kyule, M.N.; Perry, B.D. (Eds.). The Kenyan Veterinarian, 18, 382-385.

Payne, S.L. (1951). The Art of Asking Questions. Princeton University Press, Princeton, New Jersey, USA.

Schouten, J.M.; Vonk Noordegraaf, A.; Noordhuizen, J.P.T.M. (1997). The relevance of risk factors for *S.dublin* on dairy farms as assessed by conjoint analysis (Submitted).

Schukken, Y.H.; Geer, D. van de; Grommers, F.J.; Brand, A. (1989). Assessing the repeatability of questionnaire data from dairy farms. Preventive Veterinary Medicine, 7, 31-38.

Smits, M.C.J.; Frankena, K.; Metz, J.H.M.; Noordhuizen, J.P.T.M. (1992). Prevalence of digital disorders in zero-grazing dairy cows. Livestock Production Science, 32, 231-244.
Steenkamp, J.E.B.M. (1985). The Construction of Profile Sets for the Estimation of Main Effects and Interactions at Conjoint Measurements. Yearbook of the Dutch Association of Marketing Research, pp. 124-154 (in Dutch).
Vriens, M. (1995). Conjoint analysis in marketing: developments in stimulus representation and segmentation methods. PhD thesis, University of Groningen, The Netherlands.

Index

Printed in the United States
by Baker & Taylor Publisher Services